Children's and Your ractice

Joint Education and Training Library

This book is to be returned on or before the last date stamped below. Overdue charges will be incurred by the late return of books.

Renew in person, by phone (01270 612538, or internal x2538/2705) or online at:
http://libcat.chester.ac.uk (NHS staff ask for password)

Also by the authors:

Smith, L., Coleman, V., Bradshaw, M. (eds) (2002)
Family-Centered Care: Concept, Theory and Practice
(Basingstoke: Palgrave)

Children's and Young People's Nursing in Practice

A Problem-based Learning Approach

Edited by

Valerie Coleman, Lynda Smith and Maureen Bradshaw

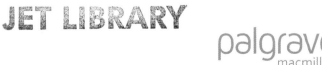

palgrave
macmillan

First published 2007 by
PALGRAVE MACMILLAN
Houndmills, Basingstoke, Hampshire RG21 6XS and
175 Fifth Avenue, New York, N.Y. 10010
Companies and representatives throughout the world

PALGRAVE MACMILLAN is the global academic imprint of the Palgrave Macmillan division of St. Martin's Press, LLC and of Palgrave Macmillan Ltd. Macmillan® is a registered trademark in the United States, United Kingdom and other countries. Palgrave is a registered trademark in the European Union and other countries.

ISBN-13: 978–1–4039–3393–5
ISBN-10: 1–4039–3393–6

This book is printed on paper suitable for recycling and made from fully managed and sustained forest sources.

A catalogue record for this book is available from the British Library.

10   9   8   7   6   5   4   3   2   1
16   15   14   13   12   11   10   09   08   07

Printed and bound in China

Contents

Foreword

Children's and Young People's Nursing in Practice is an innovative and student-centred text book, which has been written by a strong editorial team who are deeply committed to excellence in care.

In adopting a problem-based learning approach the authors are able to offer readers insights into care delivery that have firm foundations in evidence-based practice. The 12 chapters of this text book will help students appreciate the full spectrum and complexities of caring for sick children, young people and their families. In working through the various exercises embodied within the text, students and, importantly, their educators, will be able to embrace a learning strategy that is predicated on the whole being greater that the sum of the parts. In fostering the benefits of collaborative working and studying using a problem-solving approach the authors of this book will facilitate a more comprehensive learning environment that harnesses the combined efforts of both individuals and their peer groups.

At the heart of this book lies caring that is constructed around the strengths of the family, a concept which is fundamental to the art and science of children's and young people's nursing. In utilising vignettes and family scenarios the authors are able to engage with the readers in helping them explore the avenues to best practice based on personal professional reflection, an integral component of nursing.

Current government policy seeks to invest in and promote the optimum health of all children irrespective of their culture or socio-economic background. This text book will prove to be an invaluable aid for those seeking a career in the care of children and young people.

Dr Alan Glasper
Professor of Children's Nursing
The University of Southampton

Preface

The impetus for writing this book came from developing and using a problem-based learning curriculum (PBL) for a children's nursing course. The PBL approach promoted deeper and more interactive learning than traditional approaches and it was clearly focused on the reality of clinical practice. PBL also enabled the students to develop transferable key skills for lifelong learning about children's and young people's nursing. These skills are invaluable in contemporary nursing practice, which is constantly evolving and changing to provide optimum care for children, young people and their families.

The book will be of interest to student nurses and also qualified nurses working with children, young people and families both in hospital and community settings. Our intention is to provide a text that mirrors the PBL approach to learning. *Children's and Young People's Nursing in Practice: A Problem-based Learning Approach* addresses the demands of contemporary nurse education by encouraging readers to engage in the learning process in most chapters, by investigating the 'problem' for themselves to develop knowledge, understanding and transferable key skills in the first instance. Readers may then access the feedback sections at the end of each chapter to find potential answers to the 'problems.'

The concept of problem-based learning is introduced in Chapter 1 and in Chapter 2 independence in learning for problem-based learning is explored. Contemporary family-centred care is the focus of Chapter 3 because this philosophy is integral to children's and young people's nursing in practice. Chapters about promoting child health and safeguarding children follow. They encourage the readers through use of problem-based learning to develop knowledge and skills which are transferable and applicable to numerous nursing situations. Subsequent chapters enable readers to learn about the care of children and young people across a variety of different care settings, including ambulatory, acute, long-term, paediatric intensive care units and neonatal intensive care units. The concluding chapter recognises that the student nurse reading this book will make a transition to being a qualified nurse at the end of the course. This chapter therefore encourages the reader to learn theory and practice about the professional role of the nurse caring for children and young people. The reader is also encouraged to develop a personal development plan to facilitate lifelong learning. The overall aim of this book is that, through the process of PBL, children's nurses will have developed life-long skills in HOW to learn, which equips them well to meet the challenges of children's and young people's nursing practice in the twenty-first century.

Valerie Coleman, Lynda Smith, Maureen Bradshaw

Contributors

Helen Bailey has worked in Paediatric Critical Care for 13 years. She spent five years teaching this subject at the University of Sheffield and is now Clinical Nurse Manager of PICU at Sheffield Children's Hospital.

Maureen Bradshaw is Children's Nursing Lecturer at the University of Sheffield. She is keen to increase the use of problem-based learning in nurse education. Her interest in family-centred care has been shared in national and international publications and conferences.

Valerie Coleman is Children's Nursing Lecturer at the University of Sheffield with experience of problem-based learning in pre- and post-registration nurse education. Her interest in family-centred care has led her to publish and present at conferences nationally and internationally on this subject.

Shirley Cutts is Children's Nursing Lecturer at the University of Sheffield. Her interest in the topic of safeguarding children has led to the interprofessional development and delivery of post-registration programmes specialising in this field.

Lynda Smith is Children's Nursing Lecturer at the University of Sheffield with experience of problem-based learning in pre- and post-registration nurse education. She has worked extensively in the field of children's nursing practice both as a practitioner and lecturer. Her publications and conference presentations reflect her interest in family-centred care.

Angela Thurlby is Lecturer in Neonatal Nursing at the University of Sheffield. She has worked extensively in the field of neonatal intensive care nursing both as a practitioner and lecturer.

Julia R. Twigg is currently Nurse Lecturer in the School of Nursing and Midwifery at the University of Sheffield. She has wide ranging interests and a breadth of experience in Children's Nursing having worked in Sheffield, Birmingham and London. She also holds a Diploma in Counselling and is a member of the British Association for Counselling and Psychotherapy.

Introduction to Problem-based Learning

Valerie Coleman

1

Learning outcomes

- Understand what problem-based learning (PBL) is and is not.
- Appreciate the benefits of using a PBL approach to learning about children's and young people's nursing in practice.
- Utilise a PBL approach to learning in the context of this book.

Introduction

This is an important chapter because it introduces you to using a PBL approach in the context of this book, in order to maximise your learning about children's and young people's nursing practice in the other chapters. This book uses a PBL approach to cover in depth some of the core content of a children's nursing course. Using a PBL approach will help you to develop transferable key skills, such as problem solving, self-enquiry and communication, for engagement in lifelong learning. PBL enables those that use the approach to learn how to learn for life (Amos and White 1998). Burns and Glenn (2000, p. 4) explain that the skills of lifelong learning; 'Include the ability to identify a need, access and retrieve information, filter it for quality in relation to a specific client/patient problem and then use the information to provide the most appropriate care required'.

Nurses with these skills will be able to deliver optimum evidence-based practice to the children, young people and families in their care who are using the health and social care services of the twenty-first century. It is, therefore, important that you undertake the suggested work in each chapter to assist you to develop transferable key skills, especially those of analysis and problem solving, prior to reading the feedback answer sections.

A PBL medical education course set up in the mid 1960s at McMaster University in Canada is recognised as the beginning of the modern history of this approach to learning. Other PBL courses have since developed worldwide, spreading from the medical profession to other professions that have perceived the benefits of employing this learning approach (Wilkie 2000). There has been an increasing interest in using a PBL approach in nurse education since the 1990s to overcome problems of theory overload, lack of clinical practice opportunities, poor integration of theory to practice and to meet demands for lifelong learning and the development of transferable key skills (Wilkie and Burns 2003). Consequently PBL is a learning strategy that students undertaking nursing courses are increasingly encountering.

However, it is not necessary to be undertaking a PBL structured course in order to benefit from using this book. PBL is usually seen as a group venture with each member bringing different strengths and experiences to the problem and accepting responsibility for gathering particular information, suggesting questions, and providing answers as the problem is analysed (Price 2003) (See Trigger 1.1 Question One feedback). Nurses using this book may work in groups with colleagues (that is nursing or interprofessional colleagues) to analyse the presented problems or alternatively you will need to adapt the process to engage in PBL independently. What follows next mirrors the format that you will encounter in subsequent chapters of this book to enable you to take a problem-based approach, either independently or in groups, to learning about children's and young people's nursing practice. In subsequent chapters there will be more than one trigger.

! Trigger 1.1: Problem-based learning

The 'problem' is presented to you in the form of a trigger, which is the initial stimulus for learning. The intention of this trigger is to enable you to learn what PBL is in the context of this book.

The Trigger

University School of Nursing: Child Branch Pre-Registration RN (Child) and Bachelor in Nursing Degree Course Handbook. Information about learning and teaching:

This is a problem-based learning (PBL) course designed to prepare you for the future as children's nurses that are 'fit for practice' in the ever changing environments of modern health and social care services. Children's nurses that are proactive as well as reactive, critical thinkers, creative, flexible and innovative are required for practice.

The learning and teaching strategies used during this course are congruent with the PBL approach. Problems are presented to students in the form of triggers, which arise from practice and are developed in partnership with clinical colleagues. Fixed resources are identified for each trigger to assist your learning. PBL helps you to develop transferable key skills for practice as a registered children's nurse.

Situation

The 'situation' relevant to the trigger is described.
The situation for Trigger 1.1 is that you are about to commence on a child branch course. You have been sent the course handbook prior to attending the pre-course study day.

Feedback

The expected 'feedback' format on your learning is described for every trigger. Feedback may take a variety of forms for example that of a written seminar type paper, teaching package, report or a leaflet.

Your feedback for this trigger should take the form of a written seminar paper for each of the questions developed from this trigger. A seminar is a small class for discussion. The seminar papers should explore the key features of the topic and be structured in a format that would promote discussion among colleagues at a seminar presentation.

On presentation of the trigger you will need to look at the areas outlined below:

The facts

*Identify the '**Facts**' to start a problem-solving process that involves a series of cycles, these are appraisal of the problem; identifying what you do not understand and structuring hypotheses and then questions; information/evidence gathering; analysis of the information/evidence gathered; action planning for further investigation; suggesting and evaluating possible solutions; and decision-making about the 'best' solution/ response (Price 2003). These cycles may be repeated in order to gain in-depth knowledge and understanding of the trigger problem.*

Price (2003) argues that it is difficult to determine in an investigation what represents 'a fact' and identifies that individuals in groups will use different criteria regarding what represents 'a fact'. The criteria used may be scientific or circumstantial with different philosophical paradigms all treating 'facts' differently. Hence in the positivist paradigm facts are observable and measurable; in the naturalistic paradigm facts are based on the individual's experiences and understandings, and in the critical theory paradigm specific philosophical perspectives (for example social justice for disadvantaged groups) are acknowledged in relation to facts (Price 2003).

Achieving agreement on 'what is a fact' in nursing practice may be difficult to ascertain. Assessing, planning, implementing and evaluating nursing care is a complex process because all children, young people and their families are individuals and differ in their experiences, understanding and perceptions. Nurses and inter-professional colleagues may also demonstrate differences based on past experiences and their perceptions in how they interpret situations in practice.

Therefore, to engage in PBL determining the truth and what is 'a fact' is not neces-

sarily a straightforward activity. However, to move on to the next stage of the PBL process 'facts' have to be identified so you need to establish some criteria either for yourself or for the group that you are working with to agree what constitutes 'a fact'. Facts may be identified because of a body of evidence, consideration of multiple and sometimes counterclaims about available information or by theoretically testing out claims of 'facts' (Price 2003) perhaps by reflecting on practice.

The facts for Trigger 1.1 are likely to be:

- This is a handbook for a Child Branch Course.
- It is a Pre-Registration Course delivered in a University School of Nursing.
- Registered Nurse (Child) is the professional award.
- A Degree is the academic award.
- This is a problem-based learning course.
- The end product of the course is qualification as a Registered Children's Nurse who is proactive, reactive, flexible, innovative, creative and able to practice in the present climate of change and development in today's modern health and social care services.
- It identifies problems, triggers and fixed resources as learning and teaching strategies.
- Triggers arise from practice. Clinical colleagues are involved in developing triggers.
- Transferable key skills are developed for practice as a Registered Children's Nurse.

You will be required to identify 'the facts' for yourself for each trigger in subsequent chapters of this book.

The facts for this trigger are fairly obvious, but in other triggers you will need to consider very carefully what is 'a fact' to inform your subsequent learning and practice. It is likely that you may disregard some of your initial facts as being unproven and identify new ones as you engage in the problem-solving cycle in the analysis of a trigger 'problem'.

Hypotheses are speculative statements about the truth of a particular situation. A working hypothesis in practice may involve identifying what care is required now for the patient (based on the facts) and what might help in a particular situation. According to Price (2003) it involves considering what the advantages or disadvantages of action or inaction might be. Using a PBL approach enables you to 'investigate' the truth about the situation identified in the trigger, and the potential advantages or disadvantages of particular courses of action or inaction in theory to inform your future practice.

This trigger is not about patient care (triggers in other chapters will be) but what did you make of the facts for this trigger? What do they mean?

- This handbook will tell me about the course and how I am going to learn.
- Problem-based learning is different from more traditional types of teaching and learning that I have participated in before so I will need to develop new knowledge, understanding and skills.
- Problems, triggers and fixed resources are used rather than lectures from teachers so it will mean changing to a new way of learning.
- Triggers are linked closely to clinical practice, which will prepare me for practice.
- There is much change and development happening in modern health and social care services that requires registered children's nurses to develop some specific qualities and transferable key skills in their pre-registration course.

Questions developed from the hypotheses

These need to be developed from your hypotheses, taking into account what you already know. The Salford Model of the PBL process (McLoughlin and Darvill, 2001) clearly states the need for students to explore their existing knowledge in order to iden-tify their learning needs in relation to a trigger. It is fundamental to PBL that you build up your knowledge and understanding by developing questions that will facilitate you finding out new facts as opposed to 'regurgitating' what you already know. It is likely that you will choose not to ask some obvious questions that arise from your hypothe-sis because you already have this knowledge from the earlier content of this chapter. Further questions are likely to emerge from the problem solving cycles that you will undertake to determine the 'best' solutions or responses to the trigger.

The following questions may arise from Trigger 1.1:

1. What is a PBL approach to learning?
2. What are 'problems' and 'triggers'?
3. What is a fixed resource?
4. What are the benefits of using a PBL approach to learning about children's and young people's nursing in practice?

Trigger 1.1: Fixed resource material

To help you to start your inquiry there will be a list of fixed resource material identi-fied for every trigger that is current at the time of publication. You may also search and review other up to date research and evidence-based literature yourself and seek other relevant resources to provide you with answers to your questions.

Reading some of the following material will help you to answer the questions for Trigger 1.1.

Alavi, C. (ed) (1995) *Problem-based Learning in a Health Sciences Curriculum* London: Routledge. Read the Introduction, pp.1–11.

Boud, D., Feletti, G. (eds) (1997) *The Challenge of Problem-based Learning*, 2nd edn. London: Kogan Page. Read Part One: What is Problem Based Learning? pp. 15–44.

Frost, M. (1996) An analysis of the scope and value of problem-based learning in the education of health care professionals. *Journal of Advanced Nursing* 24 (50) November, pp. 1047–53.

Glen, S., Wilkie, K. (2000) *Problem-based Learning*. Basingstoke: Palgrave Macmillan. Read Chapter 2: The nature of problem-based learning, pp. 11–36.

Price, B. (1999) An introduction to problem-based learning. *Nursing Standard*, 13 (40), 23 June, pp. 48–54.

Price, B. (2003) *Problem-based Learning, Studying Nursing using Problem-based and Enquiry-based Learning*. Basingstoke: Palgrave Macmillan. Read Chapter 2, pp. 21–41.

Wilkie, K., Burns, I. (2003) *Problem-Based Learning*. Basingstoke: Palgrave Macmillan. Read pp. 1–24.

Useful Websites

The SONIC Project (Students On-Line in Nursing Integrated Curricula) http://www.uclan.ac.uk/facs/health/nursing/sonic/index.htm

United Kingdom PBL Website: http://hss.coventry.ac.uk/pbl/index.htm

Trigger 1.1: Fixed resource sessions

Fixed resource sessions are intended to compliment your own efforts to answer the identified questions.

There are two fixed resource sessions for this trigger. The first session will assist you to answer the question: What is a PBL approach to learning? The second session is intended to help you answer the question: What are the benefits of using a PBL approach to learning about children's and young people's nursing in practice?

Defining problem-based learning (PBL)

It is difficult to succinctly define PBL because of the many misconceptions that exist about its meaning. PBL is often mistaken for other approaches to learning such as problem solving and discovery learning that are not PBL, but they resemble the approach in several ways (Alavi 1995). To confuse the situation even further the term PBL is also often used interchangeably with that of enquiry-based learning (EBL), which is a similar educational method to learning that differs from PBL in its application to student learning (Glasper 2001). Grandis et al (2003) state that it is not necessary to distinguish between the two. However, if you want to gain more clarity on the distinction between the two approaches you will find it useful to read Price (2003), who identifies that both PBL and EBL require students to 'inquire' to learn.

PBL is an active student-centred approach, which is congruent with many of the definitions that have been offered to explain this approach to learning (See Table 1.1).

Table 1.1: Definitions of PBL

- 'PBL places the student at the centre of the learning process and emphasises cooperative learning' (Alavi, 1995, p. 5).
- 'PBL is an approach to structuring the curriculum that involves confronting students with problems from practice that provides a stimulus for learning' (Boud and Feletti 1997, p. 15).
- 'A major characteristic of PBL is that the problem is presented to the students before the material has been learned rather than after as in the more traditional 'problem-solving approach' (Wilkie 2000, p. 11).
- PBL is 'A means of developing learning for capability rather than learning for the sake of acquiring knowledge' (Engel 1997, p. 17).
- The foundations for a lifetime of continuing education are laid by PBL (Barrows 1986).

The definitions in Table 1.1 identify that PBL places the student at the centre of a learning process for capability that confronts them with problems from practice prior to the learning of relevant material. The outcome of this PBL process is the laying of a foundation for lifelong continuing education. There is an emphasis on co-operative learning, which may still be achieved within the confines of this book if a 'PBL team' of readers of this book address the triggers together in order to learn, in the same way as they would in a classroom situation.

The health and social care context for problem-based learning

In the twenty-first century, it is suggested that the health and social care context for children, young people, families and nurses is a rapidly changing environment where the nature of care is often complex and more demanding than in the past. This is in part due to the changing profile of childhood illness with increasing numbers of children surviving with chronic conditions throughout childhood and into adulthood. Other children and young people with acute illnesses are now often much sicker and their families 'are forced to endure increasingly difficult situations with uncertain outcomes for prolonged periods of time' (Rennick 1995, p. 258). The context of care for children and young people in this country has also 'moved from care by the family in the home, to care by professionals in hospital and now care at home [whenever possible] or in hospital by the family and health care professionals' (Coyne 1996, p. 739). This move towards care at home has led to more children, young people and families experiencing day care admissions or early discharge home from in-patient stays in hospital than in the past, which all contributes towards a changing context of health and social care.

There have also been many new developments in treatment, technology and management that have imposed ever increasing demands on nurses and other professionals forcing them to adapt and/or change their practice. Similarly contemporary health policies such as the *NHS Plan* (Department of Health 2000); the *National Service Framework for Children, Young People and Maternity Services (NSF)* (Department of Health 2004; Welsh Assembly 2004); *Investing for Health in Northern Ireland* (Department of Health, Social Sciences and Public Safety, 2002) and *Making it Work for Scotland's Children* (Scottish Executive 2003) have impacted on the health and social care context. These policies have demanded more collaborative working, patient-centred care and partnership working for professionals, children, young people and families alike.

Some well-publicised damaging events involving the care of children and young people in the health services have emerged from the healthcare context in England. These include concerns about the management of care of children undergoing complex cardiac surgery at the Bristol Royal Infirmary between 1984 and 1995, which led to an inquiry (Bristol Royal Infirmary Inquiry Report 2001). There also was the tragic death of Victoria Climbié while in the care of relatives and the social services (Laming 2003). These events prompted the development of the *National Service Framework* (Department of Health 2004), also new recommendations and child protection guidelines/policies including *Keeping Children Safe* (Department of Health 2003); Every Child Matters (Department for Education and Skills 2003). These developments are very positive, but nevertheless they are leading to further changes for nurses and other professionals to respond to in the healthcare context.

It is apparent that capable, competent, critically thinking nurses, that have the ability to understand, not just acquire knowledge are required to practice in this changing, demanding healthcare context of the twenty-first century. *Making a Difference* (Department of Health 1999) and *Fitness for Practice* (United Kingdom Central Council 1999) are contemporary national nursing policies that emphasise the need for nurses to develop high order intellectual skills and abilities for contemporary [children's and young people's] nursing practice.

PBL is an approach that will enable nurses to develop these skills and abilities and prepare them to meet the demands of today's health and social care context. The approach promotes lifelong learning to empower nurses to cope with ongoing changes and demands in practice.

→ Trigger 1.1: Feedback

Go to Chapter 1 feedback on p. 9 below

*This identifies the section that you need to go to **after** completing your inquiry to find out the answers to the questions developed for individual triggers. (You need to try and **avoid the temptation** to simply look forward to the feedback section because this will prevent you achieving the learning skills that are considered to be key to PBL.) This section will always be found towards the end of each chapter and will give 'potential answers' to the questions in the required feedback format.*

? Chapter 1 Trigger feedback: what do you know?

Remember that students should learn what they don't know and what they themselves need to learn for practice when a PBL approach to learning is used. Therefore, the answers that are given in this book may not always completely match your own answers. The feedback given will focus on principles, related to the trigger topic area, that you are likely to have included in your own answers. The questions for Trigger 1.1 are below.

Question 1: What is a PBL approach to learning?

PBL involves both a process and an end product or outcome. The trigger used in this chapter has been developed to guide you through a process of learning about PBL. The content in the chapter has already provided information about some expected PBL outcomes in respect of the development of transferable key skills such as problem solving, self-enquiry and communication for engagement in independent and lifelong learning.

PBL places as great a value on the process of learning (in this instance about children and young people's nursing) as the outcome or end product of this learning. PBL takes account of how people learn. 'Learning to develop lifelong enquiry and learning skills is more important than remembering content' (Glen and Wilkie 2000, p. 33).

Students are required to be active in the process and to take responsibility for their own learning both in the long and the short term. Biley and Smith (1998) found that 'the buck stops here' describes the sense of personal responsibility that graduates from a PBL course experienced in terms of their learning and actions.

'PBL is an educational strategy that uses material that is as close as possible to real life as a stimulus for learning' (Glenn and Wilkie 2000, p. 33). The process involves students being presented with problems from practice in the form of 'triggers' (Boud and Feletti 1997) without them necessarily possessing any prior knowledge or understanding about the topic area, which is the opposite from traditional teaching approaches when it is more usual to give students information first and to ask questions later. Using a PBL approach students are expected to engage with the triggers presented to them, identifying facts, hypothesising and finally developing questions for their enquiry. To develop these questions students have to decide:

1. What they need to know about the trigger topic.
2. What they already know about the trigger topic.
3. What 'new learning' they are going to engage in.

Students are not expected to find a series of right answers in their inquiries. The important task is to engage in a process of learning using a variety of resources including the fixed resources that are identified for individual triggers such as the one in this chapter. Engaging in this process is required in order to develop the student's knowledge and understanding of issues relating in the context of this book to the care of children, young people and their families. Students are required to give 'feedback' on their learning. The feedback for this trigger is in the form of written seminar papers. Feedback may take a variety of forms and these have already been identified earlier in this chapter.

To be able to engage in the learning process, students have to use a variety of skills including those of decision-making, library, information technology, critical thinking and problem solving. In a classroom situation the lecturer would act as a facilitator to assist the students with the process of learning and the students would work together in a group as a 'PBL team'. Working in a 'PBL team', calls for participants to use various skills including those of communication and for individual team members to adopt certain roles and responsibilities. For example, for each trigger there should be a chairperson and a scribe to write down the facts, hypotheses and questions. Price (2003) argues that the process of collaborating, challenging and sharing responsibility within the group reduces anxiety about learning and is believed to be educationally beneficial. It has already been suggested in this chapter that students using this book may choose to work as a 'PBL team' with regard to the triggers presented in this book.

An outcome or end product of going through the PBL process is the development of high level transferable skills and the confidence needed in order to manage a 'real situation' in practice. PBL effectively links theoretical learning with practice and develops independence in inquiry, which has the potential to empower nurses to provide optimum care for children, young people and their families within the health and social care context.

PBL students to varying degrees learn in greater depth than students on more traditional courses (Newble and Clark 1986) The process of fully engaging students in learning, especially that related to the context of practice, ensures students develop deep knowledge rather than surface knowledge that is dependent on rote learning and skimming the surface of content within an educational process (Margetson 1994; Marton and Säljö 1984). The outcome of this is that students undertaking a PBL course will have gained a depth of knowledge and understanding about many aspects of children's nursing, but not necessarily the breadth of learning that students on more traditional courses possess. However, students completing a PBL course will have developed the necessary skills to enable them to learn independently about new situations as they encounter them throughout their careers.

This enquiry into 'What is a PBL approach to learning?' has explored the approach both as a process and an outcome.

Question 2: What are 'problems' and 'triggers'?

Answering this question may have been rather confusing initially because everyday words have a specific meaning in PBL (Wilkie and Burns 2003). For example the so-called problem is not the problem.

The problem is a situation that promotes learning needs for students. The problem denotes that the students have a lack of knowledge about the situation. The situation identified in this chapter is one of a future student nurse receiving a course handbook opened at a particular page in advance of a pre-course study day. The student is presumed to have a lack of knowledge about the PBL approach used on the course that she/he is soon to commence, which is a problem. The situation is, therefore, a description of the situation in which the student is expected to deal with the problem (Wilkie and Burns 2003).

A problem has two components, one of which is the situation. The other component is the trigger, which 'triggers' the PBL process and creates the initial stimulus for discussion and learning. It is important that all the triggers used are perceived as being authentic to real life practice by students (Price 2003) in order to motivate them to engage in the PBL learning process. Therefore the triggers need to deal with problems from practice (Boud and Feletti 1997) to promote learning for the health and social care context of the twenty-first century. The practice referred to in this chapter is that of education and the use of a PBL approach on a course soon to be commenced by a future student nurse. In most of the following chapters the practice referred to will be that of children and young people's nursing contextualised, for example, to ambulatory care. A trigger may take a variety of forms including cartoons, photographs, weight charts, quotes, video clips, and extracts from patient notes, audiotapes and patient scenarios. Several different forms of triggers will be used in this book and students are encouraged to develop their own 'real triggers' from reflecting on personal practice experiences.

The trigger and situation, which together are sometimes known as 'the scenario', put students in the role of decision makers and problem solvers in preparation for them assuming these roles in practice as Registered Children's Nurses. It is of paramount importance that students use evidence and research-based material to justify their decision-making for nursing care with regard to the problem.

Question 3: What is a fixed resource?

A fixed resource is additional material that is intended to assist students with learning by supporting them with their inquiry into the trigger topic. Wilkie and Burns (2003) stress the importance of students being able to relate the fixed resource material to the PBL triggers and select the appropriate information from it to enable them to answer the set questions. The fixed resources in this chapter *(and the rest of this book)* take the form of book, article and website references, and fixed resource sessions that resemble 'mini lectures'. Fixed resources may also take a variety of other forms, including lectures, tutorials, clinical skills sessions, open learning packages, computer assisted learning programmes, videos (Wilkie 2000), clinical experiences and personal interviews (Wilkie and Burns 2003). Alavi (1995) explains that an expert in a particular field of practice such as a clinical nurse specialist may facilitate a fixed resource session. While engaging with the PBL triggers in this book it may often be appropriate to approach 'an expert' to find out more about the trigger topic.

The fixed resources will not attempt to cover all the material relevant to a particular area of study, but instead focus on key concepts relating them to the PBL triggers that students are engaging with at the time (Armstrong, 1997). The fixed resource does not provide all the answers to a PBL trigger, because this would undermine the principles of PBL and not encourage critical thinking and deeper learning (Wilkie 2000).

Fixed resources assist with the development of skills for critical thinking as opposed to overloading students with facts. Students are then in a position to think about the issues involved in a PBL trigger and/or children's and young people's nursing for themselves and this is more likely to result in deep learning for practice (Wilkie and Burns 2003).

Question 4: What are the benefits of using a PBL approach to learning about children and young people's nursing in practice?

'PBL has the potential to directly mirror the messy world of practice with nursing students being exposed to a learning strategy that encourages deep as opposed to surface learning' (Wilkie 2000, p. 24). This certainly suggests that the PBL approach has benefits for learning about children's and young people's nursing in practice because it has the potential to prepare students for the challenging and demanding health and social care context of the twenty-first century that was discussed in the second fixed resource session in this chapter.

Students, through the use of a problem-based approach to learning are facilitated in the achievement of learning that actively involves them being in charge of what they learn through negotiation, sharing and application to meet both personal and professional learning outcomes. All the learning is related to the context of practice to facilitate deep learning, and is for understanding rather than the recall of isolated facts.

The literature provides support for the perceived benefits of using a PBL approach, finding that it not only fully engages students in the process of learning (Doring et al 1995), but it also results in them having a more rewarding and useful clinical experience (Alavi 1995). PBL is, therefore, viewed as an attractive strategy because the learning is contextualised to and integrated with practice (Wilkie and Burns 2003), thus promoting critical thinking and problem solving while enhancing communication skills, practice skills and team working. PBL also assists students to manage unfamiliar situations, make reasoned decisions, reason critically, adapt to and participate in change, and subsequently manage their own lifelong learning (Engel 1997) using evidence-based literature to cope with the ever changing health and social care context and increasing new demands.

Many of the studies that have been undertaken relating to PBL and health care practitioners have emerged from medical education. Nursing studies in relation to PBL evaluation are more limited (Biley and Smith 1999), leaving us to extrapolate from medical studies, such as those undertaken by Cole (1985) and Newble and Clark (1986) about deep learning, on the benefits of using PBL in nurse education.

Biley and Smith (1998) undertook a study to discover the perceptions of graduates from an adult branch nursing programme, on the effectiveness of a PBL learning programme in preparing them for the reality of being a registered nurse. Three categories were identified from the data to describe the characteristics that the PBL graduates identified that made them different from traditionally trained nurses. One of these categories was the aforementioned 'the buck stops here', which describes the sense of personal responsibility that these graduates experienced in terms of their learning and actions. This study helped to bridge the gap in existing literature concerning the outcomes of a PBL nursing programme.

Another evaluative study of one cohort of Child Branch nursing students was conducted during the last enquiry-based learning session (EBL) of a three year programme. EBL and PBL are two educational methods, which are similar but different in their application. The objective was to explore Child Branch students' perceptions of the EBL process over their programme. The students were asked two questions relating to what they liked most and what they liked least about EBL over the three years. The results demonstrated overall satisfaction with the EBL method of student learning. (Glasper 2001) The research-based literature does provide some evidence to support the proclaimed benefits of PBL for children and young people's nursing practice.

Reflect on Your Learning

This chapter has prepared you for the practice of PBL in the context of this book, by facilitating your active engagement in the process for learning.

The principle learning points about Problem-based Learning are:

- PBL involves both a process and a product.
- Students engage in active learning that includes determination of 'the facts', formulation of hypotheses and setting questions.
- The problem is a situation that promotes learning needs for students. It has two components these are the situation and the trigger, which are sometimes known as the scenario.
- The situation is a description of the situation in which the student is expected to deal with the problem.
- Triggers create the initial stimulus for discussion and learning.
- Feedback of the student's work on the trigger(s) may take a variety of forms.
- Fixed resources are additional materials identified to support the learning process.
- PBL promotes deeper learning than more traditional approaches.
- Transferable key transferable skills are developed for independent lifelong learning.
- PBL is a good strategy to use to prepare children's nurses for practice in the changing, demanding health and social care context of the twenty-first century.

In the next chapter you will learn more about the skills needed for engagement in a PBL process.

References

Alavi, C. (ed) (1995) *Problem-based Learning in a Health Sciences Curriculum.* London: Routledge.

Amos, E., White, M. J. (1998) Teaching tools: Problem-based learning. *Nurse Educator* 23 (2), pp. 11–14.

Armstrong, E. (1997) A hybrid model of problem-based learning, in Boud, D., Feletti, G. (eds) *The Challenge of Problem-based Learning*, 2nd edn London: Kogan Page.

Barrows, H. (1986) A taxonomy of problem-based learning, *Medical Education* 20, pp. 482–6.

Biley, F., Smith, K. (1998) 'The buck stops here': Accepting responsibility for learning and actions after graduation from a problem-based learning nursing education curriculum. *Journal of Advanced Nursing*, 27 (5), May, pp. 1021–9.

Biley, F., Smith, K. (1999) Making sense of problem-based learning: Perceptions and experiences of undergraduate nursing students. *Journal of Advanced Nursing*, 30 (5), November, pp. 1205–12.

Boud, D., Feletti, G. (eds) (1997) *The Challenge of Problem-based Learning*, 2nd edn. London: Kogan Page.

Bristol Royal Infirmary Inquiry Report (2001) *Learning from Bristol: The Report Of the Public Inquiry into Children's Heart Surgery at the Bristol Royal Infirmary 1984–1995*. London: Stationery Office.

Burns, I., Glen, S. (2000) A new model for a new context, in Glen, S., Wilkie, K. (eds) *Problem-based Learning in Nursing: A new model for a new context*. Basingstoke: Palgrave Macmillan, Chapter 1, pp. 1–10.

Cole, C. R. (1985) Differences between conventional and problem-based curricula in their students approaches to studying. *Medical Education* 19, pp. 308–9.

Coyne, I. (1996) Parent participation: A concept analysis. *Journal of Advanced Nursing* 23, pp. 733–70.

Department for Education and Skills (2003) *Every Child Matters*, http://www.dfes. gov.uk/everychildmatters/index.shtml

Department of Health (1999) *Making a Difference: Strengthening the nursing, Midwifery and Health Visiting Contribution to Health and Healthcare*. London: Stationery Office.

Department of Health (2000) *The NHS Plan: A plan for investment: A Plan for Reform*. London: Stationery Office.

Department of Health (2003) Keeping Children Safe: The Governments Respon*se to The Victoria* Climbié *Inquiry Report and Joint Chief Inspectors Report Safeguarding Children*. London: Stationery Office.

Department of Health (2004*) National Service Framework for Children, Young People and Maternity Services*. http://www.doh.gov.uk/nsf/children.htm

Department of Health, Social Services and Public Safety (2002) *Investing for Health*. Northern Ireland: DHSSPS. http://www.dhsspsni.gov.uk/publications/2002/ investforhealth.asp accessed 03.08.05.

Doring, A., Bramwell-Vial, A., Bingham, B. (1995) Staff comfort/ discomfort with problem-based learning: A preliminary study. *Nurse Education Today* 15, pp. 263–6.

Engel, C. (1997) Not just a method but a way of learning, in Boud, D., Feletti, G. (eds) (1997) *The Challenge of Problem-based Learning*, 2nd edn. London: Kogan Page, Chapter 2, pp. 17–27.

Frost, M. (1996) An analysis of the scope and value of problem-based learning in the education of health care professionals. *Journal of Advanced Nursing* 24 (50), November, pp. 1047–53.

Glasper, E. A. (2001) Child health nurse's perceptions of enquiry-based learning. *British Journal of Nursing* 10: (20), pp. 1343–49.

Glen, S., Wilkie, K. (eds) (2000) *Problem-based Learning in Nursing: A New Model for a New Context*, (Basingstoke: Macmillan).

Grandis, S., Long G., Glasper A., Jackson, P. (eds) (2003) *Foundation Studies for Nursing: Using Enquiry-Based Learning*. Basingstoke: Palgrave Macmillan.

Laming, L. (2003) The Victoria Climbié Inquiry: Report of an Inquiry, http://www. victoria-climbie-inquiry.org.uk/finreport/finreport.htm

Margetson, D. (1994) Current educational reform and the significance of problem-based learning. *Studies in Higher Education* 19 (1), pp. 5–19.

Marton, F., Säljö, R. (1984) Approaches to learning, in Marton, F., Hounsell, D., Entwhistle, N.J. (eds) *The Experience of Learning*, Edinburgh: Scottish Academic Press.

McLoughlin, M., Darvill, A. *(2001) The Salford Model of the PBL Process.* http://www.uclan.ac.uk/facs/health/nursing/sonic/scenarios/scenario4model.htm

Newble, D. I., Clark, R. M. (1986) The approaches to learning of students in a traditional and in an innovative problem-based medical school. *Medical Education* 20, pp. 267–73.

Price, B. (1999) An introduction to problem-based learning. *Nursing Standard* 13 (40), 23 June, pp. 48–54.

Price, B. (2003) *Studying Nursing using Problem-based and Enquiry-based Learning* (Basingstoke: Palgrave Macmillan).

Rennick, J. (1995) The changing profile of acute childhood illness: A need for the development of family nursing knowledge. *Journal of Advanced Nursing* 22 (2) August, pp. 258–66.

Scottish Executive (2003) *Making it work for Scotland's Children.* http://www.scotland.gov.uk (accessed 03.08.05).

United Kingdom Central Council (1999) *Fitness for Practice: The UKCC Commission for Nursing and Midwifery Education.* UKCC: London.

Welsh Assembly (2004) *National Service Framework for Children, Young People and Maternity Services.* http://www.wales.nhs.uk/sites/home.cfm

Wilkie, K. (2000) The nature of problem-based learning, in Glen, S., Wilkie, K. (eds) *Problem-based Learning in Nursing: A new model for a new Context.* Basingstoke: Palgrave Macmillan. Chapter 2, pp. 11–36.

Wilkie, K., Burns, I. (2003*) Problem-Based Learning: A Handbook for Nurses.* Basingstoke: Palgrave Macmillan.

Developing Skills for Independent Learning

2

Maureen Bradshaw and Lynda Smith

Learning outcomes

- Develop the skills needed for PBL
- Understand how learning styles affect the learning process.

Introduction

To engage in the process of problem-based learning (PBL) in a meaningful way, a range of skills are needed. This chapter is designed to develop the reflective, analytical and critical thinking skills that are necessary for PBL. It is also set within the context of current healthcare provision and the drive towards evidence-based practice that equally necessitates practitioners to focus on clinical problems and base their resulting decision-making on the best available evidence.

To fully encompass the needs of the individual within this type of learning approach, the chapter acquaints the student with knowledge of learning styles and their relevance to good communication, negotiation, leadership and team working skills that under-pin active engagement in learning. Although students may bring varying degrees of familiarity with such skills to their course there is much scope for expanding and enhancing these and other skills such as information technology or literature search-ing, in order to facilitate efficient and effective problem-based learning.

Learning style

Problem-based learning involves working in a group to gather and analyse a variety of evidence in order to reach conclusions about practice situations. You may choose to work either individually or in a group when working through the triggers in this book. Exploring your own learning style and those in your working group may help you learn more effectively. In nursing this has often been achieved with the aid of Honey and Mumford's (1982) Learning styles questionnaire which can be accessed on line at www.peterhoneylearning.com It takes approximately 10–15 minutes to complete and reveals predominant learning styles of activist, reflector, theorist or pragmatist. When familiar with the characteristics of your predominant style you can choose learning activities that best match your style. For example activists who like new challenges, think on their feet and enjoy variety, will learn most easily from crises, activities where they are thrown in at the deep end and where they can bounce ideas around and problem solve with others. Practically, they may respond well to learning in accident and emergency units where the next challenge is uncertain. In teams and groups they are optimistic innovators and visionaries who will easily rush into things and possibly do too much themselves. They are pioneers rather than settlers and will eagerly move on to the next project without tying up the details and loose ends of the previous one.

Reflectionists, who like to think and research before making decisions or acting, will learn best from activities where they can stand back, listen, observe and gather information before carefully reaching decisions in their own time without pressure of tight deadlines. Practically, they may be comfortable learning in wards where there is an obvious routine that repeats and attention can be given to detail. As good listeners, they assimilate information well and often make good counsellors. They are settlers rather than pioneers and, therefore, add grounding and stability to the groups and teams that they belong to.

Theorists who like logical, analytical, sequential approaches to problems that stretch them intellectually, will learn best from activities where they have time to be methodical and analyse complex situations, exploring associations like cause and effect. Practically theorists are good researchers who like things to be black and white. Their nursing policy and procedure manuals are held in high regard. Flexibility is sometimes difficult for them and they may struggle with ethical issues where there is uncertainty and many shades of grey. The science of nursing may therefore be more appealing to them to learn, rather than the art.

Pragmatists, who like practical situations where they can problem solve and see the relevance of their work, learn best from activities (demonstrated by credible role models) that have practical relevance. In nurse training pragmatists favour the practical component of their course rather than the theoretical. In practice they are more interested in learning the 'how' and focus on getting the task done rather than the 'why', and if all else fails will finally read the instructions. The art of nursing may, therefore, be more appealing to them to learn, rather than the science.

Getting to know your predominant learning style and that of others is not a labelling exercise. Insight gained, however, can be used to good effect personally when we deliberately recognise and consciously choose learning opportunities that best suit our predominant styles. Conscious, self-aware decisions can also be made to develop by strengthening under-utilised styles in order to become a more balanced holistic learner.

Insight into the learning styles of others can be of major benefit if we are to learn effectively alongside them in groups or teams. Once the learning styles of others are recognised, activists for example, who easily lead and hog the limelight, may learn to not *always* volunteer their answers, thoughts or ideas first. Instead they may learn to intermittently take a back seat by actively inviting the more reluctant reflectionists to speak first and contribute their thoughts and ideas, for example, 'What do you think'? Or, 'What's your experience of . . .'? Conversely reflectionists may have to learn to push themselves to share snippets of their thoughts and ideas early on in group or team discussions (even if they don't feel that they have had enough time to think through every possible consequence of their suggestions). When contributing individual work to group learning or presentations, activists may have to train them-selves to make more effort with attention to detail, for example, read it through one last time double-checking for spelling, grammar and referencing errors. Conversely reflectionists may have to be satisfied that when the time to research information for group presentations is short, then they may have to be satisfied with only consulting 80 per cent of what's available if they are to meet the presentation deadline, not hold things up, and allow the group to move on.

Reflective Practice

Some of the triggers or problems that you encounter within problem-based learning will encourage you to reflect on associated practice experience in order to learn from it. 'Oh you know . . . X . . . , she just never learns' is not an uncommon comment over-heard when a colleague is seen to repeat unhelpful behaviours, apparently unaware that anything is amiss or that an alternative may exist and possibly be more helpful or effective. So in order not to stimulate such comment, nurses need to learn from their experiences. Jasper (2003, p. 2) describes reflective practice as 'one of the ways that professionals learn from experience in order to understand and develop their practice'. It's a process through which we actively (rather than passively) learn. There are a variety of reflective models available that students can follow. Using specific ones or a hybrid of several can be equally useful. The framework suggested to guide reflection in this text is loosely based on the reflective cycle described by Gibbs (1988).

Some of the questions raised within problem-based learning will involve you think-ing about experience or incidents that you have been involved in and learning from them. The 'critical incident' that you choose to reflect on does not have to be dramatic! While much can clearly be learnt from reflecting on your participation in cardio-pulmonary resuscitation for the first time, what you learn from reflecting on doing a bed bath with your mentor for the first time is equally valid. You may simply choose to reflect on why a patient looked so comfortable when you had finished helping him or her with several aspects of care.

Description: begins the reflective cycle. It is a précis of what you experienced and can be written down or told to 'trusted' others. It is important here that professional confidentiality is maintained so do not use the names of patients, families, colleagues, wards or hospitals. They can be referred to in general terms, for example, 'a four year old patient on a medical ward' or given fictitious names. When you first start reflecting the description phase can tend to be rather lengthy because it encompasses the details of the incident, for example what you and others were doing as well as what actually happened. Skilled reflectors eventually manage to do this stage quite succinctly but this is not essential because some would argue that 'getting the story out' and sharing it either verbally or on paper is in itself a therapeutic exercise as in 'a problem shared is a problem halved'.

It's important to finish off the incident description with what it left you *thinking or feeling*. Did you for example feel upset, angry, frustrated or confused by the incident? It is, therefore, essential at this point that we are prepared to 'bare our souls' and become vulnerable if we are to be honest about our emotions. It is necessary to try to be as objective and self-aware as possible if we are to gain quality insight.

Evaluation: is often seen as a concluding exercise so it may initially seem strange to include it next. However, it helps us to be objective about the incident we've been describing if we can try to stand back and do some initial weighing up of the incident's experience value. What for example was good or helpful about the experience and what appeared to be bad or hindering?

Having discharged the above, we can then get down to making some sense of it all in the *analysis stage of reflection*. Some of the things that we choose to reflect on have straightforward single themes like a communication issue, however other incidents described can be quite complex, for example, a chaotic morning on the ward, so perhaps the first part of the analysis may involve you breaking the incident down into its component parts to reveal what appear to be key issues. You may already have an inkling that the chaos had something to do with communication, management and leadership issues, so there is then potential for each of these issues to be broken down and analysed more fully.

When we've time to stand back and think reflectively, it's relatively easy to look at the various issues and come up with some 'common sense' reasons as to why aspects of the incident followed the course that they did. However professional practice demands more of us than this and we have to examine the issues in greater depth to search out the truths of what was actually happening in the incident. It's only when we are satisfied that we have found evidence-based reasons for what we described earlier that we will be able to draw satisfactory conclusions about the incident. So, we are required to make sense of what was described in the light of the currently available associated professional literature. This will mean consulting a plethora of resources like professional texts, journals and websites. The attitude in which this is done is worth considering at this point. It's really important that you consult the literature open-mindedly, with a view to letting its detailed, honest exploration surprise you. The danger otherwise is that you may only seek out literature that supports your pre-analysis thoughts or attitudes on the incident and thus further learning and insight will be restricted.

Once you have let the literature give you evidence-based insight into the critical incident's various issues you will then be in a position to make informed judgements and *draw conclusions* from it. The literature should have given you insight not only into the behaviour of others in the incident but also the behaviours of yourself. Sometimes revelations about ourselves, our undesirable behaviours and attitudes can be threatening or painful but the purpose of reflection is to learn from our experience and analysis thereof. It would be pointless to end the reflection here because we may meet similar critical incidents in the future and in order to practice confidently and professionally we need to know if it would be appropriate to repeat current behaviours in the next such incident.

We are, therefore, *planning ahead or 'action planning'* and as a result of the critical incident analysis this may take one of three forms. First the literature may indeed support the behaviours of yourself and others in the given incident, so you can conclude that this was satisfactory and feel professionally confident that you could explain with reference to the literature why you would do the same things and act in the same way in a similar incident in the future. You have, therefore, affirmed current practice. Second, while the literature may have supported the current behaviours, your extensive literature searching may have revealed other actions that may also be helpful or appropriate to use in such incidents, so you can plan to add these evidence-based alternatives to your repertoire of skills and behaviours for future use in a similar situation. In the future you now have a choice of using 'plan A' as before but you also have an alternative that you are confident with to use as backup if plan A doesn't work so well next time. Third, the literature may have demonstrated why your original plan of action or elements of it was inappropriate and so you can make a new action plan according to the evidence for use in similar situations in the future.

It is important that action plans are expressed in terms of self, not others, because although reference to literature in the analysis section may have revealed wrong/undesirable practice/behaviours in others, they can choose to change, but you cannot make them. All you can do is plan appropriate evidence-based personal responses to their practice/behaviour, for example, an action plan to:

- Speak out when witnessing wrong/undesirable practice/behaviours.
- Offer evidence for why you believe the practice to be wrong/undesirable.
- Suggest evidence-based alternative practice/behaviour commensurate with professional standards. You may find it helpful to discuss this in a clinical supervision session (see Chapter 12).

Even if the analysis of your critical incident revealed inappropriate practice, in terms of learning this should not be seen as negative because the ability to generate a more appropriate evidence-based action plan is a positive outcome and demonstrates that learning has taken place.

Evidence-based practice

The drive towards evidence-based practice is explicit within NHS policy and part of the larger agenda to improve quality of care to all patients. It is important that our decisions about care are based on the best available evidence. Nurses, therefore, have to articulate the basis of their decision-making which is part of being an accountable professional (NMC, 2004) and it is no longer sufficient to rely solely on tacit knowledge (that is our intuition and expertise).

Nursing practice is informed by a range of sources of evidence including clinical expertise. Le May (1999) lists a number of these sources, and these are given in Table 2.1.

Table 2.1 Sources of evidence

1. Evidence from research: This may be your own or other's research including quantitative and qualitative approaches.
2. Evidence-based experience: This may include reflecting on practice with accompanying discussions and searching of literature.
3. Evidence based on theory that is not research based: This may be learning from others through educational programmes, contact with experts and discussions, searching the literature.
4. Evidence gathered from patients/clients/carers: These may be available from research and audit data, experiential writing patient satisfaction surveys and even following complaints.
5. Evidence passed on by role models/experts: Consulting expert opinion directly or indirectly through searching the literature. Delphi surveys for example consult those best able to comment on a subject area and ultimately determine a consensus position on that topic/sphere of practice.
6. Evidence based on policy directives: Examples include clinical guidelines.

In order to provide a rationale for the care being planned and implemented nurses need to develop skills in locating their sources of evidence, analysing the quality of that evidence and evaluating its usefulness for their practice. Le May (1999) proposes three questions to ask of the evidence

1. Is it valid?
2. If valid, is this evidence important for clinical practice?
3. If valid and important, can you use this evidence to improve patient care?

To help you develop or enhance existing skills in this process the following sections will enable you to adopt an analytical approach to using the rest of this book.

Your starting point is to identify what you already know about the subject area under consideration and how you know that. You should then be left with residual unanswered questions that you seek to explore and analyse. This is a similar process to PBL where you start by acknowledging your starting point for learning about the trigger by identifying what you know so that the focus can be on new knowledge.

Step 1: What is the question?

Context
I have been asked to collect a urine sample from a nine month old baby as part of an infection screen following a febrile seizure. Different practice areas where I have worked have used a number of different approaches to collecting a urine specimen. Contamination of urine samples means that a number of repeat samples are needed which is inconvenient for the family and not cost effective in terms of resource utilisation.

Question
Does the use of the urine collection pad reduce the contamination rate in non toilet trained children?

Step 2: Searching for the evidence

If you are new to literature searching find out what help and support is available. Libraries usually have printed material to help guide you through searching manually and electronically. Often libraries also offer tutorial sessions to help you develop electronic searching skills. If you are a student at a university this type of session is often included as part of your course. Chapter 3 of Craig and Smyth's book is written in a practical and user friendly way on searching the literature (Craig and Smyth, 2002). Price (2003) also offers useful chapters on accessing and gathering information and using the internet.

As I have already indicated there are a number of sources of evidence and the goal in searching the evidence is to locate this. I have included a number of websites that you might find useful, there are many others and you can add to the list. The internet can also be used using search engines such as google (www.scholar.google.com).

Your first starting point might be to see if there is a systematic review of evidence covering your question. www.cochrane.org or try the National Electronic Library for Health www.nelhs.nhs.uk/nurse which also contains a number of databases to search, including a link to the Cochrane library.

Further searching can incorporate a number of databases such as CINAHL and MEDLINE which focus generally on nursing, allied professions and medicine.

Additionally there may be specialist databases for some subject areas for example the FSID (Foundation for Sudden Infant Death) would be a useful site for Sudden Infant Death research (www.sids.org.uk/fsid).

When accessing the databases you need to have a clear idea of what you are searching for. For example urine collection as a search term would generate many thousands of matches, the vast majority of which would not be applicable to your question. You will need to use a range and combination of search terms to locate the information and, therefore, narrow the matches to the areas you are interested in.

For the purposes of this example I have located a number of sources of evidence for this question using the databases described above. In this instance it is useful to collate the evidence in a user friendly way to be able to see at a glance the range of evidence. It is one way of organising your collection if there are a number of sources of evidence. In research these are thematic and methodological matrices and form part of the literature review. A good example of this can be found in Crookes and Davies (1998, chapter 10). It is also the start of appraising the quality of the evidence.

As the evidence I have located is all based on research findings I will develop a methodological matrix (see Table 2.2). This is not an essential requirement for appraising evidence but I think it's a useful starting point as you can feel overwhelmed as you gather your evidence and it does start to make you think analytically about the strengths and weaknesses.

Table 2.2 Methodological matrix

Author/Year	Type of evidence	Methodology	Findings	Limitations	Strengths
Lewis J 1998	Research	Quasi experimental comparing urine collection pads to clean catch	No significant difference between methods	Short trial findings not generalisable	Direct relevance to practice
Feasey 1999	Research	Quasi experimental comparing urine collection pads to urine bags n = 50	Pad showed lower contamination rates than bag White blood cells collected from pad lower than bag	Lower contamination but if cell collection lower implications for findings?	Collected 2 Samples, I for each method from each child Adds to body of evidence in supporting use of pad

(*Continued*)

Author/Year	Type of evidence	Methodology	Findings	Limitations	Strengths
Farrell 2002	Research pilot study	Concurrent specimen collection from bag and pad n = 20	Differences between WBC counts for pad and bag may lead to false negative diagnosis of UTI	Pilot study will need large scale study for findings to be tested and be statistically significant	Highlights needs for further research
Liaw 2000	Research	Comparison study of bags pads and clean catch by parents at home n = 44	All equally effective in excluding infection Contamination rates similar with pad or bag and lower with clean catch	Can give false positive and further sample required Small sample size	Parents found pads easy to use, pads cheaper

Step 3: Appraising the evidence

In appraising the evidence you will find a number of resources useful to you. All research books will have a section on critiquing research and provide frameworks to enable you systematically to identify the studies' strengths and weaknesses. Additionally there are now a number of books written specifically about evidence-based practice. The *Nursing Times* monograph *Evidence-based Practice* by Le May (1999) offers frameworks to appraise both research and non-research based papers; and Price (2003, pp. 124–7) offers an evaluative framework and criteria for appraising research evidence. Abridged versions of these are included in Tables 2.3 and 2.4. They will guide you in questioning and analysing the content of this type of evidence, but they are not to be used as a checklist. It is not enough to determine whether a paper achieves for example reliability and validity in the conduct of a study, one must also explore and question '*So what does this mean?*' in the context of the study being reviewed, and ask '*Does it have implications for practice?*'.

Table 2.3 Analysing research-based papers

Research papers
The questions you ask of the paper are pertinent to the type of research being undertaken.

Philosophical approach or research paradigm:
What is this in the context of the study – Thus what do the researchers see as their goal?

- Is it objective truth leading to generalisation of findings? (quantitative or positivist research)
- Is it a portrayal of the search for meaning from the interpretation of individual/group experience of healthcare (qualitative or naturalistic research)?
- Is it critical theory which uses naturalistic enquiry with a concern for example social justice or inequality?

Study purpose:
- Who undertook the research?
- Did they have the appropriate experience and skills?
- What was the purpose of the study?
- Is the purpose of the study clearly outlined?
- Are the research questions or hypothesis clearly stated?
- Was the literature review relevant to the purpose of the study?
- Does the literature review evaluate all the relevant issues?

Study design:
- Were the data collection procedures described in sufficient detail?
- Did the research design and methods of data collection fit the research questions and the research paradigm?
- Are ethical considerations outlined and does it produce knowledge that can be morally used?
- Were issues of reliability and validity stated for quantitative studies?
- Do the results represent what the participants said (authenticity in qualitative studies)?

Study findings:
- Was the analysis clearly stated?
- Do the findings address the research questions?

Conclusions and recommendations for practice:
- Do the conclusions fit with the data presented?
- Are implications for clinical practice discussed?
- Are any weaknesses in the study identified?
- Who funded the work (if applicable)?

Source: Abridged from Le May (1999), Price (2003)

Table 2.4 Analysing non-research-based papers

Non-research based papers

Purpose:
- Who wrote the paper?
- Why did they write the paper?
- What is the purpose of the paper?
- Is the paper clearly presented?

Findings:
- What are the sources of knowledge in the paper?
- What new ideas are presented?   (*Continued*)

Table 2.4 (*Continued*)

- Does the paper confirm existing ideas?
- What are the strengths and weaknesses of the paper?

Implications for practice:
- What is the relevance of this paper for you?
- Do practice issues emerge from the paper?
- Do research questions emerge from the paper?

Source: Abridged from Le May (1999)

In appraising the evidence from a number of studies you are making an overall judgement based on the strengths and weaknesses of the evidence in terms of what it means for practice. You are analysing how the findings cohere with other studies, audits, papers, policy guidelines to inform your practice. Returning to the question about urine collection methods, the small number of studies presented suggests the need for more large scale robust studies and that there may be some unanswered question about the reliability of the collection pad. For demonstration purposes it has to be remembered in presenting this judgement that I have only considered a small number of the studies that are available on this subject.

Step 4: Utilisation of the evidence

Having appraised the evidence you will come to a conclusion about what it means for practice whether that is your own evidence-informed practice or making recommendations for the development of practice in the clinical area. To do this you will have made a judgement in the light of strengths and weaknesses and a consideration of the clinical relevance. Moving forward with practice can be challenging and is not the subject of this chapter. This will involve a change management strategy (see Chapter 12). Putting evidence into practice and the barriers to that has in itself been extensively researched, but for now it is important that you concentrate on honing your search and appraisal skills so that you can give the rationale behind your professional practice.

You are now ready to tackle the demands of a problem-based approach to learning about the practice of nursing children and young people and their families. Before you make a start if you are new to studying or it is a long time since you studied, the following section provides a few pointers to help you with general tips for study skills. Undertaking problem-based learning necessitates researching the depth and breadth of issues in order to come to some conclusions about the evidence you have located about a particular practice. To maximise your time and make the best use of the resources available to you there are a number of techniques you can use. These include mind mapping and structuring your reading skills for effective reading.

Mind maps

Originated by Tony Buzan this technique can help with problem solving. Further information is available at www.mind-map.com

Effective reading

Faced with a number of articles, research reports and books to read through, it is important that you are able to identify quickly those that will be of most use to you in answering the questions. Websites provide a range of study skills online, including: www.jcu.edu.au/studying/services/studyskills/effreading/ (accessed October 2005). These are likely to be helpful to you.

Summary

In this chapter you have been presented with a range of information that aims to develop your study skills, self awareness with regards to learning styles, reflective practice and evidence based practice. These will enable you to engage in a problem-based learning process as you work through this book. You will need to utilise all of these skills to maximise the potential this book has for developing your critical thinking across the range of subjects that present in children's nursing.

Suggested resources for reflective practice

Atkins, S., Murphy C. (1993) Reflection: a review of the literature. *Journal of Advanced Nursing*, 18 (8), pp. 1188–92.

Boud, D., Keogh, R., Walker, D. (1985) *Reflection: Turning Experience into learning.* London: Kogan Page.

Gibbs, G. (1988) *Learning by Doing: A Guide to Teaching and Learning methods.* Oxford: Further Education Unit Oxford Polytechnic.

Johns, C. (2000) *Becoming a Reflective Practitioner.* Oxford: Blackwell Science.

Suggested resources for study skills

Northedge, A. (1990) The Good Study Guide. (Milton Keynes: Open University Press. www.psychwww.com

Suggested resources for evidence-based practice

Callery, P. (1997) Using evidence in children's nursing. *Paediatric Nursing* 9 (6), pp. 13–17.

Craig, J., Smyth, R. (2002) *The Evidence-Based Practice Manual for Nurses.* Edinburgh: Churchill Livingstone.

Crookes, P. Davies, S. (1998) *Research into Practice.* London: Bailliere Tindall.

Glasper, E. A., Ireland, L. (2000) *Evidence-based Child Health Care: Challenges for Practice*. Basingstoke: Palgrave Macmillan.

Le May, A. (1999) *Evidence-based Practice*. London: Nursing Times Books.

McSherry, R., Simmons, M., Abbott, P. (2002) *Evidence Informed Nursing: A Guide for Clinical Nurses*. London: Routledge.

Price, B. (2003) *Studying Nursing Using Problem-based and Enquiry-based Learning*. Basingstoke: Palgrave, Chapter 5, pp. 83–103; Chapter 6, pp. 104–20.

Electronic sources

http://www.eboncall.co.uk (EBM website provided by Oxford Centre for Evidence Based Medicine)

http://www.jr2.ox.ac.uk/Bandolier/ (Print and Internet Journal about Health Care using evidence-based medicine techniques)

www.evidencebasednursing.com

www.york.ac.uk/depts/htsd/centres/evidence (Centre for evidence-based nursing)

www.cochrane.co.uk (Cochrane Centre for systematic reviews)

www.york.ac.uk/inst/crd (NHS Centre for reviews and dissemination)

www.fons.org (Foundation of Nursing Studies)

www.joannabriggs.edu.au Joanna Briggs Institute for Evidence Based Nursing

www.nelh.nhs.uk/nurse

References

Craig, J., Smyth, R. (2002) *The Evidence-based Practice Manual for Nurses*. Edingburgh: Churchill Livingstone.

Crookes, P., Davies, S. (1998) *Research into practice*. London: Bailliere Tindall.

Gibbs, G. (1988) *Learning by Doing: A Guide to Teaching and Learning Methods*. Oxford: Further Education Unit Oxford Polytechnic.

Honey, P., Mumford, A. (1982) The Learning Styles Questionnaire, www.peterhoneylearning.com (accessed January 2005).

Jasper, M. (2003) *Beginning Reflective Practice*. Cheltenham: Nelson Thornes.

Le May, A. (1999) *Evidence-based Practice*. London: Nursing Times Books.

NMC (2004) *The NMC code of professional conduct: standards for conduct, performance and ethics*. London: NMC.

Price, B. (2003) *Studying Nursing Using Problem-based and Enquiry-based Learning*. Basingstoke: Palgrave.

3

Contemporary Family-centred Care

Maureen Bradshaw and Valerie Coleman

Learning outcomes

- Understand the concept of contemporary family-centred care.
- Explain the use of the 'Family-centred Care Practice Continuum Tool'
- Assess the cultural needs of children, young people and their families in the planning of family-centred care.

Introduction

Using a problem-based learning approach this chapter aims to introduce students to contemporary family-centred care, which is 'the professional support of the child and family through a process of involvement, participation and partnership underpinned by empowerment and negotiation.' (Smith et al 2002a, p. 22).

The term 'contemporary' is used because the concept of family-centred care is a social construct and hence it continues to evolve and expand in Britain and other countries (Coleman 2002). Callery (2004) suggests that when a term such as family-centred care is so familiar it is all too easy to assume that it's meaning is obvious which is not necessarily true. It is, therefore, a professional responsibility for nurses and other healthcare professionals delivering family-centred care to familiarise themselves frequently with the expectations for family-centred care according to contemporary health policy, and in response to evidence-based studies.

Inevitably and appropriately family-centred care will be implemented in different ways in practice according to the demands of different clinical environments and the assessed needs of individual children and their families. Generally though there is a move in contemporary practice and policy towards a holistic approach to family-centred care as opposed to the functional approach (Hutchfield 1999) that was more apparent in the early evolution of the concept. The triggers in this chapter will distinguish between these two approaches.

Contemporary family-centred care is clearly outlined in the *National Service Framework for Children, Young People and Maternity Services* (Department of Health, 2004) standards. Standard Three of the framework which is 'Child, Young Person and Family-centred Services' states:

> Children and young people and families receive high quality services, which are co-ordinated around their individual and family needs and takes account of their views. (Department of Health 2004, p. 6)

To achieve this standard it is emphasised that both services and care need to be child-centred. In this chapter the focus will primarily be on individual child/family-centred care as opposed to the provision of child-centred services. However, this focus on child-centred services as well as care denotes the contemporary evolvement of the concept of family-centred care (to find out about earlier evolvement of the concept you should read Trigger 3.1). Contemporary child-centred services are to:

- Provide appropriate information to children, young people and the family.
- Listen and respond to them.
- Be respectful to children and young people, involving them in seeking consent according to developmental age.
- Improve access to services.
- Provide robust multi-agency planning and commissioning arrangements.
- Provide safe quality systems for child-centred care.
- Provide a common core of skills, knowledge and competencies that should be applied to all staff who work with children and young people across all agencies. Staff training and development programmes are required.

(Department of Health, 2004)

To achieve the National Service Framework Standard Number Three it is apparent that contemporary family-centred care delivery requires a multi-agency/multi-professional approach. This standard also identifies that children and young people are central to the delivery of family-centred care and that we must listen to them and encourage their involvement and participation in their own care (see Chapter 11).

The implementation of contemporary family-centred care is not without its difficulties due to the complex nature of this evolving concept that involves working in partnership (see Chapters 4 and 11) with different families/individual family members, multi-professional colleagues and also responding to contemporary health and social care policy. Lee (2004) for example identifies that more child health care is now being delivered in the child's home and school environment, which places an increasing burden on the child's family to deliver health care. The nature of treatment is also changing so that the care that a hospitalised child receives is more intensive, which subsequently impacts on the care that families may provide in this setting.

Callery (2004) argues that family-centred care is not a straightforward concept and nor is it only relevant to nurses. He suggests that children's nurses may take family-centred care for granted and that it is useful for multi-professional colleagues to 'talk' to become aware of others' perspectives on this approach to care. Bradshaw et al (2003) agree with this arguing that family-centred care should be viewed as a multi-professional philosophy and that inter-professional education is a key strategy to use to bring about a shared philosophy.

Franck and Callery (2004) conclude from a critical literature review and discussion that a re-thinking of family-centred care is required to develop a coherent research programme into the application of theory to practice in child health care. Lee (2004) relates to the barriers to successful implementation of family involvement in care clearly outlining the diverse contemporary role of the nurse as a facilitator of care and the positive or negative attitudes held by individual nurses. She concludes that greater negotiation and recognition that each child and family is unique with unique health and social care needs is required to ensure that family involvement in care is appropriate.

It is evident that it is important for children's nurses to have an up-to-date knowledge and understanding of the concept of family-centred care for optimum care delivery. The triggers within this chapter are designed to enable you to develop this knowledge and understanding about the concept of contemporary family-centred care, and to explore the use of a tool. The Practice Continuum Tool (Smith et al 2002) can be used to assist nurses to communicate about family-centred care overtly and accurately. The triggers transcend cultural boundaries and are applicable to primary and secondary care situations.

! Trigger 3.1: The Concept of Family-centred Care

This trigger is intended to familiarise you with the concept of family-centred care.

The Trigger

Transcript of a conversation on the paediatric ward

Staff Nurse: So how are you finding children's nursing compared to your previous experience in adult nursing?

Student Nurse: I like the children and I expected their parents to visit or sometimes stay with them but the whole family come often. Brothers and sisters tend to run round and play noisily. Some parents seem to do lots for the child and others not much. I find that a bit confusing and can't it be unsafe if they start doing the nurse's job?

Staff Nurse: I know what you mean, but didn't you do anything about family-centred care in school before your clinical experience here? Giving some thought to and discussing the merits of our philosophy of care beforehand can usually help you to know what to expect before you arrive.

Student Nurse: Yes, but I was off sick on the day when it was timetabled and I've still got to catch up on that lesson.

Staff Nurse: Well, we've articles on family-centred care for you to read in the office, in fact the ward sister has asked us to come to the next ward meeting with ideas for creating a poster about it to display on the ward for families to read. I suggest we make that one of your objectives too, what do you think?

Student Nurse: That's fine, I'll look those articles out today.

Situation

You are an adult branch student nurse in the first week of your allocation to the children's ward. This conversation takes place during your initial interview with your staff nurse mentor.

Feedback

This trigger requires you to produce a draft poster about the philosophy of family-centred care for the children's ward notice board.

The facts

What are the main facts in this trigger? Make a list.

Hypotheses: What may these facts mean?

- Parents visiting or staying with their hospitalised children is part of family-centred care philosophy.
- Siblings are a consideration of family-centred care philosophy.
- It might be unsafe for parents to do 'nursing' care for their child in hospital.
- Reading about and discussing family-centred care helps us to understand it.
- Communicating the philosophy of family-centred care to families and other visitors to the ward is important.

Questions developed from the hypotheses:

Answering the following questions will inform the poster you design

1. What does family-centred care philosophy comprise?
2. Why are siblings considered within family-centred care philosophy?
3. Can parents be safely involved in nursing care?
4. What information would be useful to include in a ward poster designed to communicate the philosophy of family-centred care to families visiting the ward?

Trigger 3.1: Fixed resource material

Read the following to help you answer the questions. (You may also wish to search and review other up-to-date research and evidence-based literature and seek other relevant resources to provide you with answers to your questions)

Coleman V. (2002) The evolving concept of family-centred care. In Smith, L., Coleman, V., Bradshaw, M. *Family-centred Care, Concept, Theory and Practice.* Basingstoke: Palgrave, Chapter 1, pp. 3–18.

Franck, L., Callery, P. (2004) Re-thinking family-centred care across the continuum of children's healthcare. *Child: Care, Health and Development* 30 (3), pp. 265–77.

Lee, P. (2004) Family involvement: Are we asking too much? *Paediatric Nursing* 16 (10), pp. 37–41.

Useful website

http://www.familycenteredcare.org Institute of Family-centered Care

Trigger 3.1: Fixed resource sessions

Family-centred care

Defining or labelling health care as 'family-centred' is an attempt to convey to others the way in which we envisage and, therefore, conduct our care relationships with our clients and their significant others. It says something about our belief and value systems because when we act voluntarily, we usually end up acting in congruence with our inner beliefs.

According to Coleman (2002, p. 3) family-centred care is a 'multifaceted concept that has evolved over the past 50 years'. It is now seen as a social construct that changes as society's beliefs and values change and, therefore, what it embodies will change from one decade to the next. The last five decades have seen nurses' values and understanding of the evolving concept move from an initial acceptance that parental presence might be important to the nursing care of sick children, right through to later believing that parental involvement and participation could lead to effective partnerships in care that were beneficial not only to the sick child but also the family. As control of care issues were grappled with along the way, we see thinking and beliefs change from seeing care as essentially nurse-led to openness about the possibility of it being led increasingly by the child and family if indeed that is their choice.

As the psychological and emotional needs of sick children came to be recognised as equally (if not more) important than their physical care requirements, then families came to be seen in most instances as the key stabilising factor for the child receiving some aspect of nursing or health care (Campbell and Summersgill 1993, Bradley 1996) because family presence and involvement is emotionally supportive to the child. Policy supportive of such views started with the Platt Report (Ministry of Health 1959) and later the Court Report (Department of Health and Social Security 1976) which recognised that children have different needs from those of adults and that children's nurses and parents of sick children would benefit the sick child by working in partnership. The Children Act (Department of Health 1989) emphasised parental responsibilities within such partnerships and the Department of Health's (1991) document on *The Welfare of Children and Young People in Hospital* made it overtly clear that quality care had to be family-centred, meaning not only care of the sick child but also that of parents and siblings. The family's right to be involved in the sick child's care was highlighted in *The Patient's Charter: Services for Children and Young People* (Department of Health 1996) and more recently the *National Service Framework for Children, Young People and Maternity Services* (Department of Health, 2004).

Within family-centred care philosophy parental presence and contributions to care are valued for much more than their functional value (i.e. for the tasks that they may choose to do within a care scenario). Parents are not expected to be passive but are given the choice to be active participants in care and decision-making. This means that children's nurses might at times be the principle care givers but at other times they will be involved in teaching and supporting activities with children and families in order to empower them to competently perform chosen care activities themselves.

Children's nurses therefore require competence in a broad range of skills if they are to practice family-centred care efficaciously. These will include the good communication and interpersonal skills necessary for interviewing, assessing needs, sharing information and negotiating with the child and family. Not only do nurses need to be skilled planners, deliverers and evaluators of patient care themselves, but they also have to be effective teachers and encouragers when empowering children and families to be involved in decision-making and sharing or leading their own care, or aspects of it. Children's nurses need to become well soaked in family-centred care philosophy if they are to be comfortable and conversant in discussing family-centred care with children and families in their care.

Siblings

Siblings require consideration within family-centred care because clearly they are part of the family. The illness or hospitalisation of one child in a family may have varying degrees of effects on other family members including the sick child or young person's siblings. If the nurse is aiming to deliver holistic family-centred care then inevitably siblings must be included in this.

A variety of studies indicate that hospitalised sick children sometimes miss their brothers and sisters. Siblings on the other hand, can feel resentful (Ferrari, 1984) towards the sick child in hospital because of the amount of attention they receive which appears to be unevenly divided. This can also happen when children are nursed at home in the community. In this setting siblings can also feel resentful about care demands being made of them as well as the parents or demands that include doing the sick child's normal allocation of household chores, for example walking the dog.

Some sibling responses may depend on their age, understanding and the nature of the sick child's illness. Black (1994) for example, discusses findings where a two-fold increase in emotional disorders had been found in siblings of children with life-threatening diseases. Other studies indicate that siblings with few coping mechanisms may exhibit more physical symptoms like gastrointestinal disturbances, headaches or symptoms similar to those of the sick child.

From a family-centred care point of view, everyone in the family requires information and understanding about the nature and implications of the sick child's illness. Information giving needs to be age appropriate to aid understanding, and Taylor et al (1999) suggest that for siblings especially, this is safer than them making up their own explanations, which may be more frightening than the actual facts. Siblings can easily carry unvoiced fears that they might develop or genetically carry the same affliction as the sick child, so family-centred care would underpin provision being made for these fears to be voiced and alleviated or confirmed and dealt with in a supportive manner.

In order to appreciate the inclusion of siblings within family-centred care philosophy, it is suggested that during your clinical ward and community placements, that you talk with siblings of sick children about their thoughts and concerns. Talk too with parents, focusing this time on the siblings rather than the sick child. Explore for yourself if there is any specific provision made for the siblings of sick children within your ward/hospital.

→ Trigger 3.1: Feedback

Go to Chapter 3 Trigger feedback on p. 52

! Trigger 3.2: The Practice Continuum Tool

This trigger is intended to introduce you to the Practice Continuum Tool, and through the use of a scenario, show how it can be used by nurses to facilitate accurate communication about family-centred care.

The Trigger

You are caring for ten month old Megan, who has had surgery, with your mentor on the children's surgical ward using the Practice Continuum Tool for family-centred care.

Situation

Megan's parents had rushed her to the accident and emergency department. Following triage in the department Megan was seen immediately and following investigations was transferred straight to the operating theatre for surgery.

Feedback

This trigger requires you to choose a patient from your current clinical placement (who shall remain anonymous) for a care study presentation during your next study day seminar. Using a family-centred approach to care and the Practice Continuum Tool (Smith, Coleman and Bradshaw, 2002), identify where you would report your chosen family to be on the Continuum at significant points throughout their health care journey. This may include movement back and forth along the Continuum. Be prepared to discuss your rationale in support of the statements that you make in a seminar on your next study day.

The facts

What are the main facts in this trigger? Make a list:

Hypotheses: What may these facts mean?

● Nurses need a tool to communicate about family-centred care to families and colleagues
● Children are seen immediately in urgent situations

Questions developed from the hypothesis

1. What do the terms functional and holistic frameworks mean in a family-centred care context?
2. Are the terms involvement, participation, partnership and parent-led care synonymous with family-centred care?
3. What is the Practice Continuum Tool?
4. How can the Practice Continuum Tool be used to enhance family-centred care in a children's nursing environment?

Trigger 3.2: Fixed resource material

Read the following to help you answer the questions. (You may also wish to search and review other up-to-date research and evidence-based literature and seek other relevant resources to provide you with the answers to your questions.)

Smith, L., Coleman, V., Bradshaw, M. (2002) Family-centred care: A practice continuum, in Smith, L., Coleman, V., Bradshaw, M. *Family-centred Care: Concept, Theory and Practice*. Basingstoke: Palgrave. Chapter 2, pp.19–43.

Coleman, V., Smith, L., Bradshaw, M. (2003) Enhancing consumer participation using the Practice Continuum Tool for family-centred care. *Paediatric Nursing* 15 (8), pp. 28–31.

Trigger 3.2: Fixed Resource Sessions

The development of the Practice Continuum Tool

As family-centred care has evolved throughout the decades there have been different understandings of what it actually is, what it comprises and what sort of an approach to care defines it. It's easy to see how especially earlier on in its evolution, views of family-centred care are rather 'functional' in nature. It may have been hard for nurses to change from the mind set of nurse as expert and main care giver. The attempt to change the way nurses practiced may well have led to a sort of transitional stage that looked like family-centred care when glancing at it from the outside, but when examined in any depth still revealed vestigial elements of former care values. Nursing at this point can be described as operating within a *functional framework* where care is still nurse-led. Here families are valued for what they do that is practical and useful. This tends to include involving them in the 'normal' care duties they would perform for children at home. Nurse's language characteristic of such a framework talks about *allowing* parents to perform tasks that contribute to their children's care. Nurses although open to having families present on the ward, are still the dominant players taking the role of gatekeeper (Hutchfield 1999) as they decide what it is appropriate for parents to participate in. The functional approach is also characterised by a tendency to focus on family problems and weaknesses, and is not particularly collaborative in nature. The power base still remains with the nurse so inevitably the family is disempowered by their inability to gain control over their situation. With the functional approach there is likely to be a lack of mutuality between nurses and families because the nursing focus is on the functional role of parents rather than family empowerment (Smith et al 2002).

Further evolution of family-centred care has often led to a more *holistic framework* for care being used. This is 'grounded in respect for and cooperation with the family' (Hutchfield 1999, p. 1181) and thus is more likely to empower them. This more collaborative model of care embraces nurses and families as equal partners in care. There is mutual respect for the nurse as expert in nursing care of the sick child or young person, and parent as expert on the child. When this expertise is harnessed together it can be a powerful force for the good of the sick child because it leads to the two-way sharing of helpful information and skills. Within the holistic framework there is more of a tendency to focus on family strengths and helpful coping mechanisms (Ahmann 1994, Shelton and Smith Stepanek 1995) which can be empowering in enabling families to have some control over their situation.

Smith et al (2002a p. 20) state that 'family-centred care is used as an all-embracing term to describe a concept with many different attributes,' and some confusion can arise from associated terminology. For example the literature contains the terms parental involvement, parental participation and partnership working as well as family-centred care. It is appropriate to explore if they all mean exactly the same thing or something different.

Parental *involvement* generally refers to parents being enabled to support their sick children or young people psychologically by being with them, and being involved in basic care giving (for example the type of daily care they would normally be doing for the child at home like feeding or hygiene care) and decision-making. However, care is still nurse-led.

Parental *participation* tends to cover parents being involved in care as above but additionally participating in chosen aspects of nursing care (care that hitherto would have been seen as firmly in the nurse's domain) following negotiation with the nurse. The nurse and parent relationship here is seen as collaborative, however the nurse still continues to lead and oversee care management. The nurse's role though now includes teaching some relevant nursing care skills to the child, young person or family.

Family *partnerships* in care describe relationships between the nurse and family that have become more equal in nature. The nurse's role is that of an empowerer, supporter and facilitator for the family. As the family become more empowered here, they resume their role as the primary care givers with assistance from the nurse.

Parent/child-led care describes those care relationships where the family are now experts in all aspects of the child or young person's care. It is also acknowledged that children and young people are capable of and may choose to lead their own care in some instances. Here the relationship between nurse and family is based on mutual respect, and the family being confident in their care skills and abilities, may simply choose to use the nurse in a consultative capacity.

> Ultimately all of these terms described with their associated attributes, offer different dimensions of family-centred care, each in their own way relevant and providing an opportunity for families to be involved in the care of their child, preferably to an extent of their choosing. (Smith et al 2002a, p. 22)

These different dimensions of family-centred care were recognised in the contemporary definition of family-centred care for the twenty-first century offered by Smith et al. (2002a, p. 22), who believe that family-centred care is: 'The professional support of the child and family through a process of involvement, participation and partnership underpinned by empowerment and negotiation'.

The themes of negotiation and empowerment are important, and are expanded upon in Chapter 11 (see Fixed resource session for Trigger 11.1, 'Negotiated Empowerment Framework').

In their daily clinical practice nurses need an efficient and effective way of communicating various aspects of a child or young person's care to each other. If needing to communicate about a child's temperature for example, verbal communications may indicate that the child is hypothermic, normothermic, pyrexial or hyperpyrexial. These descriptions have instant meaning for the nurse who has previously learnt these definitions. Temperature charts on the end of the child's bed are also used as a non-verbal tool to convey information about the child's temperature history as well as indicating exactly what is happening with the child's temperature right now.

In the same way nurses need a language with which they can communicate the various aspects of family-centred care to each other and a tool that could convey this information non-verbally. The aforementioned definitions of nurse-led involvement and participation, equal status partnerships and parent/child-led family-centred care can be the specific language used by nurses to accurately communicate about their family-centred care relationships with families to one another. Instead of a temperature chart, the non-verbal communication tool for family-centred care proposed by Smith et al (2002) is referred to as The Practice Continuum Tool, (see Figure 3.1).

This Tool is easy to use and nurses can plot on the Continuum where they are at in their relationship with the child, young person or parents at any given point in time. Nurse and family relationships are dynamic, therefore, there is likely to be movement back and forth along the Continuum according to changes in the child's condition and altering family choices for example. There is, however, no ultimate goal to be reached. Family-centred care can be achieved through nurse-led family

No Involvement	Involvement	Participation	Partnership	Parent/child-led
Nurse-led	Nurse-led	Nurse-led	Equal status	Parent/child-led

Figure 3.1 The Family-centred Care Practice Continuum Tool

involvement during a child's five hour stay on a day care ward but will also be achieved by parent-led care in a family who feel confident in managing the long term care of an epileptic child at home. The Continuum includes the descriptor of a 'nurse-led, no parental involvement' position because it is recognised that in unusual circumstances like child protection situations or times where the whole family may be unwell due to accident or illness, then care may be led by the nurse with no family involvement.

Family-centred care is a requirement of current children's and young people's health care policy. The use of the Practice Continuum Tool can not only help nurses understand more about the concept of family-centred care but it can also improve professional communications about it, and make its use more overt in professional documentation. The following fixed resource session illustrates the use of the Practice Continuum Tool when caring for ten month old Megan and her family.

Using the Practice Continuum Tool to communicate aspects of Megan's family-centred care needs

Megan's story is elicited as medical examination takes place. Hours ago Megan suddenly began screaming and drawing her knees up to her chest as if in pain. A stool passed at the time appeared normal. She responded to being comforted and changed and appeared content again for approximately 20–30 minutes, subsequently this pattern has repeated itself for much of the day. Latterly Megan had appeared increasingly distressed during attacks, not taken fluids well and vomited. Frightened parents rushed her to hospital when she went somewhat pale and lethargic. These early symptoms of shock together with tachycardia, lowering blood pressure and breathing that is becoming more rapid and shallow are still evident. Megan's abdomen is swollen and the doctor can palpate a sausage shaped intestinal mass inside. Rectal examination reveals the presence of blood and mucus which is subsequently passed as stools with the appearance of red currant jelly. It is explained that Megan's signs and symptoms are suggestive of Intussusception where one portion of bowel invaginates or slides into the next (much like the pieces of a telescope). This section of bowel becomes swollen causing intestinal obstruction and the blood supply can become cut off if the intussusception is not reduced quickly. The management plan is to treat the developing shock and continue diagnostic and therapeutic procedures.

The nurse supports Megan's parents in holding and comforting her as blood is taken for analysis and intravenous fluid is commenced to help combat the developing shock and dehydration. Megan's father leaves the department to contact relatives. Meanwhile, knowing Megan's mother's choice to stay and support her child in whatever way she could, the nurse helps her put on a lead apron to safely accompany Megan in the X-Ray department. X-Rays and ultrasound examination of Megan's abdomen are both suggestive of intussusception. During this procedure, the nurse reinforces information given previously, that as well as confirming the diagnosis, it is also hoped that the force of an air enema (pneumatic insufflation) introduced rectally into Megan's bowel will be sufficient to actually push the 'telescoped' (invaginated) portion of bowel back into its original position and cure the obstruction as the bowel unfolds. According to Pillitteri (1999) this procedure is successful in 75–80 per cent of cases but unfortunately not so with Megan. Consent is, therefore, obtained from her parents to prepare and transfer her to theatre for surgical intervention to manually reduce the intussusception. They are aware that if the blood supply has been cut off resulting in 'death' of the intestine at this point, then the non-viable portion of intestine will be resected.

Anaesthetic room procedure is explained to Megan's parents and her father chooses to stay with Megan until she is anaesthetised prior to surgery. During this time he is supported by the nursing staff who encourage him to gently comfort Megan and speak softly and reassuringly to her while the anaesthetic "puts her to sleep". The nurse then takes Megan's parents to the ward where she will receive her post-operative care and introduces them to the nurse who will be caring for Megan.

At the handover of care, Megan's parents are described as being at the Nurse-led, Parental Involvement point on the Practice Continuum Tool because they are new to the situation and unsure how to help. Care is clearly nurse-led, but the parents are involved in comforting Megan, giving her emotional support and decision-making (see Figure 3.2).

Megan's new nurse recognises the parent's anxiety and endeavours to relieve as much of it as she can at this time. She takes them to the cubicle where Megan will be nursed and over a much needed cup of tea she explains the ward's philosophy of family-centred care. Realising that they are welcome to stay with Megan and make choices about their involvement in her care is reassuring to them. They are further reassured by the nurse's interest in Megan's usual routines, likes and dislikes as she gathers

No Involvement	Involvement	Participation	Partnership	Parent/child-led
Nurse-led	Nurse-led	Nurse-led	Equal status	Parent/child-led

Figure 3.2   The Practice Continuum Tool – Involvement

information from the parents that will help her to assess all of Megan's needs on return from theatre in order to plan appropriate nursing care.

On return from theatre Megan's parents are informed that a small portion of Megan's bowel had gone necrotic (died due to lack of blood supply) and, therefore, had to be removed. Fortunately this was not a large section and the bowel had been repaired, the only visible evidence of this was now a wound dressing on Megan's abdomen.

Megan has a paralytic ileus on return from theatre, therefore, over the coming days her nurse cares for the nasogastric tube situated to drain gastric secretions until peristalsis returns. The nurse also administers the prescribed antibiotics and intravenous fluids that will keep Megan hydrated until intestinal peristaltic function returns and she can drink orally again.

The nurse has a major role in information giving at this point and answers questions openly and honestly about Megan's condition and progress. Megan's resident parents choose to continue comforting her and assist her nurse with hygiene care. As some improvement becomes apparent in Megan's condition, her father returns to his off-shore job on an oil rig.

Megan is not comfortable with strangers and is reluctant to make eye contact with them or receive care from them. The nurse, therefore, negotiates to get Megan's mother participating in aspects of care that hitherto were performed by nursing staff. For example, the nurse recognises the mother's expertise in knowing her own child well and welcomes her participating in pain assessment. Megan's mother is well attuned to the subtle, often non-verbal cues that signify discomfort in her daughter and she uses her expertise in this area to negotiate appropriate pain relief for her.

Care at this point is still nurse-led but being involved in what was hitherto nursing aspects of care suggests that the family-centred care relationship is now more participative and would be shown on the Practice Continuum Tool as in Figure 3.3.

Once Megan's bowel sounds return and gastric aspirate is minimal, the nasogastric tube is removed and her mother is delighted to be able to offer Megan first fluids and then later weaning diet again. The relationship between Megan's nurse and mother is collaborative in nature at this stage and a more equal partnership is apparent. The nurse continues caring for Megan's abdominal wound, monitors her vital signs and fluid balance but otherwise most care is given by her mother who has educated the nurses as to Megan's likes and dislikes so that their interactions with her are now becoming easier.

No Involvement	Involvement	Participation	Partnership	Parent/child-led
Nurse-led	Nurse-led	Nurse-led	Equal status	Parent/child-led

Figure 3.3 The Practice Continuum Tool – Participation

Megan doesn't like her antibiotic medication now that she is free of the intravenous infusion and it can be given orally. So the nurse has to teach her mother how to hold her and administer the medication quickly and efficiently without spilling.

Family-centred care is about caring for the whole family and this becomes evident the following day when Megan's nurse notices her mother looking particularly pale. Concerned conversation reveals that she is feeling extremely nauseous due to one of her migraine headaches. They agree that Megan's mother needs to follow her usual course of action in such circumstances which includes going home, taking prescribed medication and 'sleeping it off' in a darkened room. It's arranged that a neighbour will collect Megan's mother who is reassured that she's shared enough information about Megan for her to be appropriately cared for in her mother's absence.

Other than telephone contact over the next 24 hours, there is no parental involvement in Megan's care which is nurse-led at this point. Care is still however family-centred because the nurses are able to draw on all of the previous information that her mother was able to share with them and allow this to guide their care of Megan in her absence. The family position on the Practice Continuum Tool changes again at this point in Megan's health care journey (see Figure 3.4).

No Involvement	Involvement	Participation	Partnership	Parent/child-led
Nurse-led	Nurse-led	Nurse-led	Equal status	Parent/child-led

Figure 3.4   The Practice Continuum Tool – No involvement

Megan's mother returns refreshed the following day and is delighted to hear that Megan will soon be ready for discharge. She quickly resumes her normal parenting role with Megan and also receives teaching on how to care for Megan's healing wound at home. During the last few days of Megan's stay on the ward, the nurse's role has become much more that of teacher, supporter and facilitator within what has now become a mutually respectful, collaborative, family-centred care relationship (see Figure 3.5).

No Involvement	Involvement	Participation	Partnership	Parent/child-led
Nurse-led	Nurse-led	Nurse-led	Equal status	Parent/child-led

Figure 3.5   The Practice Continuum Tool – Partnership

This scenario has not specifically addressed the issues surrounding whether it is safe to involve parents in the nursing care of their sick children. You may wish to discuss this in one of your study day seminar groups. Foxcroft's chapter on 'Professional and Legal Issues' in Smith et al (2002) will be a helpful aid to such debates.

→ Trigger 3.2: Feedback

Go to Chapter 3 Trigger Feedback on p. 52

! Trigger 3.3: Meeting cultural needs in family-centred care

This trigger is intended to help you to assess the cultural needs of children, young people and their families, and to reflect this in your delivery of family-centred care in practice.

The Trigger

Extracts from Student Nurse Gemma Hardy's reflective learning journal:

During my community placement I accompanied the health visitor on several visits to an ethnic minority refugee family. The father is age 24 years, the mother is age 21 years and their two children are age 2 and 11 months respectively. The 2 year old boy is generally healthy. The 11 month old girl is prone to chest infections and has been admitted to the local hospital on one occasion.

This family arrived in the United Kingdom with some members of their extended family following political conflict in their own country. They had never been in this country before, and there were no relatives or friends that were already here to support them. However, the family lived with the extended family and had made links with other refugee families living in temporary accommodation in the local community that spoke the same language.

The health visitor told me that the family had been very distressed initially, but very relieved to be alive and together in a safe environment. She had found it difficult to understand their culture and the impact of this on their way of life especially in relation to child rearing practices and beliefs. The health visitor was one member of the multi-professional health and social care team working with this family. She has to be accompanied by an interpreter on her visits to be able to communicate with the family.

I observed on my visits to this family that there was a lack of play resources for the children in the accommodation. The mother kept the children close to her as she 'worked' in the house. It was Ramadan, the Muslim holy month when we visited the family. The parents were fasting, but my health visitor explained that the children were exempt because they were too young. I asked if there were any other dietary restrictions when they were not fasting. The father wanted the boy to have a circumcision for non-medical reasons. I noticed that it was father who

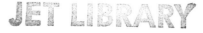

made decisions in the family and the mother always referred to him to answer questions.

I met this family again when I was allocated to the Children's Medical Ward at the local hospital. The 11 month old girl had been admitted with another chest infection. The nurses on the ward used a family-centred approach to care for the child and family and in the nursing assessment did consider cultural issues in relation to all the activities of living (Roper et al 1980). The mother seemed pleased to see me – I was a familiar face in a strange environment in which she had difficulty communicating. I did notice that on occasions a large number of visitors turned up to visit mother and child. They didn't know the family very well and some of the nursing staff were not very happy about this. I remembered that the health visitor said in some religions it was a 'duty to visit the sick'. I discussed this with my mentor.

Situation

You have reflected on your experiences with this family in preparation for a seminar session on your next study day. On this study day you presented this reflection to your colleagues and received some suggestions for further learning about meeting cultural needs.

Feedback

In response to your colleague's suggestions you should write some brief notes about 'models' or 'frameworks' that may be used to address the cultural needs of individual families such as the one described in this trigger scenario.

The facts

> **What are the main facts in this trigger? Make a list:**

Hypotheses: What may these facts mean?

- Families are individual
- Everyone has a culture

- An understanding of our own culture is essential in order to meet the cultural needs of others using a family-centred approach to care.
- A multi-professional approach to family-centred care is adopted to meet the needs of ethnic minority refugee families

Questions developed from the hypotheses

1. What is a family?
2. What are the implications of 'culture' for multi-professional working, parenting, and family-centred care delivery?
3. What guidelines are available to help nurses and other healthcare professionals meet the cultural needs of children, young people and their families?

Addressing the identified questions for this trigger will help you to complete this work and provide you with the rationale for using a 'model' or 'framework' to underpin cultural nursing care.

Trigger 3.3: Fixed resource material

Read the following to help you answer the questions. (You may also wish to search and review other up-to-date research and evidence-based literature and seek other relevant resources to provide you with the answers to your questions.)

Bradshaw, M., Coleman, V., Smith, L. (2003) Inter-professional learning and family-centred care. *Paediatric Nursing* 15 (7) September, pp. 30–3.

Hewitt, D. (2000) Child-centred care: ethnofriendly or ethnocentric?. *Paediatric Nursing*, 12 (6) July, pp. 6–8.

Holland, K., Hogg, C. (2001) Child- and family-centred care – a cultural perspective, in Holland, K., Hogg, C. *Cultural Awareness in Nursing and Health Care*. London: Arnold, Chapter 8, pp. 116–34.

Mountain, G. (2002) Parenting in society: A critical review, in Smith, L., Coleman, V., Bradshaw, M. *Family-centred Care: Concept, Theory and Practice*. Basingstoke: Palgrave, Chapter 4, pp. 62–81.

Office of National Statistics (2005) Focus on Families, http://www.statistics.gov.uk (accessed 20.10.05).

Watts, S., Norton, D. (2004) Culture, ethnicity, race: what's the difference? *Paediatric Nursing* 16 (8) October, pp. 37–42.

Trigger 3.3: Fixed resource sessions

What is a family?

It is relevant to allocate some time to considering 'what is a family?'. In fact it is imperative to have a good understanding and knowledge about the family to be able to use a family-centred approach to care. In relation to the family described in this trigger it seems that families may 'differ' due to differences in 'culture'.

The family exists in all cultures and societies in some form and it is an important institution in today's society. Abercrombie and Ward (2000) define the family as a kinship grouping of adults or adults and children, who may not necessarily have a common residence.

Suggested Activity

Undertake a literature search to find some alternative definitions of the 'family'. Compare and contrast the definitions and draw some conclusions about the definition that most accurately describes the 'family'.

Families have been divided into six different types:

1. The nuclear family consists of mother, father and child/children.
2. The extended family is a nuclear family plus other relatives of either or both spouses/partners that live together.
3. The patriarchal family is when the man has the main authority and decision-making power in the family
4. The matriarchal family has the woman as the main authority.
5. A reconstituted family consists of one divorced or widowed adult with his/her children and a new spouse/partner with his/her children.
6. Lone/single parent families consist of one adult living with his/her child(ren), usually the mother.

Hall and Elliman (2003) identify that there are also a significant number of children in the United Kingdom living in families with exceptional problems and needs including asylum seeking and refugee families. The family in this trigger is a refugee family that have left their own country 'owing to a well founded fear of being persecuted for reasons of race, religion, nationality, membership of a particular social group or political opinion' (Hall and Elliman 2003). An asylum seeker is someone that applies for refugee status. A refugee family is entitled to have the same rights to welfare benefits and health care as citizens of the United Kingdom. The family in this trigger is being supported by the health visitor and other relevant professionals because it is not easy for refugee families to familiarise themselves with local services and access them.

These different types of families should be recognised in the delivery of family-centred care. Haralambos and Holborn (1990) identify other diversities in families that may impact on family-centred care delivery (in addition to organisational diversity according to family type) These include:

- Cultural diversity
- Social class differences
- Life cycle differences (some families will have dependent children and others grown up children)
- Life experiences (the historical period when children are born may influence the length of time that they are dependent on parents)
- Regional diversity (family patterns and responsibilities vary around the United Kingdom and other countries).

Family functions include those concerned with education, economics, reproduction, sexual factors and the development of moral values. Socialisation is another function that occurs within the family and this is essential for a person to develop into a social being. Socialisation is the process by which we acquire our social characteristics and learn the ways of thought and behaviour that is considered appropriate in our society. Giddens (1989, p. 60) states that 'socialisation is the process whereby the helpless infant gradually becomes a self-aware, knowledgeable person, skilled in the way of the culture in which he/she is born.' This socialisation is a two way process because 'even the most recent new born infant has needs or demands that affect the behaviour of those responsible for its care' (Giddons, 1989, p. 60).

Mountain (2002, p. 62) questions 'the general assumption often made that the parental attitudes, behaviours and styles inherent in models of parenting and family-centred care are fundamentally altruistic and facilitative'. He also argues that practitioners working with children and their families must have knowledge and understanding of parenting within the context of childhood, family and caring for children.

Suggested Activity

It is suggested that you read Mountain (2002) Parenting in society: a critical review, to develop this knowledge and understanding of parenting. This will:

- Help you to apply the key theoretical principles and concepts to family-centred care nursing practice.
- Identify the need to understand cross-cultural perspectives in parenting.

This session provides some insight into 'what is a family'. It is suggested that you give this question further consideration to enhance your delivery of family-centred care to all families. A useful resource is the Office for National Statistics (2005) *Focus on Families* which looks at family types in the United Kingdom today and explores similarities and differences between them. For example, it identifies that the number of families headed by a married couple fell by half a million between 1996 and 2004, to just over 12 million. At the same time both lone mother and cohabiting couple families increased to 2.3 million and 2.2 million respectively. This indicates the need to establish 'who' and 'what' is the family in the nursing assessment to plan appropriate care.

Focus on Families also provides useful statistics related to ethnicity and families. Ethnicity is a concept 'that refers to the cultural practices and attitudes that characterise a given group of people distinguishing them from other groups' (Watts and Norton 2004, pp. 37–42). Families headed by a person of non-White ethnic background are more likely than White families to have dependent children living with them. Four in five Bangladeshi families had dependent children living with them in 2001 in the United Kingdom, compared with just over two out of five in White families (Office for National Statistics 2005).

Cultural issues in Children's and Young People's Nursing Practice

This session will explore what we mean by culture in general terms and make application to some cultural issues affecting children's and young people's nursing practice.

Everyone has a culture and almost everything in our behaviour is influenced by culture including health beliefs, attitudes, practices and child rearing. Culture is not limited to ethnic minority groups, but working with groups whose culture we do not share can be difficult. Culture enables members of a group, community or nation to function cohesively because of a shared set of norms, values, assumptions and perceptions (Schott and Henley 1996).

Helman (1994) describes culture as being a cultural lens through which an individual will perceive, understand and learn to live in their world. However, Herberg (1995) states that most people only have a very basic understanding of their own culture, although they function in it automatically. Most aspects of culture are invisible and intangible and it is only when we become aware of what in ourselves is cultural that we can step outside our cultural constraints to be able to promote health in other people in terms of their cultural needs (Schott and Henley 1996). However it is not easy to 'step outside' and this explains the potential to have difficulty understanding the needs of minority groups who may have a very different culture to the 'majority culture'.

'Culture is learned not only through formal study, but also through a process of cultural osmosis in which the values, attitudes, roles and behaviours acceptable to and expected by the cultural group are absorbed' (Herberg 1995, p. 9). This process begins in the family and continues in the wider community at school and through peers. This process leads to acculturation meaning that a given cultural group will adapt to or learns how to take on the behaviour of other groups (Herberg 1995). This has implications for children's and young people's nursing practice because it may be that a child's cultural needs differ to those of the adult family members due to acculturation. It is also relevant to recognise that the culture of particular groups of people does change over time. So it is important that assumptions are not made about the cultural needs of individuals. Instead an accurate nursing assessment should be undertaken of all children and families in clinical settings to be able to plan care that will truly meet their cultural needs. Smaje (1995) argues that it is important that culture is not understood as a checklist, but conversely as a dynamic active social process which is linked to broader social economic patterns.

To avoid discrimination and to ensure quality care for children and young people attention to cultural issues in healthcare is necessary (McEwing et al 2003). There is considerable cultural diversity in Britain in the twenty-first century and we need to understand our own culture to enable us to be aware that other cultures exist in our communications with children and families (Watt and Norton 2004). This is necessary for us to be able to recognise the actual and potential problems of all families in our assessment and planning of nursing care. 'Health beliefs and illness behaviours will vary across different cultures – across regions, ethnic groups and social class' (Watt and Norton 2004, p. 39). However, we need to avoid categorising these beliefs and behaviours for various groups because not only would it be difficult to remember all this information (McGee 1994) but it can lead to wrong stereotypical assumptions being made about a family's culture.

By using a family-centred approach to care and working in partnership with families cultural diversity in family structures should be recognised, and the cultural choices and needs of individual families are likely to be acknowledged and respected. This is providing that healthcare practitioners have cultural knowledge, awareness, sensitivity and competence (Papadopoulos 2003). It must be appreciated though that there may be difficulties with parents being intimidated in a strange environment (country and/or hospital) and they will be reluctant to discuss their culture (Watt and Norton 2004). There was a language barrier with the family in this trigger and the use of professional jargon and complicated medical language may be difficult for other families that do speak the same language. There are also different cultural norms in respect of non-verbal communication and misunderstandings may occur. Conversely non-verbal communication may be used positively to convey care and concern when there is not a common language.

'The method of child rearing will be dependent on the parent's values and the circumstances in which they live' (Holland and Hogg 2001, p. 120). Culture and health beliefs will influence child rearing practices. Nurses and other health care professionals should always support and help families in the way in which they wish to rear their children unless it is contradictory to health and well-being.

Suggested Activity

You will find it helpful to read some of the resources identified in the fixed resources material section for this trigger to find out more about:

1. Some of the issues raised in Student Nurse Gemma Hardy's learning diary extracts for example:
   - Ramadan
   - Non-medical Circumcision
   - The extended family
   - Play
   - Decision-making norms in families
   - 'Duty to visit the sick'
2. Diverse child rearing practices for example hygiene practices, feeding and carrying or settling children. Also to identify any differences in keeping children dependent or alternatively encouraging children to become more independent at different ages in childhood.
3. Beliefs about healthcare and responsibilities.

Holland and Hogg (2001) provide a very useful chapter focused on child and family-centred care and a cultural perspective.

→ Trigger 3.3: Feedback

Go to Chapter 3 Trigger Feedback on p. 52 below

? Chapter 3 Trigger Feedback: What do you Know?

Trigger 3.1: Concept of family-centred care

The development of your poster will be based on the answers to the questions that you are likely to have formulated for this trigger.

You may have given some thought to what the poster will look like and where to display it as well as the information it will contain. According to Ewles and Simnett (2003) it will perhaps catch most people's attention if displayed at eye level in a place where visitors would naturally have to pause for a few moments, for example whilst waiting for the lift or for security camera verification before being admitted through electronically controlled ward security doors. Displaying it in parent waiting rooms and residential facilities also has potential because here parents have a few moments to themselves away from the demands of their sick child and thus might find it a more appropriate time to pause and read the poster. Beware though of adding it to already crowded notice boards where nobody appears to have overall responsibility for updating the information displayed and keeping it uncluttered so that what really requires attention stands out.

It's worth considering other peoples posters that you can still remember and asking yourself what it was about them that drew your attention to them in the first place and what was it that created a long lasting impression. Was it perhaps the use of primary colours that really stood out or the bold use of eye-catching important words, phrases or slogans? Sometimes it's feint but emotional pictures in the background that create a lasting impression after other things have drawn your attention to the poster. Whatever it was you may be able to use some of the same 'tricks' to good effect with your poster.

The message on your poster needs to be clear and succinct so avoid excess words, jargon and abbreviations. Use lay person's language that would be suitable for a young person with a reading age of 12 years.

Following your extensive reading of family-centred care literature and from information provided in the fixed resource sessions it is likely that your poster would aim to convey such principles / key elements as:

- Parent as expert on the child.
- Nurse as expert in nursing care.
- Desire to share information.
- Desire to work in partnership with children/families.
- Desire to empower children/families.
- The non-judgemental respecting of child/family choices.
- Importance of sibling involvement.

Trigger 3.2: The Practice Continuum Tool

In your group discussions about your experiences of using the Family-centred Care Practice Continuum Tool, you may find that you and your colleagues would sometimes have positioned the family whose care history you are describing, at different points on the Continuum. The ensuing discussion of such differences is likely to lead you back to the given definitions in the first fixed resource session where the essence of involvement or partnership for example is described. Teasing out whether your relationship with the family was for example at the involvement or participation stage according to the definitions will help group members gain greater breadth and depth of understanding about the concept of family-centred care.

When using the Practice Continuum Tool you may also have become aware that sometimes family members are not all in the same place on the Continuum at the same time, so it can be used to depict different family-centred care relationships with different family members simultaneously. Also when used in conjunction with Roper et al's (1980) model of nursing where children are assessed on their ability to achieve independence in their activities of living (themselves or with family assistance), there could be situations where the child and family are at the partnership point on the Practice Continuum Tool with regard to all of the child's activities of living but then the child starts to have problems with one of those activities, eliminating for example, and becomes constipated as a side effect of drug therapy. Nursing intervention is required to rectify the situation. So for a short while the family are at the nurse-led involvement stage of family-centred care for this particular activity of the child's living because the nurse is giving prescribed aperient treatment by enema or suppository while the family comfort and support the child emotionally. However for all other activities of living the child/family remain at the participation point on the Practice Continuum.

Trigger 3.3: Meeting cultural needs in family-centred care

Addressing the questions that you are likely to have identified for this trigger will have helped you to complete this work and have provided you with the rationale for using a 'model' or 'framework' to underpin cultural nursing care.

Transcultural care

This is care provided by an individual with one culture to patients with a different culture. The fixed resource sessions identified the difficulty of stepping outside your own culture to learn about it to enable you to be in the position to promote the health of families with a different culture to your own. To help you with this process and to provide culturally congruent, sensitive and competent nursing care it may be helpful to utilise a nursing model underpinned by the philosophy of family-centred care.

Integrated nursing models for cultural care

In these models culture is viewed as an integral part of learning about another person. Cultural assessment, therefore, should be only 'one' of the factors included in the assessment of a child or young person and their family according to integrated models. The Practice Continuum Tool (Smith et al 2002) could certainly be viewed as one of these models. Negotiation with the family/child about the care they wish to engage in at any given time in terms of the continuum should be done with a recognition of culture.

The Practice Continuum Tool may be used in conjunction with Roper et al's (1980) nursing model which incorporates a socio-cultural category to enable culturally based issues in relation to each of the activities of living to be assessed leading to the development of a care plan that will meet the cultural needs of a family. This model was used to assess the cultural needs of the eleven month old girl described in this trigger when she was admitted to the local hospital with a chest infection. An appropriate cultural assessment using this model should identify different child rearing practices, which will be relevant for care planning and understanding 'why' families adopt certain approaches to child care. The assessment strategy of the Partnership Model of paediatric nursing developed by Casey and Mobbs (1988) similarly incorporates activities of living to facilitate inclusion of cultural consideration as 'one' factor in an nursing assessment.

Communication is one example of an activity affected by cultural differences that is in language, traditions, customs, behavioural norms, status position and gender relationships. Hewitt (2000) identifies that for some women major decision-making is not part of their traditional culture. This was clearly apparent in relation to the family described by student nurse Gemma Hardy. Also consultation with other family members is more formal in some cultures than others, because they have different value systems whereby joint family and/or community involvement is the norm. Eriem (1998) identifies that for some families it is expected that nurses should make decisions about their child's care because ' they [nurses] know what is best' and they [families] are unprepared to decide upon care for themselves. The nurse assessing communication and other activities of living should be prompted to consider the cultural dimensions of the child or young person and their family and use this information to plan culturally appropriate family-centred care.

Suggested Activity

If you have not already done so you should now consider the other activities of living identified by Roper et al (1980) and the cultural dimensions of care that you would assess in relation to the individual activities to enable you to deliver appropriate family-centred care.

Roper et al (1980) acknowledge that a comprehensive cultural assessment is outside the scope of their model.

Cultural specific nursing models

Theorists that advocate for cultural specific nursing models argue that this is essential because it is important to achieve a detailed assessment of culture. It is believed that a separate assessment of cultural issues will facilitate the collection of better quality information and a holistic view of the child and family.

A criticism of these models is their complexity and the depth and breadth of cultural information that they require. It is likely that a children's nurse would find them of little value to deal with the immediate problems of an acutely ill child or young person. Leininger's (1991) sunrise model for example requires assessment of technological factors, religious and philosophical factors, kinship and social factors, cultural values and 'lifeways', political and legal factors, economic factors and educational factors. The sunrise model does allow for a combination of professional health care and folk care and helpfully identifies that cultural health care may fit into one of the following categories:

- *Cultural Care preservation* meaning that the child/young person maintain their cultural norms
- *Cultural care accommodation* signifies a temporary change in cultural norms due to illness
- *Cultural care repatterning* means that the child/young person will need to make a permanent change in relation to some aspect of their usual cultural practices due to illness.

The Papadopoulos, Tilki and Taylor Model for the development of cultural competence in nursing was developed for curriculum development purposes and for guiding practice and research. The model consists of four stages: cultural awareness (e.g., self awareness and cultural identity), cultural knowledge (e.g., health beliefs and behaviours stereotyping and sociological understanding), cultural sensitivity (e.g., empathy and interpersonal skills) and cultural competence (e.g., assessment skills and challenging and addressing prejudice, discrimination and inequalities) (Papadopoulos 2003). The model also distinguishes between culturally generic competencies (that are applicable across cultural groups) and culturally specific competencies (these are particular to specific cultural groups). The model provides a structure and clearly identifies the knowledge and skills needed to provide culturally competent care. Papadopoulos (2003) argues that it is no longer tenable to treat everyone the same or to base the care we provide to individuals on the norms of the majority culture.

It can be concluded that family-centred care should certainly be individualised care that demonstrates an awareness of cultural issues, whatever model is used to assess and structure care. The Practice Continuum Tool (Smith et al, 2002) would be appropriate to use because of the reasons stated in the fixed resource session for Trigger 3.2. In your area of practice you may be using the Roper et al (1980) model and activities of living to assess and structure care and the Practice Continuum Tool could be used conjointly.

Reflect on your learning

- Contemporary family centred care involves the provision of both child-centred services and child-centred care.

- Family-centred care is seen as a range of family/child input ranging from being nurse led to parent/child care.
- Family/child input into care ranges from non-involvement, to involvement, participation, partnership and parent/child-led care.
- Negotiation with and empowerment of families and children is integral to family-centred care practice.
- Nurses and other health care professionals and the family/child work in partnership and share their expertise.
- Teaching and learning is essential to facilitate family-centred care in practice.
- The Practice Continuum Tool may be used to assess and communicate family-centred care.
- Cultural awareness should be demonstrated in the assessment and planning for family-centred care.
- Recognition of family diversity and 'who' is the family for the individual child is important.
- Siblings needs should be assessed in family-centred care provision.

References

Abercrombie, N., Ward, A. (2000) *Contemporary British Society*, 3rd edn. Cambridge: Polity Press.

Ahmann, E. (1994) Family-centred care: Shifting orientation. *Pediatric Nursing* 20 (2), March–April, pp. 113–16.

Black, D. (1994) Terminal Illness and Bereavement, in Rutter, M. Taylor, E. Hersov, L., (eds) *Child and Adolescent Psychiatry Modern Approaches*, 3rd edn. Oxford: Blackwell.

Bradley, S. (1996) Processes in the creation and diffusion of nursing knowledge: An examination of the developing concept of family centred care. *Journal of Advanced Nursing* 23, pp. 722–7.

Bradshaw, M., Coleman, V., Smith, L. (2003) Inter-professional learning and family-centred care. *Paediatric Nursing* 15 (7), September, pp. 30–3.

Callery, P. (2004) Family-centred care and fish out of water. *Paediatric Nursing* 16 (6), July/August, p. 13.

Campbell, S., Summersgill, P. (1993) Keeping it in the Family: Defining and developing family centred care. *Child Health* June–July, pp. 17–20.

Casey, A., Mobbs, S. (1988) Partnership in practice, *Nursing Times*, 84 (44), November, pp. 67–8.

Coleman, V. (2002) 'The evolving concept of family-centred care, in Smith, L.,

Coleman, V., Bradshaw, M. *Family-centred Care: Concept, Theory and Practice*. Basingstoke: Palgrave, Chapter 1, pp.3–18.

Coleman, V., Smith, L., Bradshaw, M. (2003) Enhancing consumer participation using the Practice Continuum Tool for family-centred care. *Paediatric Nursing* 15 (8), pp. 28–31.

Department of Health (1989) *The Children Act*. London: HMSO.

Department of Health (1991) *Welfare of Children and Young People in Hospital*. London: HMSO.

Department of Health (1996) *NHS: The Patient's Charter: Services for Children and Young People*. London: HMSO.

Department of Health (2004) *National Service Framework for Children, Young People and Maternity Services*. London: DoH.

Department of Health and Social Security (1976) *Fit for the Future: The Court Report* London: HMSO.

Eriem, J. (1998) Culture, ethics and respect: the bottom line is understanding, *Orthopaedic Nursing* 17 (6), pp. 79–82.

Ewles L., Simnett I. (2003) *Promoting Health: A practical guide*, 4th edn. Edinburgh: Balliere Tindall.

Ferrari, M. (1984) Chronic Illness: Psychological Effects on Siblings. *Journal of Child Psychology and Psychiatry* 25, pp. 459–76.

Foxcroft, L. (2002) Professional and legal issues, in Smith, L., Coleman, V., Bradshaw, M. *Family-centred Care: Concept, Theory and Practice*. Basingstoke: Palgrave, Chapter 8, pp 148–70.

Franck, L., Callery, P. (2004) Re-thinking family-centred care across the continuum of children's healthcare. *Child: Care, Health and Development* 30 (3), pp. 265–77.

Giddens, A. (1989) *Sociology*, 3rd edn. Cambridge: Polity.

Hall D., Elliman, D. (eds) (2003) *Health for all Children*, 4th edn. Oxford: Oxford University Press.

Haralambos, M., Holborn, M. (2000) *Sociology: Themes and Perspectives*, 5th edn. London: Harper Collins.

Helman, C. (1994) *Culture, Health and Illness*, 3rd edn. Oxford: Butterworth Heinemann.

Herberg, P. (1995) Theoretical foundations of transcultural nursing, in Andrews, M., Boyle, J. *Transcultural Concepts in Nursing Care*. Philadephia: Lippincott, Chapter 1, pp. 3–47.

Hewitt, D. (2000) Child-centred care: ethnofriendly or ethnocentric?. *Paediatric Nursing* 12 (6), July, pp. 6–8.

Holland, K., Hogg, C. (2001) *Cultural Awareness in Nursing and Health Care*. London: Arnold.

Hutchfield, K. (1999) Family-centred Care: a Concept Analysis. *Journal of Advanced Nursing* 29 (5), pp. 1178–87.

Lee, P. (2004) Family involvement: are we asking too much? *Paediatric Nursing*, 16 (10), December, pp. 37–41.

Leininger, M. (1991) *Culture Care, Diversity and Universality: A Theory of Nursing.* New York: National League for Nursing.

McEwing, G., Kelsey, J., Richardson, J., Glasper, A. (2003) Insights into Child and family health, in Grandis, S., Long G., Glasper, A., Jackson, P. (eds) *Foundation Studies for Nursing: Using Enquiry-based Learning.* Basingstoke: Palgrave Macmillan, Chapter 3, pp. 48–114.

McGee, P. (1994) Culturally sensitive and culturally comprehensive care. *British Journal of Nursing* 3 (15), pp. 789–92.

Ministry of Health and Central Health Services Council (1959) *The Welfare of Children in Hospital, Platt Report.* London: HMSO.

Mountain, G. (2002) Parenting in society: A critical review, in Smith, L., Coleman, V., Bradshaw, M. *Family-centred Care: Concept, Theory and Practice.* Basingstoke: Palgrave, Chapter 4, pp. 62–81.

Office for National Statistics (2005) Focus on Families, http://www.statistics.gov.uk (accessed 20.10.05).

Papadopoulos, R. (2003) The Papadopoulos, Tilki and Taylor model for the development of cultural competence in nursing. *Journal of Health, Social and Environmental Issues* 4 (1), pp. 5–7.

Pillitteri, A. (1999) *Child Health Nursing: Care of the Child and Family*, 3rd edn. Philadelphia: Lippincott.

Roper, N., Logan, W., Tierney, A. (1980) *The Elements of Nursing.* Edinburgh: Churchill Livingstone.

Schott, J., Henley, A. (1996) *Culture, Religion and Childbearing in a Multiracial Society.* Oxford: Butterworth Heinemann.

Shelton, T., Smith Stepanek, J. (1995) Excerpts from family centered care for children needing health and developmental services. *Pediatric Nursing* 21 (4), July–August, pp. 362–4.

Smaje, C. (1995) *Health, Race and Ethnicity: Making Sense of the Evidence.* London: Kings Fund.

Smith, L., Coleman, V., Bradshaw, M. (2002) *Family-centred Care: Concept, Theory and Practice.* Basingstoke: Palgrave.

Smith, L., Coleman, V., Bradshaw, M. (2002a) Family-centred care: A practice continuum, in Smith, L., Coleman, V., Bradshaw, M. *Family-centred Care: Concept, Theory and Practice.* Basingstoke: Palgrave, Chapter 2, pp. 19–43.

Taylor, J., Muller, D. Wattley, L., Harris, P. (1999) *Nursing Children: Psychology Research and Practice*, 3rd edn. Cheltenham: Stanley Thornes.

Watt, S., Norton, D. (2004) Culture, ethnicity, race: What's the difference? *Paediatric Nursing* 16 (8), October, pp. 37–42.

Chapter

4 Promoting Child Health

Valerie Coleman

> ## Learning outcomes
>
> - Discuss the principles of child health, health promotion and health policies.
> - Discuss strategies to reduce health inequalities for all children and young people living in poverty, through partnership working with the primary health care team and families.
> - Discuss the assessment and monitoring of child development and play to promote health.
> - Explain the principles of child growth and nutrition through preparing an example of health education material to contribute towards a health promotion programme.

Introduction

This chapter focuses on promoting child health in primary care. Primary healthcare is viewed as being of key importance in preventing ill health to ensure that children and young people have a healthy start to life. The World Health Organisation (1978) first declared that primary healthcare was essential healthcare, which should be made universally accessible to individuals and families in the community. The national health strategy in England *Saving Lives: Our Healthier Nation* (Department of Health1999) stated that primary healthcare is placed at the heart of the country's health promotion programme to modernise the health service, providing preventive services such as screening and immunisation, and forging powerful partnerships with local bodies (for example schools, employers and housing departments) to achieve shared health goals (Department of Health 1999).

This signifies that primary care programmes encompass some public health strategies that promote the health of individual children, young people and their families, and others promote the health of communities. Public health is 'the science and art of preventing disease, prolonging life and promoting health through the organised efforts of society' (Hall and Elliman 2003, p. 10).

The *National Service Framework for Children and Young People and Maternity Services* (Department of Health 2004; Welsh Assembly 2004) standards for children's services is again supportive of the need to promote both individual and community health to prevent ill health in childhood. The framework standards to prevent ill health includes those that tackle inequalities, access problems and partnership working with children, young people, families and multi-professionals, which are all integral elements of promoting health in primary care.

The new Child Health Promotion Programme (See Table 4.1) that was launched as part of the *National Service Framework* (Department of Health 2004) will be mostly carried out by members of the primary healthcare team. As part of this new programme Children's Health Guides are to be introduced to encourage children and young people to build health into the way they live. The *National Service Framework* (Department of Health 2004) is likely to identify an increasing role for registered children's nurses within primary care settings such as National Health Service Walk in Centres and General Practitioner Practices (Smith 2003/2004).

Table 4.1 Child Health Promotion Programme

The Child Health Promotion Programme encompasses

- Childhood screening.
- Immunisations.
- A holistic and systematic process to assess the individual child's and families needs.
- Early interventions to address those needs.
- Delivering universal health promoting activities.

This programme is

- Offered to all children throughout childhood and the teenage years.
- In a range of settings including general practices, children's centres, early years providers and extended schools.
- A universal service, which is individualised to meet the needs of the child and family.
- Provides more support on a targeted basis to children and families that are vulnerable or have complex needs.
- Delivered in partnership with parents to help them make healthy choices for their children and family.

Source: Department of Health (2004)

Triggers 4.1 and 4.2 are intended to prepare you for a community placement by enabling you to learn about child health and its promotion. Triggers 4.2 and 4.3 will help you to reflect on your personal community experiences with regard to promoting child development and growth.

! Trigger 4.1: Child health and health promotion

'Nurses, midwives and health visitors play a crucial part in promoting health and preventing illness' (Department of Health 1999, p. 132), because people have close contact with these healthcare professionals at key points in their lives such as infancy and adolescence thus creating significant opportunities for health promoting interventions.

The intention of this trigger is to enable you to understand the principles of child health, health promotion and health policy for use in primary care practice.

The Trigger

 Health at the beginning of life is the foundation of health throughout life. (*NHS Plan 2000*, Department of Health, 2000, p. 111)

Situation

You have a lesson next week about child health, and health promotion prior to your community placement. The lecturer has requested that you prepare by doing some reading in preparation for a discussion during the lesson.

Feedback

Your feedback for this trigger should take the form of some written notes to prepare you for the discussion

The facts

What are the main facts in this trigger? Make a list:

Hypotheses: What may these facts mean?

- Child health has physical, intellectual, emotional and social dimensions.
- Children, young people, family members and health professionals have different perceptions and understandings about health.
- An unhealthy adulthood will be the outcome of a lack of health promotion (local, national or international) in childhood.
- Health promotion in childhood means a healthy adulthood according to health policy in England.

Questions developed from the hypotheses

1. What is child health?
2. How may the perceptions and understanding about child health differ between children, young people, family members and health professionals?
3. What are the potential health outcomes of poor health in childhood for adult health?
4. What approaches are used to promote child health?

Trigger 4.1: Fixed resource material

Read the following to help you answer the questions. (You may also wish to search and review other up-to-date research and evidence-based literature, and seek other relevant resources to provide you with the answers to your questions.)

Department of Health, Social Services and Public Safety (2002) *Investing for Health*. Northern Ireland: DHSSPS, http://www.dhsspsni.gov.uk/publications/2002/invest forhealth.asp (accessed 03.08.05).

Department of Health (2004) Key issues for primary care, *National Service Framework for Children, Young People and Maternity Services*. London: Department of Health.

Department of Health (2004a) *Choosing Health: Making Health Choices Easier*. London: The Stationery Office.

Ewles, L., Simnett, I. (2003) *Promoting Health: A Practical Guide*, 5th edn. Edinburgh: Bailliere Tindall.

Hall, D., Elliman, D. (eds) (2003) *Health for all Children*, 4th edn. Oxford: Oxford University Press. Read Chapter One pp. 1–25 and Chapter 2, pp. 27–51.

Scottish Excecutive (2003) *Improving Health in Scotland – the Challenge*, http://www.scotland.gov.uk/library5/health/ihis-00.asp (accessed 03.08.05).

Welsh Assembly (2003) *Healthy and Active Lifestyles in Wales: A Framework For Action*, http://www.cmo.wales.gov.uk (accessed 03.08.05).

Trigger 4.1: Fixed resource sessions

Contemporary international and national health and/or related policy

The aim of this session is to contextualise the promotion of child health within the contemporary international and national policy framework. This is necessary for you to appreciate the current approaches to health promotion that you may encounter in primary care practice.

International policy

The underpinning philosophy for the World Health Organisation's health promotion policy is still 'Health for All' in the twenty-first century. This has been so since 1977 when the World Health Organisation identified the main social target for governments and itself in the coming decades. This target was to be the attainment of a level of health that would permit all the citizens of the world to lead a socially and economically productive life by the year 2000.

'Health for All' is a broad approach to health promotion. The approach includes health education, but it also requires political and social action with an emphasis on involving people in local communities in identifying their own health needs and working with professionals to shape their own health destiny. Political and social action is viewed as fundamental to health promotion because the major determinants of health are social, economic and environmental with individuals often having no control over these factors (Ewles and Simnett 2003).

Empowerment is a central tenet of health promotion (WHO 1984, 1986, 1998) and hence it is important that communities are enabled to have more control over factors that affect their health. This was identified in the World Health Organisation (1984) definition of health promotion that described health promotion as the process of enabling people to gain control over their own health. It was envisaged that this would lead to improvements in health. Health is seen as a resource for everyday life and not the objective of living: it is a positive concept emphasising social and personal resources, as well as physical capacities.

The Ottawa Charter (WHO 1986) identified the following key strategies for health promotion:

- Building healthy public policy.
- Creating supportive environments.
- Developing personal skills.
- Strengthening community action.
- Re-orientating health services towards prevention and health promotion.

These key strategies were reiterated by the World Health Organisation in 1997 at the Jakarta conference and twenty-first-century priorities for health promotion were added, including promoting social responsibility for health; expanding partnerships for health promotion; increasing community capacity, and empowering the individual (Ewles and Simnett 2003).

The Ottawa Charter in congruence with the 'Health For All' principles inherent in the specific European regional targets (WHO, 1985, 1993, 1998) supports the move away from focusing on individual health behaviour and lifestyles alone to the development of health promoting policies, social policies and environments and community development work (Ewles and Simnett 2003).

The United Nations Summit for Children in 1990 also developed health goals that were socially orientated for achievement by the year 2000. Unfortunately although there was some success, for example a reduction in the incidence of polio, many of these goals were not achieved. Further social goals for children were agreed by the United Nations in 2002 in an action plan for the betterment of children's health, education and well being (Kennedy et al 2002).

This broader approach to health promotion became known as the 'new public health' and manifested itself in many ways in international policy frameworks. This included the WHO identifying environmental settings for promoting health such as healthy cities, healthy hospitals and healthy schools. Healthy environments are important for promoting the health of children. The World Health Organisation (WHO2003, p. 1) is working with various groups to reduce global environmental threats to children and young people:

> Every child has the right to grow up in a healthy environment – to live, learn and play in healthy places. Acting to safeguard children's environments can save millions of lives, reduce diseases and provide a safer healthier world for our children futures.

The World Health Organisation European Region Health 21 policy (WHO, 1998) has 21 targets for achievement in the twenty-first century and most of them are relevant to children and young people. This policy is underpinned by the values of health as a fundamental human right, equity and solidarity in action, and participation and accountability in promoting health by individuals and professionals.

Health 21 (WHO, 1998) identifies four main strategies for action:

1. Strategies to tackle the determinants of health that are multi-sectoral, meaning that health promotion involves health professionals and also colleagues from other sectors such as education, transport and housing.
2. Health outcome driven programmes.
3. Integrated family and community orientated primary health care supported by the hospital systems.
4. Partnership approach.

National policy

(The focus in this part of the session is primarily on policy in England as an example of a national policy.)

The Health of the Nation (Department of Health 1992) constituted the first national health strategy in England. It focused on health and its promotion as opposed to illness and the health services, but it hardly acknowledged the socio-economic determinants of health (Ewles and Simnett 2003). Instead the Health of the Nation strategy encouraged individual lifestyle change as the impetus for health promotion.

Saving Lives: Our Healthier Nation (Department of Health 1999) the second national health strategy is a public health policy for tackling poor health and improving the health of everyone in England because too many people die young from preventable diseases, especially the worse off. It rejects the old argument that people can always make individual decisions about their own and their family's health. Instead Department of Health (1999) states that the social, economic and environmental factors pre-disposing towards ill health are potent and health inequality is widespread in England. Attainable targets have been set in priority areas for the year 2010 for:

- Cancer.
- Coronary heart disease and stroke.
- Accidents.
- Mental illness.

Saving Lives: Our Healthier Nation (Department of Health 1999) envisaged that if the targets are achieved, up to 300,000 untimely and unnecessary deaths could be prevented. Promoting health in childhood for a healthy adulthood may well lead to fewer fatalities. Three way-partnership working, comprising individuals, communities and governments are necessary to implement this policy and to achieve the targets. Much of the action to promote health is delivered at the level of local communities. Health improvement programmes set out how local agencies will achieve the national priorities through setting targets to be achieved at a local level. Additional local targets may also be developed to address particular local priorities.

The importance of implementing a public health promoting strategy is further emphasised in the *Choosing Health* White Paper (Department of Health 2004a). This White Paper reflects the public's health concerns and areas where action is required to:

- Reduce the numbers of people who smoke.
- Reduce obesity.
- Increase exercise.
- Encourage sensible drinking.
- Improve sexual health.
- Improve mental health.

Choosing Health (Department of Health 2004a) identifies how people can be empowered to make healthy choices. It identifies the support that people need, situations where they want to make their own informed choices and occasions when they want the government to intervene to help them make healthy choices. The White Paper states that the health of children is a special responsibility for families, schools, carers and government. To promote integrated planning and delivery of services it is recommended in Department of Health (2004a) that all areas will have a Children's Trust by 2008 to bring together planning, commissioning and delivery of children's and young peoples services alongside education and social care. The establishment of Children's Centres also by 2008 will bring several services together (for example, routine and non-acute children's health services; child health preventative services; parental outreach and family support) in one locality to make them more accessible especially for those children in disadvantaged areas.

There are new standards outlined by the Department of Health (2004a) in relation to food across the school day, more physical exercise and more education on nutrition in addition to the provision of better information and support. Similar strategic approaches are being employed in Northern Ireland (Department of Health, Social Services and Public Safety 2002), Scotland (Scottish Executive 2003) and Wales (Welsh Assembly 2003) towards encouraging physical exercise and healthy diets for children and young people.

> Children spend on average a quarter of their working lives in school. The school environment, attitudes of staff and other pupils as well as what children learn in the classroom, have a major influence on the development of their knowledge and understanding of health.
> (Department of Health 2004a, p. 55)

The National Healthy Schools Programme in England brings policies and approaches that foster better health into everything that schools provide, as does the Welsh Network of Healthy School Schemes (Child Policy Network 2004) and the Active Schools Network (Scottish Executive 2004). The programme currently gives priority to improving children and young people's health in the most disadvantaged areas and it is starting to have a positive effect on the health and well being of children according to recent evaluation. For example, pupils in healthy secondary schools were found to be less likely to have used drugs, and in primary schools pupils were less likely to be afraid of bullying. The results of the evaluation are to inform the next phase of the Healthy Schools Programme in England that from April 2005 provided:

- A supportive environment that includes policies on smoking, and healthy and nutritious food with time and facilities for physical activity and sport both within and beyond the curriculum; and
- Comprehensive Personal, Social, Health Education (PHSE) to include education on

relationships, sex, drugs and alcohol as well as other issues that affect young people's lives for example emotional difficulties and bereavement.
(Department of Health 2004a)

(During your community placement you are likely to spend some time with a school nurse that will afford you opportunities to see the implementation of these healthy school's programmes.)

The NHS Plan (Department of Health, 2000), from which the trigger quote arises about promoting health in childhood for a healthy adulthood, is designed to 'give the people of Britain a health service fit for the 21st century: a health service designed around patients' (p. 111). In other words it will be a patient-centred National Health Service that will bring about health improvements for patients. This philosophy underpins the NSF (Department of Health 2004) Standard 3 that promotes a child-centred service so that 'children and young people and families receive high quality services, which are co-ordinated around their individual and family needs and take account of their views'. (Department of Health 2004, p. 15).

You have already been introduced to the Child Health Promotion Programme (See Table 4.1) that has been designed as part of the National Service Framework (Department of Health 2004) to promote the health and well being of children from pre-birth to adulthood.

Summary

Contemporary international and national health policy is underpinned by the principles of health for all, equity, empowerment and partnership working in its social targets.

Children's and Young People's Perceptions and Understanding of Health

The focus of *The State of the World's Children* report (United Nations 2003) is child participation, which is intended to emphasise the need for adults to elicit and consider the views of children and young people with regard to decisions being made that will affect the individual child's life. This is in congruence with many other contemporary national and international policies including the National Service Framework, which states that 'the best wishes of the child or young person should be paramount, taking into account their wishes and feelings' (Department of Health 2003: p. 46).

In health promotion terms and this trigger, children and young people need to participate in their own preventive health care to be able to build the foundations for a healthy adulthood themselves. This is to empower them at an appropriate developmental level to be able to take some control over their own health, which is likely to be a more effective strategy than having other people do things for them. Heidi

Grande, aged 17 years expressed that children are the experts on being 8, 12 or 17 years old in today's society (United Nations 2003).

An empowerment process includes education and the giving of information (Coleman 2002). Therefore, for parents and healthcare professionals to promote successfully the health of children and young people it is necessary that they have knowledge of the children's potential perceptions and understanding about health.

Although children and young people from a sociological perspective do learn about health from close adults, their learning also relies on the cognitive development of the child. Children and young people's concepts of health and illness are often thought to be consistent with Piaget's cognitive development theory.

Suggested Activity

It is suggested that you now revise Piaget's cognitive development theory.

There are four stages to this theory:

1. Sensori Motor Stage 0–2 years;
2. Pre-operational Stage 2–6 years;
3. Concrete Operational Stage 7–10 years;
4. Formal Operational Stage 11+.

Swanwick (1990) used the question 'How do people get colds?' to illustrate children's cognitive understanding of health commencing with the pre-operational stage (2–6 years). At the start of this stage children demonstrate awareness of phenomena and, therefore, may attribute the cause of colds to the sun. Older children in the pre-operational stage develop an understanding of contamination and, therefore, are able to understand that when someone else gets near you they may give you their cold, but they do not know why and think it could be magic.

In the concrete operational stage (7–10 years) children develop their understanding of contamination further and make associations between being outside without a hat and sneezing, prior to developing an understanding of internal processes that occur in the body. Swanick (1990) suggests that the answers from this age group with regard to how people get colds will reflect knowledge about breathing too much air into their nose in winter, which blocks up the nose.

Cognitive development in the formal operational stage reflects that young people (11+ years) have developed a more adult way of thinking and will state colds come from viruses that come from other people and get into the blood stream, and that you are more likely to get a cold if you are tired or stressed.

Piaget's cognitive developmental theory has received some criticism. It should be applied with the recognition that different children and young people will have had different social and health experiences and this may affect the speed of their cognitive development, but not necessarily the sequence. Several studies, for example, Williams et al (1989; 1989a), have been undertaken to determine what children know about health and health related topics. These studies support Piaget's theory that children's perceptions and understanding change at different ages and stages of development. Williams et al (1989; 1989a) found in extensive studies of primary school children that the children produced a series of snapshots of the characteristics of each of the age ranges' perceptions of health-related behaviours.

The cognitive development of children and young people, therefore, needs to be understood and considered in the planning of health education for children and young people. Health education should enable this age group to develop some knowledge and understanding about their own bodies. However, children are likely to have limited knowledge and misconceptions about the human body (Eiser 1993). This is borne out in several studies including that by McEwing (1996) who used drawings again to determine children's knowledge about their own bodies. There were 112 children in this study (equal numbers of boys and girls) aged 4.5 to 8.5 years. This study found that many children did have misconceptions about their bodies, with regard to the positioning of internal organs and the functioning of various parts. The children knew most about the heart, brain, blood and bones in congruence with other studies because they are visible and/or can be felt. They seem to be aware of the existence of the brain, believing that it helps them to remember things. This highlights the need not to make any assumptions about a child's knowledge of their own body in a health education session, but to make an accurate assessment first.

The assessment should also take into account the social experiences (peers, parental lifestyle, family or child illnesses) and other influences on the child or young person in respect of how he/she may perceive health.

Summary

It is paramount to promoting health that children and young people are empowered to participate in this process. This requires healthcare professionals to be aware of the potential perceptions and understanding of children and young people about health.

Preventable health problems: Obesity

This session deals with one contemporary health problem that may be prevented by action being taken in childhood to lay down the foundations for a healthy adulthood. The prevalence of obesity in children and young people has risen alarmingly turning obesity into a significant public health issue and it has reached the point of endangering health (Health Development Agency 2003). The following statistics demonstrate an increase in childhood obesity:

- The National Diet and Nutrition Survey in 1997 found that the prevalence of overweight British young people (4–18 years) had increased to 15.4 per cent and that 4 per cent of these were obese.
- In 2001 8.5 per cent of 6 year olds and 15 per cent of 15 year olds were obese according to The Health Survey for England (Joint Health Surveys Unit for the Department of Health 2002).
- The prevalence of obesity in children age 2–10 years has increased from 9.5 per cent in 1995 to 15.5 per cent in 2002 (Joint Health Surveys Unit for England Department of Health 2002).
- One in three of Scotland's 12 year olds are overweight, with one in ten severely obese. And one in five toddlers are overweight before their fourth birthday (Scottish Executive 2004a)

Obese children, especially girls are more likely to come from lower social groups (Department of Health 2004a) and 'a significant proportion (between one-third and two-thirds) of obese children will go on to be obese adults' (Hall and Elliman 2003, p. 184).

Obese people are more likely to experience a number of serious chronic diseases such as diabetes Type 2, coronary heart disease, hypertension, stroke, gall bladder disease, orthopaedic problems, depression and certain types of cancer which are life limiting (Hall and Elliman 2003, Laing, 2002; Pearson, 2003/2004; The Health Development Agency, 2003). Laing (2002) argues that if the current childhood trend is unchallenged a future generation of obese adults will result with a likelihood of them developing these chronic illnesses. Hall and Elliman (2003) identify that obesity in children is associated with emotional and psychological distress. Chronic illnesses which were once only seen in the adult population are starting to present in obese children and young people, particularly Type 2 non-insulin dependent diabetes. These are all very good reasons for preventing obesity in childhood.

Laing (2002) states that the logical way to combat the increasing incidence of obesity is to prevent children becoming overweight in the first place. It is necessary to be aware of the causative factors of childhood obesity to be able to take preventive measures (See Table 4.2).

Preventing obesity is not only the responsibility of health professionals and the National Health Service (Department of Health 2004a; Pearson 2003/2004). The World Health Organisation (2000) clearly emphasised the need for collaborative working between government agencies, the food industry, farming, transport, national health services, and media and advertising agencies. This is necessary to ensure consistent messages are sent and received to facilitate effective preventative strategies being implemented. However it is stressed in Department of Health (2004a) that a

---

Table 4.2 Childhood obesity

Causative factors of childhood obesity	Preventive strategies
At Risk Groups: ● Overweight/obese parents ● Genetic disposition ● Socially deprived groups ● Low levels of education	Target these groups Allocate resources Education about nutrition Information giving about food and its availability Empower children to eat healthily
Social and cultural changes: ● Convenience food driven society ● Ability to make healthy choices limited by structural changes in society ● Overweight children believe it is not possible to achieve perfect body portrayed by media so why try ● Attitudes	Attitude change Develop coping strategies Promote self-esteem Behaviour change
Nutritional intake: ● Early experiences with food ● Family feeding practices and choices ● Marketing of food ● Positive energy balance (energy intake exceeds energy expenditure over a period of time) ● Energy dense foods are abundant ● Food portion sizes are larger ● Vending machines	Education Changing marketing regulations
Sedentary low activity lifestyle in children: ● Safety concerns ● Parental working habits ● Television viewing ● Low activity pursuits e.g., Computer games ● Eating habits ● Car journeys are routinely taken even for short distances ● Racial harassment	Education Transport policy changes Behaviour change Promoting physical exercise Provision of safe play areas

Source: Laing (2002); Pearson (2003/2004)

comprehensive response to the threats that obesity poses for individuals and society must include concerted NHS action that has to be a systematic and determined approach to the prevention and treatment of obesity. 'Children are particularly at risk and need a healthy start in life, but about 17 per cent are now obese' (Department of Health, 2004a p. 43).

The Department of Health (Department of Health 2004a) has set a national target 'to halt by 2010 the year-on-year increase in obesity among children under 11 in the content of a broader strategy to tackle obesity in the population as a whole' (Department of Health 2004a, p. 43).

The responsibility for achieving this target is to be shared by the government departments with responsibility for health, education and sport. A typical care pathway to provide a model for the prevention and treatment of obesity would involve:

Raising awareness and providing information
↓
Raising the issue opportunistically and providing advice
↓
Referral to specialist services as appropriate to consider the required type of support, for example diet and physical activity.
↓
Reviewing and maintenance of progress.
(Department of Health 2004a)

Fruhbeck (2000) suggested that childhood obesity is managed, prevented and treated in three main settings namely, the family, school and primary care:

Family setting

The early intervention initiatives namely Sure Start programmes from a preventative perspective for families are likely to include advice and skill development in respect of nutrition, purchasing food and the preparation of it for eating. Health visitors implementing the Child Health Promotion (Department of Health 2004) will also provide advice and practical support to help parents make healthy choices about their children's diet.

Health Development Agency (2003) found evidence of effective treatment programmes:

- Targeting overweight/obese children and involving at least one parent with physical activity and health promotion.
- Providing multi-faceted family-based behaviour modification programmes. Parents take responsibility for behaviour change in primary school children: diet, exercise, and reducing sedentary behaviour, lifestyle counselling, with child management, parenting and communication skills training.

School setting

The *National Service Framework* (Department of Health 2004), *Health Life and Action* (Welsh Assembly 2003) *Investing in Health* (Department of Health Social Services and Public Safety 2002) and the *Active Schools Network* (Scottish Executive 2004) all describes the role of schools in encouraging healthy lifestyles in children and enabling early identification and personalised help for children at risk of becoming overweight or obese. The emphasis on schools playing a key role in childhood obesity management is central to the *Choosing Health* public health White Paper (Department of Health 2004a). This is to be achieved through the 'Healthy Schools Programme' promoting clear and consistent messages about nutrition and healthy eating using a whole school approach including:

- Providing opportunities to learn about diet, nutrition, food safety, hygiene, food preparation and cooking as well as where food comes from.
- Actively promoting healthy food and drink. For example, 5 a Day (at least five portions of fruit or vegetables per person per day), healthy vending machines, healthier breakfast clubs, and water provision.
- Restricting the availability and promotion of other options. For example, banning unhealthy tuck shops.

There is also a need to extend the opportunities that schools provide through formal and informal opportunities for sport, play and active travel to and from school (Department of Health 2004a). This is to be achieved through partnership working in the public and voluntary sectors. Encouraging physical exercise alongside making healthy choices about diet is seen as being imperative in the management of obesity in childhood.

Primary care setting

Department of Health (2004a) states that activity on obesity prevention and management is to be co-ordinated in each Primary Care Trust for both adults and children with a range of appropriately trained staff (health trainers, school nurses, health visitors, community nurses, practice nurses, dieticians and exercise specialists). There will be a clear referral mechanism to these specialist obesity services. An explanation of what treatment programmes in Primary Care Trusts should include is to be found in Department of Health (2004a), for example regular weight checks, advice on nutrition, physical activity and weight loss by health trainers and other healthcare professionals. There should also be early identification of risk and joined up action between the health services, local authorities and schools about nutrition and physical exercise.

Summary

It is logical that preventative action is taken to prevent children and young people becoming overweight and obese in the first place because once they do their eating and activity habits are deeply ingrained and resistant to change (Laing 2002). Therefore, action needs to be taken to stop the rise of childhood obesity.

 ## Trigger 4.1: Feedback

Go to Chapter 4 Trigger feedback on p. 97

! Trigger 4.2: Inequalities in child health

The intention of this trigger is to enable you to understand some of the strategies that may be used to reduce health inequalities for children and young people living in poverty to promote their health.

The Trigger

> NOT ONE OF OUR CHILDREN LIVES IN POVERTY 3.9 MILLION DO.
> *End Child Poverty* (2002, p.1) Poverty and Child Health Briefing Paper,
> (London: End Child Poverty Group (Supported by Barnados)).

Situation

Statistics in March 2004 revealed that 3.6 million children in Britain live in poverty, which is one in every four children (End Child Poverty 2004). Prior to your community placement you are required to investigate a local area to determine how the health of children and young people is being promoted, especially with regard to the questions arising from the trigger about strategies to reduce health inequalities for children and young people living in poverty.

Feedback

You are required to write a short report about the results of your investigation into a local area. The trigger questions should act as the framework for this report. What did you find out about health inequalities, child poverty and strategies to reduce inequalities in this local area?

The facts

What are the main facts in this trigger? Make a list:

Hypotheses: What may these facts mean?

- Childhood poverty is a major problem in the United Kingdom.
- The statistics of children living in poverty have changed since 2002.
- Health promotion and other policies are advocating action through partnership working to reduce health inequalities for children living in poverty.
- Inequalities in child health are determined by social, economic and environmental factors.
- Children living in poverty experience worse health than other children that are better off materially.
- Promoting the health of children and young people living in poverty is difficult.

Questions developed from the hypotheses

1. What is the current extent of childhood poverty in your local area compared with contemporary and projected national statistics in the United Kingdom?
2. What determinants may be causing inequalities in health for children and young people living in the local area that you have investigated?
3. How may health inequalities and poverty affect the health of children and young people? Provide some examples from your local area?
4. What action is being taken to tackle child health inequalities in the local area that you investigated?

Trigger 4.2: Fixed resource materials

Read the following to help you answer the questions. (You may also wish to search and review other up-to-date research and evidence-based literature and seek other relevant resources to provide you with answers to your questions.)

Department of Health (1998a) *Independent Inquiry into Inequalities in Health (The Acheson Report)*. London: Stationary Office.

Department of Health (1999) *Saving Lives: Our Healthier Nation*. London: Stationery Office, www.doh.gov.uk

Department of Health, Social Services and Public Safety (2002) Investing for Health, Northern Ireland: DHSSPS. http://www.dhsspsni.gov.uk/publications/2002/investforhealth.asp (accessed 03.08.05).

Scottish Exceckutive (2003) *Improving Health in Scotland – The Challenge*, http://www.scotland.gov.uk/library5/health/ihis-00.asp (accessed 03.08.05).

Welsh Assembly (2005) A Fair Future for our Children: The strategy of the Welsh Assembly Government for Tackling Child Poverty, Executive Summary, http://www.wales.gov.uk/subichildren/content/summary-action-plan-e.pdf (accessed 03.08.05).

Trigger 4.2: Fixed resource sessions

Partnership working

Partnership is integral to the practice of family-centred care for children's nurses and it is also at the heart of the White Paper, *Saving Lives: Our Healthier Nation*. 'To improve health and to tackle health inequality, we need a new three-way partnership, comprising: individuals, communities and government' (Department of Health 1999, p. 8). This three-way partnership is intended to be inclusive and integrated, and at the same time comprehensive and coherent, ensuring that all involved play their part in improving health.

Individuals need to take responsibility for their own health and that of their families. Many are doing so by utilising better health information stated Department of Health (1999), but those living in poverty are likely to require support from health professionals and others to take on this responsibility. This is support in the form of accessible services, and to develop skills for empowerment.

Communities work in partnership through local organisations. Department of Health (1999) informs us that local agencies led by health and local authorities are responsible for delivering local services and local programmes to enable people to achieve better health. Hence initiatives such as healthy citizen programmes, health improvement programmes, and health action zones all provide a focus to deliver local programmes that will help individuals to improve their health and that of their families.

Government has the responsibility to provide everyone with the opportunity for better education, better housing, and better prospects for employment (Department of

Health 1999). The government to is also taking action to 'make work pay to support children and families, to promote community safety ... which will do much to improve people's health and to improve the health of the least fortunate in our country' (Department of Health 1999, p. 9).

An integrated partnership approach to tackling poor health is best according to Department of Health (1999), citing the example of smoking. It is necessary to relieve the conditions of social stress, unemployment, poor education, crime and vandalism, which cause far more people in disadvantaged communities to smoke than in other community sections. If smoking is tackled effectively the impact of cancer and heart disease may be reduced for today's children when they reach adulthood.

Suggested Activity

You will find it useful to read:

1. Department of Health (1999) *Saving Lives: Our Healthier Nation*. London: Department of Health, to find out more about the aforementioned initiatives of healthy citizen programmes, health improvement programmes and health action zones.
2. Department of Health (2004a) *Choosing Health: Making Healthier Choices Easier*. London: Department of Health, to find out about new initiatives with regard to partnerships in the community that require joint action by local authorities with business and voluntary groups to tackle local health inequalities. The initiatives include 'Communities for Health', 'Local Area Agreements and '5 A Day' initiatives for all 4 to 6 year olds in local education authority schools in England who are eligible for a piece of free fruit or vegetable every school day. In deprived communities more Primary Care Trusts are now providing support for cookery clubs and co-operatives.

Sure Start programmes

Sure Start is a major UK government programme whose main aim is to improve the life chances of young children living in disadvantaged areas. The programme supports families from pregnancy through until the children are 14 years of age and up to 16 years of age for those with special educational needs and disabilities. Early intervention research has indicated that intervention with families when children are very young is most likely to be effective (Eisenstadt 1999), ensuring that a child is ready to benefit from education when he/she starts school (Hall and Elliman 2003). This principle of early intervention is one that was built upon in the Green Paper 'Every Child Matters' (Department for Education and Skills 2003) to protect them and promote their well being.

400,000 children living in disadvantaged areas in the United Kingdom, including a third of children under four living in poverty are now being helped by 524 local Sure Start programmes (Department for Education and Skills 2005). The aim of these programmes is through working with parents and children to promote the physical, intellectual and social development of pre-school children by drawing on the best practice in early education and childcare to:

1. Provide better access for every family to a range of supportive services.
2. Provide services that respond to varying family needs.
3. Provide flexible services through a single point of contact whenever possible with regard to opening hours, location, transport and childcare.
4. Start early with services by intervening at the first antenatal visit to advise not only on health in pregnancy but to prepare for parenthood. Sure Start local programmes work with parents to be and parents to develop parenting, nurturing, early learning, play and childcare skills. Long-standing support is to be ensured by building confidence and self-esteem in parents, but also by influencing services that older children move on to so that they will be equally supportive in their work with families.
5. Customer driven, respectful transparent services should be provided.
6. Community driven services are provided that are professionally co-ordinated with professionals sharing expertise and listening to local people on a day-to-day basis to discover what their priorities are for service provision.
7. Outcome driven services, which have at their core better health outcomes for children, especially those living in disadvantaged areas, need to be developed. To achieve this the government needs to ensure a joined up approach with partnership working as we discussed in the previous session.
(Department for Education and Skills, 2005; Eisenstadt, 1999; Hall and Elliman, 2003)

Making sure that children have equal access to healthy living is one of the main action areas in *Choosing Health* (Department of Health 2004a) and new projects are to be developed for the Sure Start programme.

Another source of advice for parents is Home Start a voluntary organisation that provides trained volunteers as part of a home visiting programme to support families under stress to care for and nurture children during their early years. There will be increased funding to this programme 'so that by 2006/07 nine out of ten local authorities in England will have this service available' (Department of Health 2004a).

Working together at all levels is essential for the successful implementation of Sure Start programmes and Home Start programmes. 'It requires a commitment to collaborative planning and policy development as well as joint working at field work level' (Eisenstadt 1999, p. 27).

Summary

Therefore, Sure Start is a real challenge with regard to partnership working for health professionals and others. It may be centrally driven but it does require local innovation and ownership by both professionals and parents, whose contributions and experience must be valued (Eisenstadt 1999).

It is suggested that as part of your investigation into a local area that you find out about the local Sure Start programme and possibly Home Start Programme.

Empowering communities and individual families

Children, young people and their families living in poverty are likely to feel disempowered because they have not got the material means to take control of their lives. Disempowerment is a negative concept that engenders feelings of hopelessness and powerlessness and hence compromises psychological health for those living in poverty in addition to potentially causing physical ill health. It is not surprising, therefore, that empowerment is a central tenet of health promotion action in *Saving Lives: Our Healthier Nation* (Department of Health 1999) and *Choosing Health: Making Healthy Choices Easier* (Department of Health 2004a). This is the empowerment of both individuals and communities to enable them to assert control over factors that affect their lives. Empowerment is a reciprocal social process that helps people to participate with competence' (Coleman 1998, p. 32).

In the past health strategies have tended to focus on lifestyle issues with children and families being expected to passively change their behaviour after receiving health information from professionals. There was a failure to recognise that not all children, young people and families are in a position to adopt healthier lifestyles based on information giving alone especially those living in poverty. According to Department of Health (1999) this contributed to the widening of the health gap, because the better off are more likely to have the resources to act on health information to change behaviour and thus reduce risks to their health.

In response to contemporary health policy including *Choosing Health* (Department of Health 2004a) there has been recognition that effective health promotion involves more than just giving information or offering help (Hall and Elliman, 2003). Families that live in poverty are more likely to be suffering from depression, poor health and unhealthy lifestyles leading to low birth weight babies, children at a higher risk of illness, sudden unexpected death, neglect, abuse, dental decay, injuries and educational problems. Utilisation of medical health promotion models that aim to develop parental knowledge, skills and change attitudes are unlikely to succeed when the families are pre-occupied with difficult life circumstances and environments. These circumstances make it difficult for families to benefit from one-to-one professional expertise and advice (Hall and Elliman 2003).

Health visitors and other professionals working with families in the primary health care setting will find that alternatively relationship building is not only worthwhile for its own sake, but also as an essential prerequisite to the empowerment of these families at an individual level (Hall and Elliman, 2003). This is because within this relationship building there is the potential for the development of trust, listening, mutual valuing and respect leading to the development of coping skills and self-efficacy feelings for families. When this relationship building on an individual level is supported by accessible services, including Sure Start programmes, family empowerment is a likely outcome. Engagement in such programmes facilitates the development of social networks leading to families believing that they are cared for, loved, esteemed and a member of a network of mutual obligations. This can reduce the stress of disadvantage and social isolation (Hall and Elliman 2003). Membership of a social network of peers is in itself empowering (Rissel 1994).

Community development is the process by which people in a community identify their own health needs and with the facilitation of health professionals and others organise themselves in order to bring about change that are likely to promote the health of children and families (Hall and Elliman 2003). It is an empowering approach to health promotion due to the central autonomous role that the community plays in the process. Community development should be about empowering the pubic to work on their own agendas of heath issues, even if these are radically different from those working for those in a professional capacity' (Ewles and Simnett 2003, p. 295).

The agenda for the *Choosing Health* White Paper (Department of Health 2004a) was set by the public during a public health consultation that enabled them to express their views on key health issues and on the relationship that the government should have to society and personal responsibility. It could be argued that this is community development at a national level, but it is imperative that consultation also takes place in local communities if the public are to become empowered.

➡ Trigger 4.2: Feedback

Go to Chapter 4 Trigger feedback on p. 97

❗ Trigger 4.3: Promoting and monitoring child development for health

The *Making a Difference* Strategy for Nursing, Midwifery and Health Visiting (Department of Health 1999a) recognised the potential for all nurses to contribute to public health, which is viewed as fundamental to contemporary child health promotion.

During a community placement you are likely to be working alongside health visitors and nurses who contribute to the public's health. The nurses include not only children's community nurses but also school nurses and practice nurses. The community placement will enable you to appreciate the contributions of all these professionals to the public health of children, young people and their families.

The intention of this trigger is to enable you to understand child development, and the role of the health visitor in implementing the Child Health Promotion Programme (Department of Health 2004), and monitoring the developmental progress of children and young people.

The Trigger

Chloe is the youngest of four children aged between 2 weeks and 14 years old. Sarah and Matthew had their first child 14 year old Helen in their early twenties and then came 10 year old Tom. Joseph age 3 years was unexpected but a very welcome addition to the family. Sarah is now enjoying being at home, on maternity leave from her job as a teacher, looking after the new arrival 2 week old Chloe. Matthew is self-employed with his own small business, which keeps him very busy.

The health visitor is due to visit today to do the two week health check. Chloe is a very contented baby who is feeding well and Sarah and Matthew have no concerns about her. They are rather anxious about Joseph though because he has been very 'clingy' and quite demanding since Chloe was born. Sarah wants to discuss Joseph's behaviour with the health visitor especially as he is now reluctant to go to nursery. Helen the 14 year old is being surprisingly helpful at the moment and trying to help out as much as possible; usually she behaves like a typical teenager, which is hard work! While Tom, the 10 year old, has taken the arrival of his new sister in his stride and is getting on with his life as usual, especially playing football with his friends and a local under 11 team.

Matthew and Sarah are rather concerned about the prospect of their new daughter being immunised. Their other children were immunised without any problems, but there has been so much in the news recently about complications especially about the Mumps, Measles and Rubella (MMR) immunisation and children having autism and other problems. It's difficult to know what to believe, perhaps the health visitor will have some answers.

Situation

You have commenced your community placement. You met this family with your Health Visitor mentor during the first visit to see a 2 week old baby. After the visit your mentor asks you about the development of each child in the family. What is your assessment? It is suggested that you do some reading about child development

Feedback

Write a reflective account about your visit to this family with regard to promoting child development. The questions arising from the trigger should provide the focus for your reflection

The facts

What do the facts mean in this trigger? Make a list.

Hypotheses: What may these facts mean?

- Health visitors routinely check on children's health and give advise to promote health.
- 2 week old babies spend their time sleeping and feeding.
- Younger siblings may be upset by the arrival of a new brother or sister.
- Adolescents demonstrate typical behaviours.
- 10 year old boys like playing football.
- The MMR immunisation links to autism and other health problems.
- Immunisation is controversial and has received adverse publicity in the media.

Questions develop from the hypotheses

1. What are the expectations for child development at different ages?
2. What is the role of the health visitor in monitoring and promoting child health?
3. What are the current concerns about the immunisation programme for children?

The answers to these questions will inform your reflective account for the feedback.

📚 Trigger 4.3: Fixed resource material

Read the following to help you answer the questions. (You may also wish to search and review other up to date research and evidence-based literature and seek other relevant resources to provide you with answers to your questions.)

Bee, H., Boyd, D. (2004) *The Developing Child*, 10th edn. Boston: Allyn and Bacon.

Sheridan, M. (1997) *From Birth to Five Years: Children's Developmental Progress.* (revised and updated by Frost, M., Sharma, A.). London: Routledge.

Trigger 4.3: Fixed resource sessions

Health visitors' role in promoting and monitoring child health

A family-centred public health role is advocated by Department of Health (1999a) for health visitors who are public health practitioners. Public health according to Hall and Elliman (2003) aims to provide a collective view of health needs and health care of a population. It involves preventing disease, prolonging life and promoting health through the organised efforts of society (Department of Health 1998). The health visitor's public health role includes them contributing towards the development of communities and tackling poverty and health inequalities as well as promoting the health of individual children, using a family-centred approach. Hall and Elliman (2003) concluded from the literature that health promotion programmes where professionals have both the time and skill to establish a relationship of respect and trust with families are more likely to be successful. The child needs to be seen as a member of the family and the family as part of the community to promote optimal child health.

A universal or core programme of preventive health care and parent support accessible to every parent with additional services targeted at those that need them has been implemented by health visitors working in partnership with individual families (Hall and Elliman 2003). The contribution of an individual approach such as that recommended in the preventive health care core programme should not be underestimated in primary health care (Hall and Elliman 2003). The core programme has been used as well as community development work to prevent ill health in children. The core child health promotion programme that is summarised at the start of this chapter identifies that new birth visits are made by the health visitor or midwife usually around 12 days post birth. The health visitor then performs four developmental reviews of the child at the following times:

- 6–8 weeks old;
- By the first birthday;
- 2–3 years old;
- 4–5years old.

Before each visit there is a questionnaire for the parents to fill in about their child.

It is suggested that you now read the following to find out more about the core programme (Hall and Elliman 2003) and the new Child Health Promotion programme (Department of Health 2004):

Hall D, Elliman, D. (eds) (2003) *Health for all Children*, 4th edn. Oxford: Oxford University Press. Read Chapter 18, pp. 345–66.

Department of Health (2004) *Key Issues for Primary Care, National Service Framework for Children, Young People and Maternity Services*. London; Department of Health. Read the Child Health Promotion Programme.

Health visitors will also encourage the use of the children's 'Personal Health Guide' (PHG). These health guides are intended to encourage children and young people to build health into the way that they live their lives (Department of Health 2004a). During the child's early life the guide is to be held by their parents or carers with advice and support from health visitors, school nurses and other healthcare professionals. However, as children and young people grow up they will take on responsibility for developing their own health goals with help from parents, school staff and health professionals. Department of Health (2004a) suggests that the PHGs are to be reviewed at key transition points such as starting school, moving to secondary school or starting work. Children and young people will get support from health visitors and other professionals in order to make healthy choices about their lifestyles.

Preventing infectious diseases: Immunisation and health education

Primary care providers participating in the National Service Framework Child Health Promotion Programme (Department of Health 2004) are required to ensure that all children receive immunisation against major infectious diseases. 'Immunity can be induced, either actively (long term) or provided by passive transfer (short term) against a variety of bacterial and viral agents' (Department of Health 1996, p. 5).

Therefore, there are two main types of immunisation, which act to play their part in protecting individuals and the community from serious infectious diseases. With active immunisation, immunity to specific diseases develops in response to the injection of a vaccine or toxoid that is sufficiently powerful enough to stimulate the production of antibodies and thus build up an active immunity without causing a disease. Passive immunisation is when ready made antibodies are injected into the body to provide short term protection from disease for those that are most vulnerable (National Health Service immunisation Information 2004).

Health visitors will use contacts with children during home visits or at the clinic to provide appropriate health education advice to the family carers about the nature and purpose of the immunisation programme. The current full childhood immunisation schedule was implemented in 2004 in England.

Full immunisation schedule

The health visitor will use the Personal Child Health Record or the child's medical record, including the National Health Service Care Record Service when it is estab-

Table 4.3 NHS immunisation information (2005)

When to immunise	What is given	How is it given
2, 3 and 4 months	Diphtheria, tetanus, pertussis (whooping Cough), polio and Haemophilus influenza type b	One injection
	Meningitis C	One injection
Around 13 months	Measles, mumps and rubella (MMR)	One injection
3 years and 4 months to 5 years old	Diphtheria, tetanus, pertussis (whooping Cough) and polio	One injection
	Measles, mumps and rubella (MMR)	One injection
10 to 14 years (and sometimes shortly after birth)	BCG (against tuberculosis)	Skin test, then if needed one injection
13 to 18 years	Diphtheria, tetanus, polio	One injection

Source: NHS Immunisation Information (2004)

lished, to check immunisation uptake by individual children. Children will be referred for catch-up immunisation whenever necessary. The NSF (Department of Health 2004) also states that the immunisation history of children and young people who enter into the country or who move into the area has to be checked. If these children are either un-immunised or have an unknown history, a full course of immunisations is to be offered. The NSF (Department of Health 2004) proceeds to identify that primary care providers will follow up failure to attend for a scheduled immunisation by triggering an assessment of the reasons.

Sarah and Matthew were anxious about the prospect of Chloe commencing the immunisation programme, despite their other children's trouble free immunisation history. Hall and Elliman (2003) recognise that parents receive a great deal of confusing information about immunisation. Much of this information comes from the media who publish advertisements emphasising the importance of immunisation, but also report on apparent complications attributed to vaccines. To counteract this adverse media information and to be able to give appropriate health education advice Hall and Elliman (2003) advocate that healthcare professionals:

- Familiarise themselves with the diseases that immunisation is designed to prevent
- Develop knowledge and understanding of what the evidence actually shows with regard to effectiveness, risks and contraindications.

Suggested Activities

1. Write some brief notes about the diseases immunised against
2. Perform a literature review to establish the evidence regarding effectiveness, risks and contraindications

---

- Have a firm commitment to immunisation among all primary care staff.
- Acknowledge honestly areas of uncertainty.

The mumps, measles and rubella vaccination has been the subject of much recent controversy because of controversial links that have been made to autism and bowel disease following immunisation. These disputed links have created much debate about the safety of this vaccine and this has led to some parents seeking single vaccines for their children as opposed to the triple mumps, measles and rubella vaccine. It has already been identified that parents will receive health education advice from their health visitor and other primary care providers. There are also other sources of health education advice for parents (and healthcare professionals) from:

- Health Education Immunisation leaflets;
- Immunisation videos;
- NHS Direct http://www.nhsdirect.nhs.uk
- NHS Immunisation Information http://www.immunisation.nhs.uk

---

Suggested Activity

You should access these health education sources and evaluate how effective this material may be in allaying parental anxieties, and promoting immunisation uptake.

Ewles and Simnett (2003) suggest the following criteria for selecting material to use for health education:

1. Is it appropriate for achieving your promotion aims?
2. Is it the most appropriate kind of material?
3. Is it consistent with your values and approach?
4. Is it relevant for the people you are working with?

5. Is it racist or sexist?
6. Will it be understood?
7. Is the information sound?
8. Does it contain advertising?

The National Health Service Immunisation Website provides comprehensive information including a long list of frequently asked questions about the MMR vaccination. It also introduces the new five in one vaccination for diphtheria, tetanus, pertussis (whooping Cough), polio and Haemophilus influenza type b to be administered at 2, 3 and 4 months.

The other aspect of health education with regard to immunisation is to ensure that the parents receive appropriate advice on how to care for their children immediately following their immunisation. Check with the nurse on your community placement to find out what advice is given.

Immunisation is essential to the promotion of child health.

Factors that affect Child development

Some of these factors have been identified in Table 4.4 to create an awareness of how development may be promoted or not, and the implications of this for health promotion at primary, secondary and tertiary levels. It is not an exhaustive list and it is suggested that you may wish to add to it by reflecting on your personal experiences.

An awareness of these factors will also prepare you for your community placement, especially the developmental assessments that you will observe or participate with in practice.

Play

It is apparent from Table 4.4 that play is important for child development in all dimensions. Play is a child's way of making sense of the world and ultimately it prepares a child for adulthood. Play is a process in which the child is active, so they are likely to learn from it and are willing to engage in it because play is a pleasurable activity.

Suggested Activity

It is suggested that you read more about play to enable you to further develop your knowledge about how it affects child development, and how to use it to the best advantage with children of different ages in whatever setting that you are working with children and families.

Table 4.4 Factors that affect development

Dimensions of development	Influencing factors
Physical	Genetic
	Congenital problems – early diagnosis
	Good health
	Poor health (acute or chronic)
	Accidents
	Safety of physical environment
	Play/toys to develop posture and large movements
	Nutrition
	Hygiene
Intellectual	Education
	Play/toys
	Encouragement
Emotional	Stimulation
	Parental love and affection
	Play/toys
Social	Siblings
	Peers
	Living conditions
	Parenting skills
	Play/toys
	Socio-economic status of family
	Culture

Culture

How children play may be culturally determined. Culture has also broader implications for child development with regard to beliefs and practices (see Chapter 3). It is suggested that this is another area for further reading. You are likely to find that there are differences relating to the supervision of play and provision of toys that depends on the culture of individual families.

Early intervention for children that are disadvantaged

The Sure Start programmes have already been discussed in this chapter. These identify that early intervention in education and childcare promotes the physical, intellectual and social development of pre-school children living in disadvantaged areas so that they are ready to benefit from education at school. This suggests that some nurturing for children that have not had the best start in life may promote child development.

Nature-nurture controversy?

The nature-nurture controversy is about whether a child develops as he/she does, because the pattern is built in at birth or alternatively because of influences after the birth. Bee and Boyd (2004) argue that while virtually all psychologists would state that a child's development is a product of some interaction between nature and nurture there are important concepts on each side of the nature–nurture debate that it is useful to be familiar with.

Suggested Activity

It would be useful for you to read about these concepts in:

Bee, H, Boyd, D. (2004) *The Developing Child*, 10th edn. Boston, Allyn and Bacon. Read Chapter 1: Perspectives on development, pp. 3–13.

Implications of factors for promoting development

The Sure Start programmes are a good example of primary health promotion to prevent children having developmental problems in later life. Prevention is key to local, national and international health policies.

Early diagnosis of health problems in children is desirable so that every effort can be made to promote optimum child development for individual children. Therefore, secondary health promotion is necessary to achieve this through screening (for phenylketonuria, hypothyroidism, hearing problems, speech delay)

It is evident in Table 4.4 that some children may have continuing care needs and poor health, which could affect their development. It is important to recognise this and to promote optimum development at a tertiary level of health promotion. For example some children may have mobility problems that affect their physical development, but these do not necessarily interfere with their intellectual, emotional and social development, which should be encouraged. In the physical domain the mobility problem may interfere with their lower limbs, but they can still develop physical skills with their upper limbs.

The factors that affect child development are many and need to be seen in the context of the individual child, young person and family to be able to help them meet their needs and to promote optimum health.

→ Trigger 4.3: Feedback

Go to Chapter 4 Trigger feedback on p. 97

❗ Trigger 4.4: Child Growth and Nutrition

Children and young people grow and develop. The intention of this trigger is to enable you to find out about child growth and nutrition.

The Trigger

An extract from the Personal Child Health Record (PCHR) written by a mother.

Things I would like to discuss with health visitor/GP/other health professional at the 6–8 week visit

Baby has not been feeding very well. Still trying to breast feed but supplementing

with bottle milk feeds. Baby's weight gain is slow? To ask my health visitor's

advice about feeding. I'm worried!

Situation

This mother was asking for advice about feeding at a visit by the health visitor, and expressing concern about the babies slow weight gain. Your mentor shows you some *centile charts* on your return to the health centre and explains that children's growth measurements are recorded on these charts. Therefore, healthcare professionals are able to monitor children's growth through the use of these centile charts.

Feedback

Based on your answers to the trigger questions you are required to develop an original health education leaflet to inform mother's about infant nutrition. You should also give rationale for the development of your leaflet demonstrating knowledge and an understanding of the broad issues around infant feeding which arise from the trigger questions set.

The facts

What are the facts in this trigger? Make a list:

Hypotheses: What may these facts mean?

- The PCHR enables mothers to document information about their children.
- Health visitors (and other professionals) routinely visit children/families at specified times.
- There is an expected weight gain for babies.
- Mothers need health education about infant feeding.
- Breast feeding is best.

Questions developed from the hypotheses

1. What is a Personal Child Health Record?
2. What are the expectations for child growth?
3. What are the nutritional requirements in the first year?
4. What health education about infant feeding needs to be provided for mothers?

Trigger 4.4: Fixed resource material

Read the following to help you answer the questions. (You may also wish to search and review other up-to-date research and evidence-based literature and seek other relevant resources to provide you with answers to your questions.)

Department of Health (2004b) *Birth to Five: Your Complete Guide to Parenthood and the First Five Years of Your Child's Life*, www.dh.gov.uk (accessed 07.01.05).

Hall, D., Elliman, D. (eds) (2003) Health for all Children, 4th edn. Oxford: Oxford University Press www.health-for-all-children.co.uk (accessed 07.01.05).

Trigger 4.4: Fixed resource sessions

Personal Child Health Record (PCHR)

A model PCHR was launched in 1993 with the philosophy that parents would hold their child's record to encourage partnership between health professionals and parents and to improve communications between health professionals. This intention was that this would lead to better continuity of care and not only increase parent's understanding of their child's health and development, but it would empower them (Hall and Elliman 2003).

A review of the PCHR and wide consultation to achieve agreement resulted in the development of a new record in 2003. It is intended that this record should evolve with changing needs and findings from research. There is a lack of health promotion material in the record because the assumption is that it will be used in conjunction with *Birth to Five* (Department of Health 2004b). The parents have responsibility for keeping the record in a safe place, because it is the main record of their child's health. Parents are also encouraged to use the record jointly with the health professionals that care for their child. The child's parents should be encouraged to record any information that they believe is valuable (this trigger is an example of how a mother may use the record). These factors enable parents to take some control over their child's health monitoring and promotion, which is likely to be empowering for them. Empowerment is a central tenet of health promotion.

The PCHR should be given out antenatally whenever possible or failing this as soon as possible after birth. Health visitors have responsibility for explaining the record to parents and encouraging them to bring it to various visits such as the child health clinic and a hospital emergency or outpatient department.

The PCHR provides information about health care services and also about meeting the child's health needs in respect of immunisations, screening/routine reviews and child growth and development. It also provides record sheets for parents and health-care professionals to record information about individual children.

During your community placement you should have opportunities to judge how well PCHRs are being used in practice Remember that these records should also be available for children's nurses and other healthcare professionals in hospital if the child attends or is admitted.

Child growth and measurement

An infant will triple in weight and increase in length by 50 per cent in the first 12 months of life. After the first year of life growth slows down and continues at a steadier rate until puberty starts. At puberty an increase in growth hormone initiates a final and rapid growth spurt (Wardley et al 1997). These gains in weight and length are the primary indices of nutritional status (European Food Information Council 2004). 'Accurate measurement and the use of standard growth charts are important tools for monitoring a child's progress' (Wardley et al 1997, p. 2).

Growth monitoring and promotion is the preferred term, as opposed to growth measurement, because it can be used to assess and inform health promotion activity in respect of nutritional advice and overall quality of child care (Hall and Elliman 2003). The measurement and plotting of height, weight and head circumference on a suitable chart where there are concerns about growth or chronic health problems is good practice (Hall and Elliman 2003). It is also considered important to do growth monitoring of apparently healthy children, to detect disorders and facilitate early intervention.

Centile charts are used to plot these measurements. 'The value of centile charts is that infants and children can usually be expected to follow a genetically predetermined centile line without deviation upwards or downwards' (Wardley et al 1997, p. 2).

Suggested Activity

Discuss with your health visitor the significance of these charts in relation to the children you encounter in practice.

Effective growth monitoring is dependent on the use of growth charts; correct measurement techniques; accurate charting of measurements;

correct interpretation; appropriate explanation about the measurements to parents; initiation of appropriate action if necessary, and access to specialist advice (Hall and Elliman 2003).

The development of appropriate skills with regard to correct measurement techniques is important and it is suggested that you read: Hall, D., Elliman, D. (eds) (2003) *Health for all Children*, 4th edn. Oxford: Oxford University Press, especially Chapter 8, pp. 169–95.

Nutrition in the first year of life

To enable children to grow and develop to their optimum potential it is vital that they are provided with nutritionally sound diets (European Food Information Council, 2004). Childhood diet and exercise patterns are likely to make the difference between health and ill health in adulthood. Children of different ages have different nutrient needs. The nutritional needs in the first year of life will now be considered (see Table 4.5).

It is essential that nutritional needs be met in this first year because of the rapid growth that occurs.

Table 4.5 Infant nutritional requirements

Infant requirements in the first year	Function
Protein	Used by infants almost entirely for growth.
Carbohydrates	The main energy source
Fat	Stored by infants as an emergency energy food and it insulates them from the cold. Fatty acids are essential for normal growth
Minerals	The infant's iron store will last for approximately 6 months after birth. It is essential for an iron source to be provided when weaning is introduced.
Calcium	This is needed for the development of bones and teeth
Trace elements (Copper; zinc)	Essential for normal development
Vitamins	Requires a full range for normal development

Source: Adapted from McEwing et al (2003)

The Department of Health (2004c) recommendations on feeding infants state that:

- Breast milk is the best form of nutrition for infants;
- Exclusive breastfeeding is recommended for the first six months of an infant's life;
- Six months is the recommended age for the introduction of solid foods for infants;
- Breastfeeding (and/or breast milk substitutes if used) should continue beyond the first six months, along with appropriate types and amounts of solid foods.

Breast-feeding

Breast-feeding on demand remains the ideal form of feeding for healthy babies born at term. Human milk provides all the energy and nutrients the infant needs for optimum growth and development and maintenance. It also contains proteins, antibodies and white blood cells, which help to protect the infant against infection (British Nutrition Foundation 2005).

> *Suggested Activity*
>
> You should now refer to:
>
> 1. Chapter 9 to learn more about breast milk and breast-feeding.
> 2. Find out about the United Kingdom Baby Friendly Initiative http://www.babyfriendly.org.uk
> 3. Royal College of Nursing (1998) *Breast Feeding in Paediatric Units: Guidance for Good Practice*. London, RCN.

Weaning

It is stated by the World Health Organisation (2001) and the Department of Health (2004c) that the best nutrition for babies is provided by exclusive breastfeeding to 6 months. Introducing solids earlier than six months can increase the risk of infections and the development of allergies such as eczema and asthma. Infants require solid food from six months of age for nutritional and developmental reasons. This is because infant's need more iron and other nutrients than milk alone provides.

World Health Organisation (2001) recommends that the food is in addition to breast milk and initially it should be given 2–3 times a day between 6–8 months, increasing to 3–4 times daily between 9–11 months and 12–24 months with additional nutritious snacks offered 1–2 times a day. The pace of the introduction of quality, number and variety of solid feeds can be increased gradually as dictated by individual infants (European Union Food Information Council 2004).

At about five months infants are usually able to take soft pureed foods from a spoon, form a bolus and swallow it (Department of Health 2004c). When infants are about six months they are then able to be actively spoon fed with the upper lip moving down to clean the spoon. Infants at six months are also able to chew, move the food around the mouth from the back to the front; finger feed and are curious about other tastes and textures. Department of Health (1994) advise that the older the baby the more readily will they accept a diet that varies in texture, taste and amount.

Bottle feeding

Milk delivered to the infant from a bottle and teat is generally safe provided that an approved infant formula is used under strict hygiene conditions (European Food Information Council 2005). Infant formula milk must comply with guidelines from the European Union and the World Health Organisation. Infant formula does attempt to mimic as far as possible the composition of mature human milk, however they cannot mirror the complex immunological, hormonal and enzyme content (Wardley et al 1997). Bottle fed infants should be demand fed to enable them to regulate their own volume of intake similar to breast fed infants. An average intake of 150–200 ml/kg/day is a useful guideline for calculating the required fluid intake of infants. However infants will differ greatly in their requirements (Wardley et al 1997).

It is stated in the Department of Health response to the consultation exercise for the 'Healthy Start: Reform of the Welfare Food Scheme' that health professionals will continue to have an important role in advising beneficiaries about health and nutrition, including breast feeding and in promoting the appropriate use of vitamin supplements (Department of Health 2004c). The advice giving is likely to include the use of leaflets such as the one you are being asked to produce for this trigger.

Useful Websites

European Food Information Council http://www.eufic.org (accessed 24.01.05).
British Nutrition Foundation http://www.nutrition.org.uk (accessed 24.01.05).
World Health Organisation: Child and Adolescent Health and Development http://www.who.int/child-adolescent-health (accessed 24.01.05).

Trigger 4.4: Feedback

Go to Chapter 4 Trigger Feedback on p. 97 below

Chapter 4 Trigger feedback: what do you know?

Trigger 4.1: Child health and health promotion

Question 1: What is child health?

To answer this question you may have started by considering your own definition of health now and as a child. You may have found out that you put more value on your physical health than the intellectual, emotional and social dimensions of health or vice versa. Discussion with some of your colleagues about what is child health may have revealed that they valued one of the other dimensions of health more than you. On the other hand yourself and your colleagues may equally value all the possible dimensions of personal and child health. A diversity of views on what constitutes child health suggests that different meanings are given to it, which may have consequences for how child health is promoted.

The World Health Organisation with regard to all age groups has provided some international definitions of health:

The World Health Organisation (1946) described health as a state of complete physical, mental and social well-being and not merely the absence of disease and infirmity. This definition is still used by the World Health Organisation. It is often criticised for being too idealistic, because it is difficult for individuals to achieve and or maintain a state of complete, physical, mental and social well being. Prior to this World Health Organisation definition, health seems only to have been viewed from the physical dimension. Therefore, this definition is important because it recognises that there is more than one dimension of health and that these dimensions are inter-related. In other words this definition provides a holistic view of health in relation to individuals. The next definition, part of which was identified in the fixed resource session about health policy, is a much broader one that is applied to groups of people as well as individuals.

According to the World Health Organisation (1984) health is the extent to which an individual group is able on the one hand to realise aspirations and satisfy needs and on the other hand to change or cope with the environment. So, therefore, health is seen as a resource for everyday life, as opposed to an object for living. It is a positive concept that emphasises social and personal resources as well as physical capacities. This definition identifies that social and personal resources are required for health. This means that individuals and groups need appropriate social environmental support for health. How this is interpreted reflects on the context of living in both developed and developing countries. To have health there should be social support to ensure that the basic survival needs identified by Maslow (1987) are met, that is air, food, water, shelter and warmth. Social targets for health are now developed by the World Health Organisation to ensure that people have these social resources for health. Personal resource development has become central to promoting health with an emphasis on empowering people to take some control over their lives.

The definition that underpins the World Health Organisation (1998) Europe policy stresses that the enjoyment of health is one of the fundamental rights of every human being. Health is viewed as a pre-condition for well being and quality of life. World Health Organisation (1998) sees health as a benchmark for measuring progress towards the reduction of poverty, the promotion of social cohesion and the elimination of discrimination. This definition is different again reflecting the beliefs and values of society in the twenty-first century. Health is being viewed in collective terms as opposed to individual terms in this definition to some extent signifying the current emphasis on public health promotion.

It is likely that you have tried to find some specific definitions about child health. Several of them refer to the need to promote 'normal' growth and development of children for health (Open University 1985). A broad, holistic definition is:

> Health in childhood is affected not only by biological factors, but also by the lifestyle and problems of the parents, including unemployment, low income, and poor housing. Individual and community relationships therefore play a major role in health. (Hall and Elliman 2003, p. 6)

The contemporary definitions that are used to explain child health have a tendency to reflect the quote used in this trigger from the *NHS Plan* (Department of Health 2000,

p. 111): 'Health at the beginning of life is the foundation of health throughout life.' An example being:

> People's patterns of behaviour are often set early in life and influence their health throughout their lives. Infancy, childhood and young adulthood are critical stages in the development of habits that will affect people's health in later years. (Department of Health 2004, p. 41)

You are likely to have concluded that child health is not only defined on an individual basis, but also more holistic definitions are provided in recognition of all the factors that may influence children's health in both the long and short term.

Question 2: How may the perceptions and understanding of children, young people, family members and health professionals about child health differ?

It has already been identified in the fixed resource session that children's and young people's perceptions and understanding of health will change dependent on their developmental age and social experiences.

It is likely that the perceptions and understanding of adult members of the family in relation to child health are going to be influenced by their own social experiences and upbringing. The responsibility taken by individual parents and/or carers for promoting their children's health may be influenced by their social-economic circumstances, with the better off having more resources to promote health and those less well off looking to health care professionals and others to take on this responsibility. The locus of control theory of Rotter (1966) seems to link in with this issue of responsibility suggesting that whatever the parents and or carers understand about child health those with an external locus of control will look to others to take on responsibility for their child's health or leave it to fate, which is a negative approach to promoting child health. On the other hand those adults with an internal locus of control will take positive health preventative action to promote their child's health.

There is also the potential for conflict between professional and lay beliefs due to different perceptions and understanding. You may observe this happening in practice in the community and should reflect on these situations. The emphasis in contemporary health policy with regard to working in partnership may help to overcome some of these differences to ensure that child health promotion is effective.

Question 3: What are the potential health outcomes of poor health in childhood for adult health?

It was recognised several years ago in *The Health of the Nation* (Department of Health 1992) that health in childhood is likely to have consequential benefits for health in adulthood. This national strategy (Department of Health 1992) outlined the potential ill health outcomes in adulthood for children whose health was not effectively promoted in childhood stating that the consequential health problems in adulthood may include:

- Coronary heart disease and strokes: lack of exercise or a balanced diet in childhood may cause health problems in adulthood.
- Cancer: reducing smoking among young people is crucial to reducing smoking in later life. Smoking in pregnancy may lead to low birth weight infants with resultant health problems. Parental smoking may cause infant respiratory problems.
- Mental Illness: early effective intervention in childhood can be important in promoting adult mental health.
- Accidents: some childhood accidents may lead to lifelong disability or a pre-disposition to ill health later in life.
- Sexual health: family planning and pre-conception care is needed so that pregnancies can be planned and teenage pregnancies reduced.

The Public Health White Paper *Choosing Health* (Department of Health 2004a) is about taking action to ensure that children and young people have the healthiest possible start to life as a major priority because many and it seems an increasing number of children are in 'danger' of having poor health outcomes in adulthood. The areas that are identified in Department of Health (2004a) as being top of the agenda for action are obesity (see the fixed resource session for this trigger), sexually transmitted diseases, alcohol abuse and smoking. The identification of these action areas focuses us on the relevant contemporary health issues to target our child health promotion work.

You should be able to add some examples of initiatives in your own locality to promote health in childhood for a healthy adulthood during your community placement.

Question 4: What approaches are used to promote child health?

Health promotion is an umbrella term that involves several activities (Ewles and Simnett 2003). Health education is a major activity and programmes may include 'Providing information, exploring values and attitudes, making health decisions and acquiring skills to enable behaviour change to take place' (Ewles and Simnett 2003, p. 29).

Health education may take place on a one-to-one basis or within a group. It has the potential to promote self-esteem and empower people to take positive action in relation to their health, but this may be dependant on the resources and support that individuals have available.

The other activities described by Ewles and Simnett (2003) are:

- Preventive health services, for example, immunisation;
- Healthy public policies such as transport and housing policy;

- Environmental health measures that could include smoke free areas;
- Economic and regulatory activities involve political activity in relation to policies, lobbying for legislative changes and advertising codes of practice about alcohol or smoking and such financial measures as an increase in tobacco taxation;
- Organisational development to promote the health of staff and possibly customers. It may include offering healthy food choices in staff dining rooms;
- Community-based work is about communities identifying their own health needs and concerns and with the support of professionals taking action to improve their health. It is a bottom up approach that may involve forming self-help and pressure groups.

Health promotion, therefore, is 'any planned and informed intervention, which is designed to improve physical or mental health or prevent disease, disability and premature death' (Hall and Elliman, 2003, p. 6).

The Child Health Promotion Programme that was launched as part of the *National Service Framework* (Department of Health 2004) is a planned and informed intervention that will be used to promote child health. The implementation of this plan may involve the use of several of the aforementioned health promotion activities and using more than one approach to promote health at one of the following preventive levels:

- Primary aims to prevent ill health occurring in the first place.
- Secondary aims to diagnose health problems early so that treatment may be instigated early and restoration of health is then more likely.
- Tertiary aims to educate patients and their family about how to achieve optimum health when ill health cannot be prevented or completely cured.

Ewles and Simnett (2003) provide a useful framework of five approaches to health promotion that encompasses most of the values inherent in the international and national health policy that was explained in one of the fixed resource sessions for this trigger. The framework is also inclusive of the underpinning philosophies of most models of health promotion and education. The five approaches are:

1. *Medical*: medical intervention to prevent or cure ill-health.
2. *Behaviour change*: encouraging attitude and behaviour change leading to healthy lifestyles being adopted.
3. *Educational*: information giving, exploring values and attitudes and developing skills.
4. *Empowerment*: working with health issues, choices and actions identified by the child/family.
5. *Societal change*: social targets and action to change the physical and social environment.

The medical and behavioural approaches to health promotion tend to focus on the determinants of disease at the level of the individual, appearing to blame the victims and ignore the social and economic factors, which often prevent people from making appropriate choices, for example, some parents may be too poor to buy healthy foods or recommended safety equipment (Hall and Elliman 2003). The public health policy, *Choosing Health* (Department of Health 2004a) however states that practical support will now be provided to enable children and families to make healthy choices in the future.

A modern view of the educational approach includes information giving, consumer information on services and benefits and personal strategies to cope with stress, loneliness, unemployment and poor housing for example (Hall and Elliman 2003). Therefore, skill development may include assertiveness and other coping skills.

The empowerment approach is about empowering people to take control over factors that affect their lives, 'while recognising and affirming their personal responsibility for their own health' (Hall and Elliman 2003, p. 7). This again involves developing assertiveness skills, self-esteem and self-efficacy beliefs to deal with barriers to becoming empowered at both the individual and community level.

Hall and Elliman (2003) seem to suggest that better health is potentially achieved by societal change, which promotes healthy physical and social environments and public policies that affect benefits, finance or employment.

The approaches taken to promote child health are wide and varied and as stated by Ewles and Simnett (2003) there is no one right approach for promoting the health of children. The approaches chosen are dependant on accurate assessments of the needs of individual children, young people and their families.

Trigger 4.2: Inequalities in child health

The feedback for this trigger is in the form of a report of an individual investigation into a local area to find out about child health inequalities and poverty. Therefore, the answers that you provide in your report to the questions you formulated are likely to differ, from the example provided in this chapter. Some of you may have conducted your investigation in an area of deprivation and others in areas where the population is a mixture of affluent and deprived families. The example report provided here will focus on national information and strategies to reduce child health inequalities and poverty and make some suggestions about what you may have found out in your local area.

Inequalities in Child Health Report: Local Area

Focus of the report

The trigger stated that 3.9 children live in poverty in the UK (End Child Poverty Group 2002). Further reading informs us that childhood poverty is a worldwide problem.

The local area that you have been investigating may be a deprived area with statistics showing some of the determinants of health inequalities. Alternatively you may have found that within a community of relatively well of families that there are some families living in poverty.

Background

Numerous studies have identified determinants that are associated with health inequalities for example the Black Report (Townsend et al 1988); the Acheson Report (Department of Health 1998a). These determinants are in the main inextricably linked with children, young people and families that are living in poverty. Department of Health (1999) states that the determinants are personal, social and environmental. They include low wages, unemployment, poor education, substandard housing, polluted environments, social class, geographical, occupation, gender, ethnicity, stress and undesirable living conditions.

The health of children living in poverty is often characterised by their families being able to make less use of the health services, especially preventive health services than others, which results in them experiencing poorer health and social outcomes than their counterparts (Department of Health, 2003) with material wealth. There is a marked social gradient in the prevalence of poorer health and social outcomes (Department of Health, 2003). This is reflected in some of the following outcomes:

- High infant mortality rates;
- Low birth weight babies;
- Poor nutrition;
- Higher incidence of accidental injury;
- Child protection issues;
- Prevalence of dental caries;
- Poor mental health;
- Incidence of substance misuse;
- Smoking;
- High teenage pregnancy rates;
- Delayed development;
- Poor education.

Your investigation into a local area is likely to reveal specific outcomes for that area. For example in your area there may be a high rate of teenage pregnancies or alternatively dental caries. It will vary from area to area, but the outcomes identified above are the ones that are likely to present when children and young people are living in poverty.

Current situation

There may be some of the following initiatives happening in the area that you have been investigating (you are likely to be able to add other ones to this list):

- Health Action Zones;
- Early intervention programmes: Sure Start: Home Start;
- Children's Centres;
- Teenage pregnancies programmes;
- Fluoride dental care;
- Community development and empowerment projects.

Key issues

- It is difficult to reduce the incidence of childhood poverty.
- Children and young people living in poverty experience inequalities in health.
- Inequalities in health result in poorer health and social outcomes for children and young people.
- Governments target children, young people and families living in poverty to improve their health experiences and subsequently health outcomes.

Recommendations

1. Provide health promotion for individuals and communities to empower them.
2. Implementing initiatives to give children and young people a good start to life is important for health in later life.
3. Develop social targets to promote health of children and young people living in poverty and to reduce inequalities in health.
4. Children's nurses should assess the needs of children and young people in hospital and give appropriate health education advice based on their social status.
5. Children's nurses should not be judgemental with regard to the circumstances necessitating hospitalisation for children and young people living in poverty (Fatchett 1995).

Trigger 4.3: Promoting and monitoring child development for health

The student nurse's reflective account: (Your account may be similar to this example)

This is a reflective account of a visit I made with my health visitor mentor to a family with four children. It was a first visit to see the youngest member of the family, a two week old baby called Chloe. My mentor also asked me a lot of questions after the visit about child development in relation to the other children in the family. I am going to use Gibbs (1988) reflective cycle to reflect on this experience. This involves, describing the visit, reflecting on my feelings both positive and negative prior to analysing the key issues and then concluding and identifying what this reflection means for my future practice.

Description

We visited this family during the first week of my community placement. The purpose was for my health visitor mentor to undertake the initial visit to the new baby Chloe that should occur when the baby is between 10–14 days old. Sarah the mother already knew the health visitor because of previous home and clinic visits with Joseph her 3 year old son. Joseph is in the room playing with his toys when we arrive keeping a watch on his mother with the new baby. I spend some time playing with him and trying to keep him occupied so that Sarah can concentrate on the baby and answer questions. The older children 14 year old Helen and 10 year old Tom are at school. Sarah tells us that they are both doing important exams this year and she is finding herself nagging them to revise. Her husband is very busy at work at the moment. This means that he is often late home and is not seeing as much of the new baby as he would like and is not able to help out with the children very much.

The health visitor asks Sarah how she is, about the new baby and the rest of the family. Sarah states that she is feeling well although a bit tired. The older children, particularly Helen, are being very helpful around the house, which is a pleasant change. According to Sarah, Helen is being a typical adolescent most of the time, so this unexpected help is a real bonus. Sarah is slightly worried about 3 year old Joseph who has become very clingy since Chloe was born and he is wetting himself again during the night. He was just becoming dry prior to the birth.

The health visitor asks how Chloe is feeding and if she is sleeping all right. Sarah expresses no concerns about Chloe in respect of these activities. She also gives some information to Sarah about immunisation and child health clinics prior to us departing.

Feelings (Good)

It was really good that I could be helpful during this visit. I enjoyed playing with Joseph and eventually seemed to gain his trust. I was really impressed to see how well

Sarah was managing with the new baby and three other children with minimal support from her husband due to his work commitments. It was evident that my health visitor had built up a good relationship with Sarah and her family that enabled her to communicate effectively. I also felt this helped with Sarah accepting me as a visitor in her home and being open to me observing the visit as well as playing with Joseph.

Feelings (Bad)

I was concerned about my level of knowledge and understanding about child development. We have had lessons about it in school, but the reality is different. Although I had enjoyed playing with Joseph I was rather apprehensive at first. I also wasn't sure what were the answers that my health visitor was wanting when she was asking Sarah about Chloe. I then thought about the developmental stages of the other two children in the family and what characterised children of those ages. What did Sarah mean by stating that Helen was a typical teenager?

Analysis of key issues

The key issues that emerged for analysis were child development at two weeks, 3 years, 10 years and 14 years old, which are obviously the ages of children in this particular family. It will be helpful to me to explore the expectations for development at these specific ages to contextualise my visit.

I am going to identify some of the key physical, social, psychological and intellectual developmental characteristics for each child according to their age after establishing the expectations for the common pattern of development.

Pattern of Development: Development may be seen in terms of progressing from head to toe. There are expectations when milestones should be reached in child development, but it is important to recognise that all children may not reach them on time and it does not matter as long as they arrive at them in reasonable time. There are individual differences in progression.

Neonates: At 2 weeks old babies are neonates, which describes the age range from birth to one month. Therefore, I am going to describe briefly the characteristics that denote the neonatal period of development (*Also see Chapter 9*).

Neonates are born with a large collection of reflexes. These are physical responses triggered involuntarily by a specific stimulus. Bee and Boyd (2004) explain how some of these are lifelong reflexes such as the knee jerk, but additionally the neonate has a set of primitive reflexes controlled by the more primitive parts of the brain. When the brain has developed more fully with regard to controlling perception, body movement, thinking and language the primitive reflexes (for example tonic neck reflex) begin to disappear at about six months as if superceded by the higher level brain functions (Bee and Boyd 2004). Some of the primitive reflexes are essential for survival such as breathing and sucking reflexes for feeding, while others have less obvious usefulness.

> ### *Suggested Activity*
>
> You probably found out about primitive reflexes as you wrote your own reflective account. You should write a short description of each of the following:
>
> - Moro;
> - Rooting;
> - Palmar grasp;
> - Asymmetrical tonic neck response;
> - Walking-stepping.

At age four weeks the neonate will in the supine position lie with head to one side with the arm and leg on face side outstretched or both arms flexed. The knees will be apart and the soles of the feet turned inwards. There are large jerky movements of the limbs with the arms being more active than the legs. The head falls loosely when the neonate is lifted from the cot unless it is supported and also the head lags when pulled to sit until the body is vertical. The head in this vertical position is only held for a moment erect prior to falling forwards. When the neonate of four weeks is held in a sitting position the back is one complete curve. The head will be in line with the body and hips when holding the neonate in ventral suspension and in the prone position the head turns immediately to one side with the arms and legs flexed, elbows away from the body and the buttocks in quite a high position. The neonate will make a forward reflex walking movement when held standing on a hard surface. A stepping up over the curb will occur against a table edge when the dorsum of the foot is stimulated (Sheridan 1997).

The neonate at four weeks will turn head and eyes towards a light source and eyes will follow bright moving objects. There will also momentarily be visual fixation on objects and adult faces. Sheridan (1997) states that from about three weeks mother's nearby face will be watched when she feeds or talks to the neonate with increasingly alert facial expressions. Chloe should be doing this by next week.

Neonates at four weeks are startled by noise and will be momentarily 'frozen' when a small bell is rung at ear level and then may move eyes and head towards the sound source. Neonates usually turn towards the sound of a soothing human voice, providing that they are not screaming or feeding. They will cry lustily when hungry or uncomfortable and alternatively utters little guttural noises when content.

Socially at four weeks the neonate will sleep most of the time except when being fed or handled. It was apparent from the responses to the health visitor's questions that

Chloe was following this pattern. Neonates will stop crying when picked up and spoken to and turn to regard a nearby speaker's face. The social smile and responsive vocalisation come later at about five to six weeks. Sarah, Chloe's mother, was asking about this during the health visitor's visit.

Three year old children: Children at this age are able to walk alone upstairs with alternating feet and downstairs two feet at a time. They are able to walk forwards, backwards, sideways and so on hauling large toys with confidence. Three-year olds are able to ride a tricycle using the pedals and can steer round corners. They have the ability to stand on one preferred foot. Children of this age can also throw a ball overhand and catch a large ball on or between extended arms. They are able to kick a ball forcibly. Children aged three are able to build a tower of nine or ten bricks, cut with scissors, paint with a large brush and draw a man with a head indicating one or two other features or parts.

At this age children have a large vocabulary that is intelligible even to strangers, but their speech still has some unconventional grammatical forms. Three year old children will give their full name, sex and sometimes age. They will carry on simple conversations and briefly describe present activities and past experiences. Three year olds will ask many questions that begin with what, where and who. They are able to count by rote up to 10 or more with little appreciation of quantity beyond two or more.

Socially three year olds are able to eat with a fork and spoon, wash their hands with supervision, but they need help with buttons and other fastenings in dressing. These children like make believe play that includes invented people and objects and will do this with other children. They enjoy floor-play with bricks, boxes, and so on alone or with siblings, because at this age they understand about sharing your things with others (Sheridan 1997).

They may be dry with regard to urinary continence through the night, however this is variable. This is probably why Joseph has started to be incontinent of urine again during the night. He has regressed in this behaviour due to the birth of the new baby, which has unsettled him at this time in his development. Three-year old children are pre-operational as described by Piaget and in this stage of cognitive development they are still egocentric in thought and behaviour and hence regression occurs in stressful situations such as a new sibling. It may also occur on admission to hospital especially if parents are unable to be resident with their child. Regression means that a child will temporarily stop using newly acquired skills in an attempt to retain or regain control of a stressful situation (Brunner and Suddarth 1992). This may explain why Joseph has also become clingy. He is stressed and needs to ensure that he has some control over his mother's attention. It is important that sibling's feelings and needs are not overlooked when a new baby arrives if their health is to be promoted.

Ten year olds: Physically ten year olds will be losing their childish appearance facially and begin to take on features that will characterise them as adults. Growth spurts occur and some secondary sexual characteristics begin to appear in females 10–12 and later in males at age 12–14 years old.

Children in this age group are likely to be energetic, restless and to develop active movements (Brunner and Suddarth 1992). Tom invests this energy into playing for the under eleven year olds football team. Playing football will provide him with the opportunity to use the skilled manipulative movements that this age group have developed. Children of this age work hard to perfect their physical skills and want to take on challenges, doubtless Tom will be doing this to contribute to his football teams success.

Ten year old children like to reason and enjoy learning. Their thinking is still concrete operational (Piaget). They are matter of fact, which would explain why Tom took the arrival of his new sister in his stride. This age group like to memorise and identify facts, but their attention span may be short.

Young people age 14 years: Adolescence is a period of great change both physically and psychologically for young people. The age range given for the adolescent period varies. In this reflection it is identified as 11 to 19 years (Department of Health 2004). This is a wide age range, which Jacobs (1985) divides into three stages that have been adapted by Taylor and Cooper (2003) into:

- Early adolescence and sexuality;
- Middle adolescence: authority and independence;
- Later adolescence: faith and responsibility.

Helen the 14 year old in the family could be either in the early or middle stage of adolescence. Adolescence is a dynamic process according to Taylor and Cooper (2003) as opposed a series of steps or stages to go through prior to arriving at adulthood. The implication of this is that it is likely that adolescents will pass through these adolescent stages identified by Jacobs (1985) at different ages.

Physical changes in adolescence are due to the effect of hormones that trigger puberty, with oestrogen production rising in girls and testosterone production increasing in boys. This results in growth spurts and a changing body image. Physical changes for girls are associated with the commencement of the monthly menstrual cycle and for boys changes include deepening of the voice.

Psychologically the young person learns to think abstractly, to idealise and develops an identity of their own and independence. This is supported by Piaget's cognitive development theory that suggests adolescent's are in the formal operational stage signifying that they have moved onto a more adult way of thinking, which is perhaps why Helen is willing to help her mother more after the birth of Chloe. It is a confusing time though for young people. Erikson's psychological theory identifies that the task for the adolescent stage of development is identity versus confusion. Adolescents need to establish their own identity but it is confusing with the physical and social changes that they are contending with in their transition to adulthood.

Socially adolescence involves experimentation noted in extremes of dress, hair and social behaviour. Adolescents are likely to resent interference from their parents and it can be a challenging time for young people and parents alike. Schoolwork and education at this time are important in preparation to transition to adulthood and employment in the near future.

Different cultures view adolescence in different ways.

Conclusion

This reflection has enabled me to develop my knowledge and understanding of child development. It was evident that the children in this family were developing in line with the expected 'norms' for their age. I know that this may not always be the position, but in this family there were many positive factors that would promote development, including a loving family, siblings, play/ toys, and financial security.

Future practice

I will be more confident when I accompany my health visitor on visits to other families. I will prepare for these future visits by reading about child development at different ages, either before or after the visit. This learning about child development will also be really useful for my future practice in the hospital setting. I will need to remember though that children may regress in stressful situations like hospital admissions. This is similar to Joseph who regressed after the birth of Chloe and a brief separation from his mother.

Trigger 4.4: Child growth and nutrition

Producing a health education leaflet

Ewles and Simnett (2003) suggest that you need to take into account:

- Who is the target group?
- An assessment of the needs of this target group for information.
- The accuracy of the information in your leaflet,
- Colour, layout and print size.
- Use of pictures.
- The use of plain English.
- Presentation of statistical information in a visual way.
- How the leaflet will be used to promote health and educate?
- How the leaflet will be evaluated?

Figure 4.1 is the template for a leaflet that you may have designed for your feedback for this trigger. The wording that goes under the main headings of breast-feeding, bottle-feeding and weaning should be written in plain English. The pictures are

Feeding Your Baby	Breast Feeding	Weaning
Helping your Baby to Grow!	Bottle Feeding	*Personal Child Health Record*: Use to record how well your baby is feeding for discussion with your health visitor *For Further Information Contact:*
Front Cover	Inside Page	Back Cover

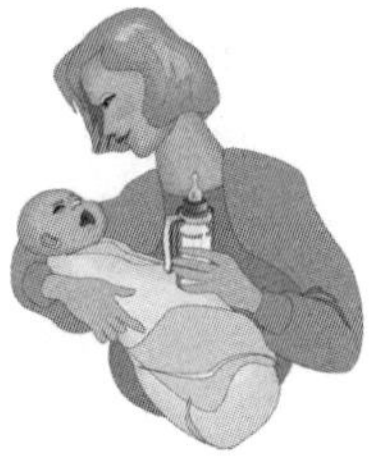

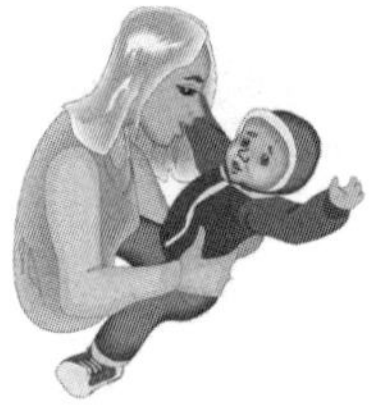

Figure 4.1 Health education leaflet: Infant nutrition

intended to make the leaflet visually attractive. There is space for a contact number for further information, which is always useful, and a reminder about using the Personal Child Health Record.

Reflect on your learning

- Apply national and international health promotion principles to promote child health in primary health care settings.
- Use public health strategies to reduce inequalities in child health.
- Promote child growth, development and play for health.
- Educate and support children, young people and families to make healthy choices.
- Transfer learning about health promotion principles in primary health care to promoting the health of children and their families in the hospital setting.

The next chapter continues to deal with promoting child health with the focus being on safeguarding children.

References

Bee, H., Boyd, D. (2004) *The Developing Child*, 10th edn. Boston: Allyn and Bacon.

British Nutrition Foundation (2005) *Welcome to the British Nutrition Foundation*, http://www.nutrition.org.uk/information/dietthroughlife/babies.html (accessed 07.01.05).

Brunner, L., Suddarth, D. (1992) *The Lippincott Manual of Paediatric Nursing*, 3rd edn. London: Harper and Rowe.

Child Policy Network (2004) *Child Policy Review 2004: Summary of Key Policy Developments Across the FOUR Nations of the UK*, http://www.childpolicy.org.uk (accessed 03.08.05).

Coleman, V. (1998) *What is the meaning of the concept of empowerment and do nurses use it to promote the health of children with a chronic illness*. Unpublished Master's Dissertation, Sheffield: Sheffield Hallam University.

Coleman, V. (2002) Empowerment: Rhetoric, reality and skills, in Smith, L., Coleman, V., Bradshaw, M. (eds) *Family-centred Care: Concept, Theory and Practice*. Basingstoke: Palgrave, Chapter 5, pp. 85–113.

Department for Education and Skills (2003) *Every Child Matters*, http://www.dfes.gov.uk/everychildmatters/index (accessed 07.01.05).

Department for Education and Skills (2005) Welcome to Sure Start www.surestart.gov.uk, (accessed 07.01.05).

Department of Health, Social Services and Public Safety (2002) *Investing for Health*. Northern Ireland: DHSSPS, http://www.dhsspsni.gov.uk/publications/2002/investforhealth.asp (accessed 03.08.05).)

Department of Health (1992) *The Health of the Nation: A Strategy for Health in England*. London: HMSO.

Department of Health (1994) *COMA Working group on the Weaning Diet: Weaning and the Weaning Diet*. London: Department of Health.

Department of Health (1996) *Immunisations against Infectious Diseases*. London: HMSO.

Department of Health (1998) *Our Healthier Nation, A Contract For Health Consultation Paper*. London: The Stationery Office.

Department of Health (1998a) *Independent Inquiry into Inequalities in Health (The Acheson Report)*. London: The Stationery Office.

Department of Health (1999) *Saving Lives: Our Healthier Nation*. London: The Stationery Office.

Department of Health (1999a) *Making a Difference: Strengthening the Nursing, Midwifery and Health Visiting Contribution to Health and Healthcare*. London: Stationery Office.

Department of Health (2000) *The NHS Plan, A Plan for Investment, A Plan for Reform*. London www.nhs.uk/nhsplan.

Department of Health (2003) *Getting the Right Start: National Service Framework for Children – Standard for Hospital Services*. London: Department of Health). www.doh.gov.uk/nsf/children.htm (accessed 07.01.05).

Department of Health (2003a) *Emerging Findings*. London: Department of Health.

Department of Health (2004) *The National Service Framework for Children, Young People and Maternity Services*. London: The Stationery Office.

Department of Health (2004a) *Choosing Health: Making Healthy Choices Easier*. London: The Stationery Office.

Department of Health (2004b) *Birth to Five: your complete guide to parenthood and the first five years if your child's life*, www.dh.gov.uk (accessed 07.01.05).

Department of Health (2004c) *Infant Feeding and Child Nutrition Resource Pack*. London: Department of Health.

Eisenstadt,N (1999) Sure Start: A New Approach for Children under Four, *Primary Health Care*, 9 (6), July–August, pp. 26–7.

Eiser, C. (1993) *Growing up with a chronic illness: the impact on children and their families*. London: Jessica Kingsley.

End Child Poverty (2002) *Poverty and Child Health Briefing Paper*, 16.8.02., http://www.ecpc.org.uk (accessed 01.02.04).

End Child Poverty (2004) *End Child Poverty News*, at http://www.ecpc.org.uk (accessed 09.01.050).

European Food Information Council, Children Nutrition, http://www.eufic.org/en/quickfacts/child_nutrition.htm 2004 (accessed 07.01.05).

Ewles L., Simnett I. (2003) *Promoting Health: A Practical Guide*, 5th edn. Edinburgh: Bailliere Tindall.

Fatchett, A. (ed.) (1995) *Childhood to Adolescence: Caring for Health*. London: Bailliere Tindall.

Fruhbeck, G. (2000) Childhood obesity: Time for action, not complacency. *British Medical Journal*, pp. 20, 328–9.

Gibbs, G. (1988) *Learning by Doing : A Guide to Teaching and Learning Methods*. Oxford: Oxford Further Education Unit, Oxford Polytechnic.

Hall D., Elliman, D. (2003) (eds) Health for all Children, 4th edn. Oxford: Oxford University Press, www.health-for-all-children.co.uk (accessed 07.01.05).

Health Development Agency (2003) *The Management of Obesity and Overweight: An Analysis of Reviews of Diet, Physical Activity and Behavioural Approaches*. London: NHS.

Jacobs, M. (1985) *The Presenting Past: An Introduction to Practical Psychodynamic Counselling*. Milton Keynes: Open University Press.

Joint Health Survey Unit on behalf of the Department of Health (2002) *Health Survey for England 2001*. London: The Stationery Office.

Kennedy, M., Ferri, R., Sofer, D. (2002) United Nations summit resolves to improve children's lives, *American Journal of Nursing*, 102 (8), August, p. 21.

Laing, P. (2002) Childhood obesity: a public health threat. *Paediatric Nursing*, 14 (10), December, pp.14–16.

Maslow, A. (1987) *Motivation and Personality*, 3rd edn. New York: Harper Row.

McEwing, G. (1996) Children's understanding of their internal body parts, *British Journal of Nursing* 5, pp. 429–33.

McEwing, G., Kelsey, J., Richardson, J., Glasper, A. (2003) Insights into child and family health, in Grandis, S., Long, G., Glasper, A., Jackson, P. (eds) *Foundation Studies for Nursing: Using Enquiry-Based Learning*. Basingstoke: Palgrave Macmillan, Chapter 3, pp. 48–114.

National Health Service Direct (2004) http://www.nhsdirect.nhs.uk (accessed 07.01.05).

National Health Service Immunisation Information (2004) *Immunisation for Life*, http://www.immunisation.nhs.uk (accessed 07.01.05).

Open University (1985) *Birth to Old Age: Health in Transition*. Milton Keynes: Open University Press.

Pearson, D. (2003/2004) Weight Management. *Primary Health Care* 123 (10), December/January, pp. 43–9.

Rissel, C. (1994) Empowerment: the Holy Grail of health promotion?. *Health Promotion International*, 9 (1), pp. 39–46.

Rotter, J. B. (1966) Generalised Experience for internal versus external control of reinforcement. *Psychological Monographs* 80, (1 Whole No 609).

Royal College of Nursing (1998) *Breast Feeding in Paediatric Units: Guidance for Good Practice*. London: RCN.

Scottish Excecutive (2003) *Improving Health in Scotland – The Challenge*, http://www.scotland.gov.uk/library5/health/ihis-00.asp (accessed 03.08.05).

Scottish Executive (2004) *The Active Schools Network*, http://www.scotland.gov.uk/Topics/Health/health/Introduction/ActiveSchools (accessed 08.08.05).

Scottish Executuve (2004a) *Health Indicators Report: December 2004*. Scotland: NHS Quality Improvement.

Sheridan, M. (1997) *From Birth to Five Years: Children's Developmental Progess* (revised and updated by Frost, M., Sharma, A.). London: Routledge.

Smith, F. (2003/2004) The children's NSF in primary care, *Primary Health Care* 13 (10), December/January, p. 17.

Swanwick, M. (1990) Knowledge and Control. *Paediatric Nursing* June, pp. 18–20.

Taylor, C., Cooper, M. (2003) Insights into adolescent health and eating disorders, in Grandis, S., Long, G., Glasper, A., Jackson, P. (eds) *Foundation Studies for Nursing: Using Enquiry-Based Learning*. Basingstoke: Palgrave Macmillan, Chapter 4, pp. 115–37.

Townsend, P., Davidson, N., Whitehead, M. (1988) *Inequalities in Health*. Harmondsworth: Penguin Books.

UNICEF UK Baby Friendly Initiative, http://www.babyfriendly.org.uk (accessed 24.01.05).

United Nations (2003) *The State of the World's Children*. New York: UNICEF.

Wardley, B., Puntis, J. W. L., Taitz, L. S. (1997) *Handbook of Child Nutrition*, 2nd edn. Oxford: Oxford University Press.

Welsh Assembly (2003) *Healthy and Active Lifestyles in Wales: A Framework or Action*, http://www.cmo.wales.gov.uk (accessed 03.08.05).

Welsh Assembly (2005) A Fair Future for our Children: *The Strategy of the Welsh Assembly Government for Tackiling Child Poverty, Executive Summary*, http://www.wales.gov.uk/subichildren/content/summary-action-plan-e.pdf (accessed 03.08.05).

Welsh Assembly (2004) *National Service Framework for Children, Young People and Maternity Services*, http://www.wales.nhs.uk/sites/home.cfm (accessed 03.08.05).

Williams, T., Wetton, N., Moon, A. (1989) *A Picture of Health. What Do You Think makes you Healthy?* London: Health Education Authority.

Williams, T., Wetton, N., Moon, A. (1989a) *A Way In. Five Key Areas of Health Education*. London: Health Education Authority.

World Health Organisation (1946) *Constitution*. Geneva: WHO.

World Health Organisation (1978) *Report on the International Conference on Primary Health Care, Alma Ata, 6–12 September*. Geneva: WHO.

World Health Organisation (1984) *Health Promotion: A WHO Discussion Document on the Concepts and Principles*. Geneva: WHO.

World Health Organisation (1985) *Targets for Health For All*. Geneva: World Health Organisation.

World Health Organisation (1986) *Ottawa Charter for Health Promotion: An International Conference on Health Promotion*. Geneva: WHO.

World Health Organisation (1993) *Health for All Targets the Health Policy for Europe, Updated Edition*. Copenhagen: WHO, Regional Office for Europe.

World Health Organisation (1998) *Health 21: An Introduction to the Health For All Policy Framework for the WHO European Region, European Health For All Series, No 5*. Copenhagen: WHO.

World Health Organisation (2000) *Obesity: Preventing and Managing the Global Epidemic, WHO Obesity Technical Report, Series 894*. Geneva: WHO.

World Health Organisation (2001) *The Optimal Duration of Exclusive Breastfeeding: Report on an Expert Consultation*. Geneva: WHO.

World Health Organisation (2003) *Health Environments for Children*, www.who.int/features/2003/04/en (accessed 07.01.05).

5 Safeguarding Children

Shirley Cutts

Learning outcomes

- Discuss the recognition of, categorisation of and appropriate response to each type of child abuse.
- Examine the legal framework, which underpins safeguarding children.
- Analyse the role and responsibilities of the nurse in safeguarding children.
- Analyse the knowledge base required by the nurse.
- Discuss the roles of the professionals who may be involved.
- Recognise risk factors, which can give cause for concern.

Introduction

Children are our future and safeguarding children is the responsibility of us all. What an obvious statement! It seems almost bizarre that living in a civilised and highly sophisticated society as we do that we should even have to make that statement, but the reality is that not all members of our civilised society regard children in this positive way. In this chapter you are going to have the opportunity to examine the concept of safeguarding children and how you can begin to meet your responsibilities as both a member of society and as a professional with the added responsibilities that go along with that. The four triggers will aid you in the recognition of abuse and to identify actions, which may be appropriate in the four, categories of child abuse, that is emotional, physical, sexual and neglect.

'Unfortunately, there is no absolute definition of abuse' Dartington Social Research Unit, 1999). In this chapter definitions for each type of abuse will be taken from the Department of Health (1999) to enable continuity.

As a professional with clear responsibility and accountability for safeguarding children it is important that you are aware of the strategies and information used in your own decision-making. Munro (2002) suggests that we make decisions in a number of ways and are reliant on different types of knowledge to inform the decisions that we make. This could be described as a decision-making continuum (see Figure 5.1).

Intuition ——————————————————————————— Formal knowledge

Figure 5.1   Decision-making continuum

In this chapter the intention is to encourage you to move along the continuum from reacting intuitively to information to using existing knowledge and gaining new knowledge to enable you to analyse a situation before coming to a conclusion. The outcome should be that you could present an objective and rational argument based on current available evidence which promotes the safety of the child.

! Trigger 5.1: Neglect

This trigger requires you to consider a case study, which describes two siblings admitted to the ward in an emergency. Department of Health (1999, p. 6) defined neglect thus,

> Neglect is the persistent failure to meet a child's basic physical and/or psychological needs, likely to result in the serious impairment of the child's health or development. It may involve a parent or carer failing to provide adequate food, shelter and clothing, failing to protect a child from physical harm or danger, or the failure to ensure access to appropriate medical care or treatment. It may also include neglect of, or unresponsiveness to, a child's basic emotional needs.

The signs of neglect in this case study are relatively easy to recognise, the intention is for you to consider the whole family, including a focus on parenting skills and capabilities.

The Trigger

Josh and Lauren Martin have been on your medical ward for seven days. Josh is aged 15 months and Lauren 5 years. They were originally admitted, as the Practice Nurse was concerned that Josh was displaying signs of a chest infection when he attended for his Mumps, Measles and Rubella vaccine. There was also some concern about the neglected state that the children were in, so both were admitted for observation.

On admission physical assessment revealed:

- both were slightly underweight for their age;
- both showed height below 50th centile;
- their skin was in a poor condition;
- both had severe head lice;

- Josh had a chest infection, temperature 38.5 degrees centigrade, pulse 118 beats per minute, respirations 20 per minute, with coryza and a cough; and
- both were wearing clothes that were too small, inappropriate for the weather, and in Josh's case for his gender (a Barbie t-shirt and trousers which had presumably been Lauren's originally).

Ms Martin arrived with the children but her visits during the seven days of their admission have been spasmodic and very brief. Staff have commented that her physical appearance was as neglected as the children's.

Social services have concerns regarding the welfare of both children should they return home. They have been working with Ms Martin since the birth of Lauren, arranging parenting classes, nursery places and ensuring appropriate financial support is received. Her attendance at classes is haphazard and her participation is minimal.

During their stay on the ward both children have gained weight and the head lice have been successfully treated, Josh's chest infection has responded well to treatment. Both are very co-operative with staff and like nothing better than a cuddle while they listen to a story or watch TV.

Both children are always pleased to see their Mum, but do not seem concerned when she leaves. The staff have noticed that Ms Martin shows very little interest in the children, she doesn't play with them or enquire about their progress, she hasn't commented on their improvements or asked when they can come home, in fact it is very difficult to engage her in conversation at all. One day she confides in the staff nurse that she feels that she can't cope any more and it would probably be best if the children were taken away from her.

A case conference is to take place before the children are discharged.

Situation

You have been involved in caring for the two children during their stay and have built up a good rapport with them and their mother.

You have been called to attend the case conference where a decision will be made to secure Josh and Lauren's long-term future. The ward staff has been asked to perform an assessment on the children to assist in the decision-making at the case conference.

Feedback

You have been asked to complete the initial assessment for discussion with a more senior member of staff. The document *Working Together to Safeguard Children* (Department of Health, 1999) provides an assessment framework in appendix one, which will help you in this task.

The facts

What are the main facts in this trigger? Make a list.

Hypotheses: What may these facts mean?

- It is better for Josh and Lauren to stay with their Mum.
- Ms Martin cannot cope with the children.
- Ms Martin is depressed.
- If her depression is treated then she will be able to cope.

Questions developed from the hypotheses

1. Is Ms Martin's care of the children 'good enough'?
2. What are the possible options available for the children?

Trigger 5.1: Fixed resource material

Read the following to help you answer the questions. (You may also wish to search and review other up-to-date research and evidence-based literature, and seek other relevant resources to provide you with the answers to your questions.)

Department of Health (1991) *The Children Act: An Introductory Guide for the NHS.* London: Department of Health.

Department of Health (1999) *Working Together to Safeguard* Children. London: The Stationary Office.

Howe, D. et al (1999) Attachment *Theory, Child Maltreatment and Family Support, A Practice and Assessment Model.* Basingstoke: Macmillan Press Ltd.

Smith, M. (2004) Parental mental health: Disruptions to parenting and outcomes for children, *Child and Family Social Work* 9, pp. 3–11.

Trigger 5.1: Fixed resource sessions

Risk factors associated with safeguarding children

In the scenario information is given which implied that Ms Martin might be suffering from depression, which may in turn be affecting her ability to care for her children. It is now widely recognised that there are a number of parental problems and behaviours, which can impact on their ability to care for their children. Professionals working with these families must be able to recognise if and when these risk factors exist and subsequently make a judgement as to whether the risk factor(s) is impacting on parenting capacity. Commonest risk factors are mental health problems, substance misuse and domestic violence. The presence of a risk factor does not necessarily mean that children are at risk. Parents can successfully care for their children when these risk factors are present, so care must be taken when assessing parenting capacity, that any risk factor is seen in context. Each family's situation must be looked at individually and appropriate help and support provided.

As previously suggested there are indications that Ms Martin may be suffering from depression, and this must be sensitively considered as part of the assessment process.

Assessing the situation

Assessing the whole situation is a complex and demanding process but one that is extremely important. As mentioned in the introduction a number of skills and a range of knowledge is required if the assessment is to be objective and informative. To help the process it can be useful to use a structured model, just like you would use a nursing model when assessing a patient in hospital. The Department of Health framework previously mentioned requires that a holistic approach be taken by requiring that aspects of child development, parenting capacity and environmental factors be considered (Department of Health 1999). (At the time of writing the United Kingdom government is advocating the development of a generic assessment framework to be used by all professionals involved).

As a nurse on an acute ward it will not be possible to consider all the elements, but you will have important information to contribute about many aspects.

→ Trigger 5.1: Feedback

Go to Chapter 5 Trigger feedback on p. 130

! Trigger 5.2: Emotional abuse

Emotional abuse can be difficult to recognise so read the following quote from the Department of Health (1999, p. 5), who define emotional abuse as

> the persistent emotional ill treatment of a child such as to cause severe and persistent adverse effects on the child's emotional development. It may involve conveying to children that they are worthless or unloved, inadequate, or valued only insofar as they met the needs of another person. It may feature age or developmentally inappropriate expectations being imposed on children. It may involve causing children frequently to feel frightened or in danger, or the exploitation or corruption of children. Some level of emotional abuse is involved in all types of ill treatment of a child.

The intention of this trigger is to help you to recognise emotional abuse.

The Trigger

Helen Cooper has arrived at the baby clinic with her daughter, Amy. Emily Dobson, the health visitor running the clinic is pleased to see them as they have been out on her last few visits to the home. Amy is now 15 months old, and on looking at the records, Emily realises with some shock that it is six months since she last saw Helen and Amy.

Emily's assessment of Amy is outlined in the notes below:

Posture and large movements	Can walk independently, quite steadily but cannot get to feet alone. Cannot pick up toys from floor.
Vision and fine movements	Pincer grip is well developed, can pick up small bead with no problem. Can hold crayon and scribble, when shown. Quickly lost interest in looking at a book, although did point when requested.
Hearing and speech	Makes very few sounds, did not respond at all to questions, and has no recognisable words. Mum says she does not attempt to say anything. Startles in response to loud noises.
Social behaviour Play	Sits quietly unless given a command. Shows in no interest in available toys and no curiosity regarding environment. When Helen left the room to go for a cigarette Amy remained sitting on the floor and showed no signs of distress or even interest.

When Helen got Amy ready to leave there was no talking or playing as Amy passively let Helen put on her coat and sit her in her buggy.

Situation

Helen Cooper has arrived at the baby clinic with her daughter, Amy. The health visitor running the clinic is your mentor,

Feedback

When you have completed the trigger you should develop an action plan with your mentor to assist Helen in recognising and meeting Amy's emotional needs.

The facts

What are the main facts in this trigger? Make a list:

Hypotheses: What may these facts mean?

- Helen understands how to meet Amy's physical needs.
- Helen does not appear to communicate with Amy.
- Amy does not appear to have formed an attachment to Helen.
- Helen might be meeting her own needs before Amy's.

Questions developed from the hypotheses

1. Why doesn't Helen talk to Amy?
2. Why wasn't Amy upset when Helen left the room?
3. What course of action should Emily take?

Trigger 5.2: Fixed resource material

Read the following to help you answer the questions. (You may also wish to search and review other up to date research and evidence-based literature, and seek other relevant resources to provide you with the answers to your questions.)

Bee, H., Boyd, D. (2004) *The Developing Child*, 10th edn. Boston: Allyn and Bacon.

Sheridan, M. (1997) *From Birth to Five Years: Children's Developmental Progess* (revised and updated by Frost, M., Sharma, A.). London: Routledge.

Smith, P. K., Cowie, H., Blades, M. (2003) *Understanding Children's Development*, 4th edn. Oxford: Blackwell Publishing. Chapter 4, Parents and Families. www. early-development-childhood.com

Trigger 5.2: Fixed resource sessions

The importance of emotional nurturing

If children are to grow into caring, supportive, responsible adults then meeting their emotional needs is crucial. It is the responsibility of parents to meet these needs. The Department of Health (1999) definition is clear regarding what it regards as emotional abuse. In practical terms none of us are perfect, and neither are children! If we reflect on our own attitudes with children and consider the behaviours we see everyday in the supermarket or on the street, we could identify many incidents of emotional abuse. The key word is 'persistent'. Many of us may say something or act in some way that could be interpreted as emotionally abusive but these are usually isolated situations, and would not be seen as persistent. In the scenario above there might be concern that the approach to Amy is persistent and ongoing. What we should remember is that the effects of emotional abuse are also long term. This is recognised by Department of Health (1999) in the same document (p.7).

The Role of the health visitor in safeguarding children

The role of the health visitor has grown and developed since its introduction in the early 20th century. At that time the focus was on hygiene in the home and the physical and material well being of the child, with work being focused on the poor.

Today, health visitors have a responsibility to monitor children's development and support parents in their parenting. This support includes planned assessment of children's developmental milestones, with a responsibility to identify developmental concerns and take appropriate action.

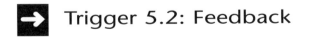 Trigger 5.2: Feedback

Go to Chapter 5 Trigger feedback on p. 130

! Trigger 5.3: Sexual abuse

For most of us sexual abuse is a topic that we do not feel comfortable thinking about, much less talking about and maybe having to become involved in. The Department of Health (1999, p. 6) states that,

> Sexual abuse involves forcing or enticing a child or young person to take part in sexual activities, whether or not the child is aware of what is happening. The activities may involve physical contact, including penetrative (e.g., rape or buggery) or non-penetrative acts. They may include non-contact activities, such as involving children in looking at, or in the production of, pornographic material or watching sexual activities, or encouraging children to behave in sexually inappropriate ways.

In this next scenario you are going to read about some very vague suggestions made by a 12 year old girl. These were made to a School Nurse, Julie Spencer.
Faller (2003, p. 4) recognised that

> school staff are first among professionals in the number of cases they report to child protection agencies (USDHHS, Children's Bureau, 1998). Cases are usually discovered when children reveal their abuse to persons they trust, often in school.

This trigger is intended to help you to recognise sexual abuse.

The Trigger

Julie Spencer is a School Nurse based in Uppertown Comprehensive School. Twice a week she holds a 'Trouble Shared' Clinic at lunch time. Today she was given some information which she will have to act on quickly. Claire Jones, form 7L, told Julie that she was having a hard time settling in to school. She could not make friends, all her friends from her old school had gone to Newtown, but as Uppertown had a Sixth Form her Mum and Dave (her Mum's boyfriend) wanted her to go there. Claire was upset, but she also became angry when she talked about Dave, saying things like 'It's none of his business, he's not my real Dad'. In her anger she also blurted out to Julie the information which worried her. Claire said 'He's not my Dad and he's not my boyfriend either, and if he carries on coming to my room when Mum's at work I'm going to tell her what he does'.

At this point Claire refused to say any more so Julie comforted her. They agreed that Claire would see Julie again in one week. Claire then insisted on going to mathematics as it was her favourite lesson and she thought she would do well in the quiz.

Situation

This young person obviously trusts Julie and you need to think about what Julie must do in the time between hearing the worrying information and when she meets with Claire again in one week's time.

Feedback

On completion of the trigger you should prepare information and an action plan which Julie may use at her next meeting with Claire.

The facts

> **What are the main facts in this trigger? Make a list:**

Hypotheses: What may these facts mean?

- Claire is unhappy at the moment as she appears to have no friends.
- Claire does not like Dave being involved in the decisions made about her future.
- Claire is angry with Dave.
- Claire is confused. She is unhappy at school but was happy to go back to lessons.
- Dave is 'doing something' which Claire does not like.
- Claire's Mum does not know what is happening at home.
- Claire's Mum does not know that Claire is unhappy at school.

Questions developed from the hypotheses

1. What should Julie do?
2. Why hasn't Claire made any friends at this school?
3. What is Dave doing to make Claire think he is acting like her boyfriend?
4. Is Dave doing anything?
5. Does Claire's Mum know?

Trigger 5.3: Fixed resource Material

Read the following to help you answer the questions. (You may also wish to search and review other up-to-date research and evidence-based literature, and seek other relevant resources to provide you with the answers to your questions.)

Bray, M. (1997) *Sexual Abuse: The Child's Voice: Poppies on the Rubbish Heap.* London: Jessica Kingsley.

Faller, K. C. (2003) *Understanding and assessing child sexual maltreatment*, 2nd edn. London: Sage.

Trigger 5.3: Fixed resource sessions

Recognising the impact of sexual abuse on a child's behaviour

Sexual abuse can result in effects on a child that last a lifetime. These effects can be minimised by early intervention and support. They can manifest themselves in many diverse ways including behavioural and emotional changes.

School nurses are ideally placed to recognise these changes as they have contact with children over a period of time and can get to know them and their families well.

Behavioural changes are many and varied and can include, a deterioration in school performance, withdrawal from peer group activities, apathy or inattention to what is happening, and falling asleep at inappropriate times. In younger children regression to a previous stage of development may also be seen as well as inappropriate sexual behaviour and language.

Emotional changes include mood swings, animosity towards friends and family and lack of interest in peer activities. Fairly normal teenage behaviour! The important thing is to build up a picture of *changes* in behaviour and to interpret them.

Communicating with children who have been sexually abused.

Children generally find it extremely difficult to disclose sexual abuse. When they do it is important that the person receiving the information acts sensitively and honestly. The listener must make it clear that disclosed information cannot be kept secret, in accordance with the Nursing and Midwifery Council Code of Professional Conduct (2004). This enables the child to be in control of whether they 'tell' or not, recognising that there will be consequences to any disclosure.

The listener must allow the child to disclose as much or as little as they are comfortable with, and must not fall into the trap of probing for more information. If the police become involved at a later stage such probing can taint any evidence gathered.

The listener must also accept that what is said is the truth. Any doubts or concerns regarding the legitimacy of the information disclosed must not be voiced to the child. These should be raised with the appropriate professional at a later date.

➜ Trigger 5.3: Feedback

Go to Chapter 5 Trigger feedback on p. 130

❗ Trigger 5.4: Physical abuse

Many children regularly suffer from physical harm which may be inflicted deliberately or accidentally.

The Department of Health (1999, p. 5) defines physical abuse in the following way:

Physical abuse may involve hitting, shaking, throwing, poisoning, burning or scalding, drowning, suffocating, or otherwise causing physical harm to a child. Physical harm may also be caused when a parent or carer feigns the symptoms of, or deliberately causes ill health to a child whom they are looking after. This situation is commonly described as Munchausen syndrome by proxy.

This trigger is intended to help you to recognise physical abuse.

The Trigger

A conversation between two Staff Nurses in the Accident and Emergency (A&E) Department.

Staff Nurse Brown:	Have you seen James in cubicle four? He's five and looks so cute in his school uniform . . . a cap as well! And he's been really brave.
Staff Nurse Green:-	What makes you say that?
Staff Nurse Brown:	Well I took him to X-ray and he never made a murmur when we positioned his arm. And he's let me do all his observations.
Staff Nurse Green:-	Oh! What's he done?
Staff Nurse Brown:	He said he fell off the swing playing before he went to school. He's got a fractured radius and ulna. His Mum's really upset, I bet he's being brave to make her feel better.
Staff Nurse Green:	Is his Mum the lady in the navy suit?
Staff Nurse Brown:	Yes that's her. She's had to miss work and she's a bit worried about it . . . I know she's been trying to phone James's Dad to see if he can come and take over.

Staff Nurse Green: Only I heard her on the phone earlier and thought she said that James had fallen off his bike.

Situation

The two Staff Nurses have gone for their break. James is waiting for Plaster of Paris to be applied to his injured arm. You are worried that the staff nurses will not pursue the inconsistencies between James' and his mum's stories. As a senior student nurse you feel that there are some issues which need some clarification.

Feedback

Write down your concerns, together with rationale, so that you can voice them to the two staff nurses when they return from their break.

The facts

> **What are the main facts in this trigger? Make a list:**

Hypotheses: What may these facts mean?

- James is too co-operative for a 5 year old boy.
- Either Mum or James is not telling the truth.
- Neither Mum nor James is telling the truth.
- The two staff nurses need more information.

Questions developed from the hypotheses.

1. Does it matter whether James fell off his bike or from the swing? He's still broken his arm.
2. Is it normal for a five year old to be so co-operative?

3. Is James's injury consistent with either of the stories told?

4. What should the two staff nurses do?

Trigger 5.4: Fixed resource material

Read the following to help you answer the questions. (You may also wish to search and review other up-to-date research and evidence-based literature, and seek other relevant resources to provide you with the answers to your questions.)

Bee, H., Boyd, D. (2004) *The Developing Child*, 10th edn. Boston: Allyn and Bacon.

Browne, K. (1995) Child abuse: Defining, understanding and intervening, in Wilson, K., James, A. T*he Child Protection Handbook*. London, Balliiere Tindall. Chapter 3, pp. 43–65.

Department of Health (1999) *Working Together to Safeguard Children*. London: The Stationary Office.

Trigger 5.4: Fixed resource sessions

The 'normal' five year old

Of course there is no such thing as a 'normal' five year old, or 'normal' child of any age. But when assessing a child, developmental milestones provide useful guidance.

The suggested reading should provide some of this information. This reading in addition to finding your own information should enable you to create some developmental parameters to assist in your assessment of James, using the clues in the given trigger to answer 'Question 2: Is it normal for a five year old to be so co-operative?'.

Causes for Concern

There are a number of causes for concern which you should be able to identify. Some involve James's behaviour and link with the previous fixed resource session, for example James's compliance with treatment.

The other major cause for concern is around the different explanations which have been given. Of course, it is inevitable that stories change during repeated telling, and this is more likely in stressful situations. What is important in this situation though is that James and his Mum have given different stories, it is not a change due to repetition. Therefore, this needs some clarification.

→ Trigger 5.4: Feedback

Go to Chapter 5 Trigger feedback on p. 130 below

? Chapter 5 Trigger feedback: What do you know?

Trigger 5.1: Neglect

Question 1: Is Ms Martin's care of the children 'good enough?

Defining what is 'good enough' care is difficult, but it is important that an objective assessment is performed. In order to perform an objective assessment *The Assessment Framework* (Department of Health 1999) will be used to provide a structure which will help us to think about the question objectively.

Let's start by considering Josh and Lauren's developmental needs, the following headings are given to guide the assessment:

Health: it is obvious that Ms Martin is not ensuring that the children remain healthy. Their physical condition is poor, they are both small for their age and their head lice has been left untreated for some time, suggesting that their nutrition and hygiene needs are not being met. It is also unclear whether Ms Martin recognised that Josh had a chest infection as it was the practice nurse who expressed concern. On the plus side Ms Martin had taken Josh for his immunisation.

Education: Josh is too young to have begun formal education and we have no information regarding Lauren's attendance at school. The school nurse and the teacher will be able to supply this information to inform the case conference. On the ward it would be useful if the nurses worked with the play specialists to determine whether the children are meeting their cognitive developmental milestones.

Emotional and behavioural development: there are a few clues regarding this which can be gained from the trigger, particularly about Josh and Lauren's emotional development. They are pleased to see their Mum which is encouraging as it suggests that the parent and child relationship is a positive one. But we should be concerned that the children do not respond negatively when Mum leaves. Howe et al (1999, p. 13) suggest that 'attachment behaviour is activated whenever young children feel distressed and insecure.' Josh and Lauren are not displaying the attachment behaviours first described by Bowlby (1984) as protest followed by despair followed by detachment. This acceptance of Mum's departures may suggest that their attachment to her is not strong, which has implications for their future emotional maturity and stability. Children need close relationships to give them the opportunity to learn about themselves and others.

These close relationships provide the foundation for their ability to build future relationships (Howe et al 1999).

Identity: again, a difficult area to be certain about with the information that we have, and this area has links with emotional security, so some knowledge of Bowlby's theory may be useful here.

However there are some points to think about. One way of portraying a sense of self is through dress. Admittedly both Josh and Lauren are too young to have much control over this, but Lauren will be aware of how her peers present themselves and that her clothes are different to theirs. We do know that on admission both were dressed in clothes that were too small which could suggest that Ms Martin takes no pride in how the children are presented, or cannot afford new clothing. It could also be argued that 'Barbie' clothes are inappropriate for a boy and are not helping him to develop a sense of male identity. As he has no constant male role model this could be particularly important. Of course the reasons for this may well be financial, but we do know that Ms Martin has had help to make sure she receives all her entitlements. Perhaps she is unable to manage her finances efficiently, or maybe she does not attach much importance to clothing, either the children's or her own.

Family and social relationships: the children do not appear to struggle to make social relationships, they have demonstrated this with the staff. We should consider how usual this is for children of their ages. At 15 months Josh should be wary of strangers but he seems to have developed relationships very quickly with staff which may raise questions about the strength of his attachment to his mother. Lauren will obviously have more regular contact with others, including her peers. It might be useful to observe her interactions with other children and parents as well as the staff.

Social presentation: this links in with the previous section and requires that you observe and make judgements about the children's adherence to cultural norms and values regarding behaviour. For example their use of communication, not just use of verbal language but also their understanding of 'rules', for example personal space and turn taking in a conversation. This would also have to be appropriate for their age.

Self-care skills: because of his age Josh's self-care abilities will be limited but what you can do is observe his feeding and whether he tries to feed himself. Also observe how he co-operates when being dressed, bathed, toileted etc. as this is where independence in these skills begins. Lauren should of course be quite independent, possibly requiring help with more complicated tasks like tying shoe laces.

An important point to note is whether they are too independent for their age and expected stage of development. For example does Lauren take on a 'mothering' role with Josh? If the answer is in the affirmative this could suggest that Ms Martin is not actually fulfilling her parenting responsibilities and Lauren is taking over. This again is also detrimental to her psychological development.

Parenting capacity: is possibly more difficult to assess on the ward but by observing Ms Martin with the children you can certainly add to the assessment which will be made by others, for example health visitor, social worker, teacher, school nurse. Understanding of attachment theory could be useful again in assessing this dimension as it encourages us to focus on the mother's responses to her children's basic cues.

Basic care: this dimension gives us something more concrete to focus on. You might comment on the children's appearance when they arrived on the ward and make comparisons with how their weight and appearance has changed while on the ward. You could also comment on Ms Martin's involvement in the children's care while they are with you.

Ensuring safety: again this might be difficult to judge during a hospital stay unless there are obvious breaches of safety such as leaving a cot side down or inadequate supervision during play. In Ms Martin's favour, she did take Josh for his immunisations suggesting that she is aware of more global safety issues.

Stimulation: when Ms Martin visits you could observe the type of play she encourages, or does entertainment involve simply having the TV on in the corner of the room and leaving the children to their own devices?

Guidance and bounds: this part of the assessment is concerned with identifying whether Ms Martin is able to ensure that the children learn what behaviour is accept-able and what is not. We have very few clues about this from the scenario, but your observations regarding their social presentation and social relationships should contribute to this section.

Emotional warmth and stability: are the other elements to be considered within the dimension of parenting capacity. Some of the observations which will help to assess this are included in other sections. Again, understanding of attachment theory and psychological development will assist you in identifying key areas for observation using the clues in the scenario.

The final element of the *Assessment Framework* (Department of Health 1999) is that of *Family and Environmental Factors*. This includes obtaining information regarding:

- Family history and functioning;
- Wider family;
- Housing;
- Employment;
- Income;
- Family's social integration; and
- Community resources.

On the ward it is inappropriate for you to gain information for this part of the assessment. Workers involved with the family in the community will be able to gather this. You do need to know that this information will be used to inform decisions made regarding the welfare and the safety of the children, and that you will be part of the decision-making process at the conference.

Question 2: What are the possible options available for the children?

The Children Act 1989 is clear that when any decisions are made they must be made in the best interest of the child, and that the welfare of the child is paramount. In this situation professionals have had long-standing involvement in supporting Ms Martin and have to decide what will be best, long term for the children.

The information gathered in the assessment as discussed above will be important in informing the decision, and your report will give another dimension, that is how Ms Martin copes in an acute emergency situation.

Another factor that is likely to be given consideration is Ms Martin's own health. One thing to think about is Ms Martin's appearance. Does it reflect that of the children i.e., neglected? Or is she always clean, smart, and well dressed? If it is the former then there should be concerns about her ability to look after herself, as well as the children, she may be depressed and unable to cope. If it is the latter it suggests that she cares for herself more than the children and may not have their best interests at heart.

A clue in the scenario is that she has disclosed that she feels unable to cope. This, coupled with her apparent disinterest (if not non-co-operation) with the support offered could also indicate some form of depression. According to Smith (2004) the association between parental mental health problems and negative outcomes for children has been long known, illustrating that this cannot be ignored and treatment is essential for the sake of her and the children.

So what are the options? Again the Children Act 1989 makes it clear that the best place for children is with the biological family. The support given to this family so far suggests that this has been adhered to. But what might force a different decision to be made?

If Ms Martin is suffering from depression then compliance with treatment for this may be a condition of the children remaining with her. If not, then it may be decided to remove the children as it could be seen that this in their best interests. This may not necessarily be a permanent solution. A short term placement, preferably with other family members, may give Ms Martin the opportunity to improve her ability to care for herself, ultimately leading to her caring for the children again. In accordance with the Children Act 1989, she would maintain contact with and responsibility for Josh and Lauren. Permanent removal of the children would be a last resort, only taken if it was felt that Ms Martin would not be able to parent them 'well enough' to ensure that all of their developmental needs are met.

Trigger 5.2: Emotional abuse

Question 1: Why doesn't Helen talk to Amy?

Emotional abuse is possibly the most difficult type of abuse to recognise and substantiate, but it is also potentially the most damaging (Department of Health 1999). Parents may unknowingly harm their child's emotional development, possibly through ignorance of child development and / or lack of understanding regarding their child's emotional needs. Of course there are also parents who deliberately harm their children through witholding affection. The aim of this discussion is to determine how we can attempt to differentiate between the two.

In this trigger we have identified that Amy's physical needs are being met. She is well nourished, clean and appropriately dressed and is achieving many of the developmental milestones for her age. It can be assumed then that Helen is able to recognise some of Amy's needs and how to met them. The more difficult task is to discover why Helen is apparently not recognising and therefore not meeting Amy's emotional needs. In the response to question 3 the assessment process will be discussed, but here we will take the opportunity to explore some possible reasons for why this can happen.

One possible explanation might lie in Helen's own experiences as a child, which according to socialisation theory, will contribute towards forming Helen's own skills as a parent. Perhaps Helen herself was raised in an emotionally 'cold' environment. The majority of us today learn our parenting skills from our own parents, although some may argue that we instinctively know how to be parents. What is evident from our trigger is that while we might know how to meet some needs we may not know how to meet them all. If as children we did not learn from our parents how to express emotions positively, then we may find it difficult to do so ourselves as parents. If this is the case, then Helen's omission is through ignorance rather than a deliberate attempt to deny Amy affection. Emily, therefore, needs to have some detailed discussions with Helen to determine the facts.

Of course it could be that Helen uses emotional distance as a form of discipline. She may believe that denying warmth will result in Amy developing into a strong, capable, independent adult, which of course it may. But we should also remember that 'emotional abuse has an important impact on a developing child's mental health, behaviour and self-esteem. It can be especially damaging in infancy' (Department of Health 1999, p. 7). This statement should leave us in no doubt that Emily has to discover the origins of the lack of warmth from Helen to Amy in order to protect Amy from further harm.

A third possibility may be that Helen believes that she is doing her duty as mother by meeting Amy's physical needs and by providing an environment which meets her physical needs. Howe et al (1999) suggest that mother's who ignore their children's signals tend to be absorbed in their own pursuits, an aspect that may be worthy of further investigation.

The final cause for lack of warmth could be Helen does not feel any attachment to Amy. This may be through lack of bonding following birth or to other difficulties that Helen may be experiencing in her own life and relationships.

It is clear that Emily has a complicated task ahead of her which will be discussed in response to question three.

Question 2: Why wasn't Amy upset when Helen left the room?

To begin to answer this question we need to look at attachment theories as we did for the previous trigger. Bowlby was the first psychologist to identify both the importance of mother and child attachment and the consequences of the attachment not being formed. Smith et al (2003) provide us with an overview of attachment relationships which will help us towards some understanding of the mother and child relationship, and the development of attachment. Howe et al (1999, p. 24) also provide an explanation of how children respond to 'parents who are insensitive, rejecting, interfering or emotionally unavailable present their children with a psychological problem', which is worth further reading.

According to Howe et al (1999, p. 10),

> Attachment behaviour brings infants into close proximity to their main carers. It is within these close relationships that children learn about themselves, other people and social life in general. Young children interact with their parents and other family members and, in so doing, develop an understanding of both themselves and other people.

This rather lengthy statement should leave us in no doubt of the importance of Emily intervening to encourage Helen to interact socially with Amy.

Question 3: What course of action should Emily take?

Emily has to inform Helen of her concerns regarding Amy's lack of emotional response so that they can together develop a plan that will enable Helen to support Amy and facilitate her development.

Her discussion with Helen will need to be tactfully managed requiring excellent communication and interpersonal skills and have a fairly structured format. The environment in which the assessment takes place is crucial as Emily needs to be able to build up an accurate picture of what is happening within this family. This will ensure that she is able to initiate appropriate actions that are supportive rather than punitive for Helen and protective and stimulating for Amy. Ideally then an appointment should be made for Emily to visit Helen and Amy at home. This should ensure that Helen feels relaxed and comfortable and, therefore, not threatened, and it will give Emily the opportunity to observe Amy in a familiar environment which will add to her understanding of Amy's development.

The Department of Health's (1999) Assessment Framework was used in Trigger 5.1 to assist in the assessment of that situation. It will also be a useful tool for Emily to use in this situation. The first of the three elements of the assessment is the child's development, which in this trigger has been the starting point of Emily's concern. The second element is parenting capacity, potentially a very sensitive area of discussion and Emily will need to be aware of the importance of recognising Helen's strengths as a parent, as well identifying her weaknesses. The final element is that of family and environmental factors. Conducting the interview at home will allow Emily the opportunity to observe how appropriate their home is to foster Amy's development. Emily could observe whether there are age appropriate toys available, whether they are tidied away and if Amy is encouraged to play with them. Enquiries could be made asking if Amy has her own room and how much time she spends there.

Munro (2002) also identifies a framework that can assist in the assessment of a situation, (pp. 84–91), and highlights the complexities of these situations. This framework looks at the professionals' use of knowledge in assessing a situation. In these situations it would be expected that Emily would use formal knowledge rather than intuitive knowledge to make an objective, professional assessment.

It is clear that Emily has a responsibility to act and to ensure that Amy is protected from the long term effects of emotional abuse. Ideally she will do this with the co-operation of Helen and other family members who may be available to help.

Helen has to recognise that Amy has emotional needs and needs to be shown love and warmth and she also needs to make a commitment to provide this. Emily can support her in this by making use of services which may be available in their area, for example Sure Start, mother and toddler groups or a neighbourhood nursery. By working together, Emily and Helen should be able to enable Amy to develop the confidence and happiness which stems from secure attachment.

Trigger 5.3: Sexual abuse

As discussed previously Julie the nurse has a responsibility to act on information that leads her to be concerned that a child's safety might be threatened. The discussions around the issues raised by the questions are what Julie will need to have before she meets again with Claire and subsequently decides what the most appropriate course of action might be.

Question 1: What should Julie do?

The responses to this question begin before Claire returns to her mathematics lesson. They also focus on what Julie must not do.

Before Claire returns to her lesson she needs to be clear that 'doing nothing' is not an option for Julie. Julie must be honest with Claire about this and must not promise to keep this information secret. Ideally Julie would have had the opportunity to clarify this before Claire spoke any further thus leaving Claire in control of what and how much information she gave Julie. Unfortunately conversations rarely conform to a given script and information. That which is difficult to say, is often disclosed before ground rules can be established. Julie must also convince Claire that it is *she*, *Claire*, who is important and not the suspected abuse. As Fitzgerald (1991, p. 47) states it is essential that 'children and young people are seen as such, first and foremost, and that where sexual abuse has occurred it is but one part, albeit a very significant part of their lives'. Perhaps this is illustrated by Claire's eagerness to return to her mathematics lesson once she has disclosed what was troubling her.

Julie therefore, needs to be honest and open with Claire about what she will be doing before they meet again, and hope that Claire will keep the appointment. While Julie might feel uncomfortable about Claire going home, her suspicions that something potentially harmful is happening are *only* suspicions, and these suspicions are based on one small sentence uttered by Claire which was 'and he's not my boyfriend either. And if he carries on coming to my room when Mum's at work I'm going to tell her what he does.' The implication of course is that Dave is behaving inappropriately toward Claire, certainly as far as Claire is concerned. He *appears* to be acting as her boyfriend when he should in fact be acting more as a surrogate father.

First of all Julie must make a record of her concerns. Laming (2003, p. 379) recommended that 'when concerns about the deliberate harm of a child have been raised, a record must be kept in the case notes of all discussions about the child, including telephone conversations.' Julie then needs to speak to Claire's form teacher. It is important that at this stage Julie finds out more about Claire, her friendships and her behaviour. Her form teacher should have knowledge regarding all of this and about whether Claire's behaviour has changed. The teacher has an important role to play, both in providing information regarding Claire's behaviour and school performance and in supporting Claire in the long term. See Dent (1991) for more detailed discussion regarding the role of the teacher.

Claire implied in her conversation with Julie that Dave went to her room when her Mum was at work. Anticipating his visits may, therefore, affect Claire's ability to sleep. For many children their bedroom is their 'safe place', they keep their private and secret things in there and can usually escape the pressures of school, parents, etc. In this situation it might be that this safety is being violated. If Dave is entering her room uninvited and performing acts with which she is uncomfortable then she is likely to be feeling very vulnerable and probably unable to relax and subsequently fall asleep. She now has no 'safe place'. This impact on her sleep pattern is likely to affect her behaviour and her performance at school. If she is unable to relax because she can't get Dave's behaviours out of her mind then she will find it difficult to respond naturally to her peers and they might interpret this as her being 'stand-offish' and, therefore, begin to isolate her. In a worst case scenario they may also begin to bully her. Claire's teacher will be able to give Julie information regarding Claire's academic performance and her levels of concentration in class. She may even have fallen asleep on occasions!

Question 2: Why hasn't Claire made any friends at this school?

There are lots of possible explanations to this question, and we must begin by recognising that for someone of Claire's age their peer group is extremely important. In many ways more important than parents, especially regarding developing a positive self-image and high self-esteem. It could be argued that if a child has received positive and stable parenting in the early years, enabling the development of a positive self-image, then this will enable them to continue in this positive way in adolescence. We need to acknowledge that for many young people adolescence is a turbulent time of physical, emotional and structural changes. Claire has been separated from her familiar peer group, and although she may have opportunities to meet with them outside school, the school day is long and she needs to have positive social contact during lessons and break times.

Initiating this contact and making new friends is not always easy. Friendship groups may already be established from previous schools and becoming part of these requires confidence and for want of a better word, courage. If Claire is being sexually abused then it is likely that this will have psychological consequences (Johnson 2004), which in turn are likely to affect her behaviour and her ability to interact with her peers. If Claire is unhappy, confused or angry about events at home she may find that her confidence is low and her courage is lacking. This is turn may affect her ability to respond naturally to her peers and they might interpret this as her being 'stand-offish' and, therefore, begin to isolate her. In a worst case scenario they may also begin to bully her. There are a number of texts which provide information and analyses on the psychological impact of sexual abuse. See Hoier et al (1992) for an analysis of the impact of sexual abuse and Lipovsky and Kilpatrick (1992) who provide an interesting analysis of the long-term effects of child sexual abuse.

Question 3: What is Dave doing to make Claire suggest that he is acting like her boyfriend?

In a sense the only people that this information is important to are Claire and Dave. Julie certainly does not need to know. Julie will have to decide what action to take, if any, based upon the information gained through answering the previous questions. For those who will support Claire it is the impact on her behaviour and her psychological well being that it is important, and how that can be managed in the long term.

If Claire does disclose to Julie the nature of any abuse which may be taking place, then Julie must immediately inform social services who in turn may have to inform the police (See Department of Health 2003, *What To Do If You're Worried A Child Is Being Abused*, for details of the referral process). Julie should not be tempted to probe for information as this may taint the evidence gathering process if the police are involved and intend to pursue a criminal prosecution.

Question 4: Is Dave doing anything?

As with the discussion regarding the previous question this is not for Julie to find out. It is Julie's responsibility to make a judgement based on what Claire has said and the results of her investigations. The need for this judgement has been initiated by Claire due to information disclosed during a confidential consultation. Claire has been informed that Julie has a responsibility to act, and is aware that Julie will be seeking out information. Claire can do nothing to stop that happening, nor can she influence the teacher's judgements. Claire can, however, decide how much more she is willing to disclose. If she attends the planned meeting with Julie, Julie should inform her of what is happening and what will happen next. If the decision is to contact social services then Mrs Jones (Claire's mother) will also be informed. If it is decided that no further action is needed, perhaps Claire confesses that Dave merely sits on her bed but she does not like it and has not given him permission to do so, then it will be agreed with Claire how to make sure that Dave changes his behaviour and whether her mother is informed or not.

Trigger 5.4: Physical abuse

Question 1: Does it matter whether James fell off his bike or from the swing? He's still broken his arm.

What a good question, and a complicated one. With regards to the injury sustained then it doesn't really matter as the treatment will be the same and his arm will heal in a few weeks.

The more complicated questions we need to ask are around why Mum and James have given different accounts of how the injury has occurred. We would always begin with the assumption that the majority of parents care for their children and want the best for them, but we must also remember that in the year 2000 the names of more than 34,000 children were put on the child protection registers in England (National Society for Prevention of Cruelty to Children 2000.) So what we need to think about is why their stories are different, and possibly most importantly, what really happened?

So why might their stories be different? One explanation is that Mum might be confused. She is in a stressful situation for a number of reasons. She is late for work and we have evidence that this appears to be worrying her from the staff nurse's report of her overheard phone call. To us this may not seem to be a priority at the moment, but we should try to remember that James's injury is one acute episode in this family's life while work is an ongoing obligation. We do not know what kind of work Mum does, and it does not really matter, but it is obviously important as it seems to be taking priority over James's needs at the moment. Neither do we know her motives for going to work, they may be financial, she may be pursuing a professional career or they may be social. Our concern at this moment should be the impact that Mum's work is having on the care that James is receiving, both in hospital and at home. Having children is a big responsibility and parents have responsibility for ensuring their children's safety (see Hendrick, 1993, for an explanation of the scope of parental responsibility). If we suspect that James's safety has been compromised then we have a professional duty to act.

So what explanations might there be for Mum changing her story? Well, she might not have seen what happened if she was busy with her preparations for work and school, so she might have made up a story rather than admit the truth. Or a more sinister explanation might be that yes, James had gone outside to play . . . and refused to come in when shouted . . . Mum goes out to fetch him in . . . pulls him off the swing/off his bike . . . he falls awkwardly . . . his arm is broken. Rather than admit this, Mum thinks she can make life easier for herself and so makes up a story. Unfortunately James has made up a different story. An even more sinister version might be something like James was being slow in getting ready for school . . . Mum shouts at him to hurry up . . . this makes him anxious and clumsy . . . he drops something . . . it breaks . . . Mum grabs his arm and swings him round . . . she lets go . . . he falls awkwardly . . . his arm is broken.

At this point we do not want to make judgements about parenting skills and attitudes, but we do need to be sure that James will be safe.

Question 2: Is it normal for a five year old to be so co-operative?

The instinctive response to this question is 'No, most five year olds will object to and probably refuse treatment and investigations.' This can be so for a number of reasons. The majority will be frightened and almost certainly in pain. Let us begin to examine possible explanations for James's co-operative behaviour using a range of developmental theorists to inform our debate.

As far as his gross motor development is concerned, James is apparently a physically active little boy. We know this because he seemed to be outside playing when his injury occurred, either on his bike or on the swing, depending upon which story is correct. This would be acceptable as being within the range of 'normal' activities for a five year old. Active and vigorous play is beneficial and important for health and well being, and it would not be unusual for a boy of James's age to be more interested in being outside playing than co-operating in getting ready for school. Presumably physical observations within the A&E department would also support these observations. With regard to cognitive development he would be classified as being in Piaget's pre-operational stage, which means that James's will have started to internally represent objects by the use of images or words. However these internal representations are not yet organised in a coherent manner.

With regard to his social development it appears that he is an articulate little boy, he's persuaded Staff Nurse Brown that he's cute and brave. This seems to be largely due to his behaviour rather than his actual communication ability, but presumably there has been some dialogue between them. But it was James's behaviour that raised this question. We have ascertained that the very active behaviour which is being seen as the cause of his injury is not out of the ordinary but we have some questions about the 'normality' of his co-operation with the investigations. First of all he has to cope with a completely alien environment, or does he? One possible explanation for his co-operation might be that the environment might *not* be alien, but may be quite familiar. If he has attended this hospital before then this will quickly become apparent as his notes are seen, but he may not have. This will be discussed further when answering question 4, and is an important point to remember. Also, let us look at what we know about James. He attends school. He wears a uniform, which includes wearing a cap. These two facts give us quite a lot of information and can help us make some deductions. All five year olds in the United Kingdom should attend school. Many schools have a uniform. Not many school uniforms include a cap, especially for five year olds. It would, therefore, be reasonable to assume that James attends a private school, which may have implications regarding his social development. Class sizes at his school may be lower than those in state schools, meaning that support and attention from the teacher gives children confidence in their own abilities and in the world around them. This in turn may mean that while in an alien environment James is confident and sure that all around are doing their best for him. You might have questions around the nature of discipline in the school but we could assume that if his parents are happy to keep him in the school, then they are confident that James is safe in the school.

Browne (1995) identified that there are five important aspects to consider when assessing violent parent and child relationships. Although, at the moment, we have no reason to believe that this is a violent relationship, these factors below may help us to organise our thoughts as we assess the situation.

1. Caretakers knowledge and attitudes towards child rearing: In a situation like this, an emergency when you have no prior knowledge of the family, attitudes can be difficult to assess. You have to utilise a range of interpersonal skills to build up a relationship with this family which may be difficult in this anxious situation in a pressurised environment. You also need to utilise your theoretical knowledge and understanding of parent and child relationships and child development. Munro's decision-making continuum, previously described, is a useful tool here (Munro 2002). All nursing decisions should err towards the formal analytical end of the continuum and it is particularly important in child protection situations that we assess situations objectively. It is important in this situation that staff are honest and open with mum and give her the opportunity to talk about what has happened in a safe and open environment. We will discuss this further when answering the question 'what should the two staff nurses do'?

2. Parental perceptions of the child's behaviour: Parents who have little or no understanding of children's development may have unrealistic expectations of how they should behave, (previously mentioned in Trigger 5.2), and perhaps expect them to behave like adults. This in turn can lead some parents to believe that the child is being deliberately difficult and may lead to them punishing the child inappropriately. It is appropriate at this point to take time to consider some aspects of child development in order for us try to understand James's behaviour before discovering his mum's perceptions.

At five years old we would expect James to be physically active, keen to explore and have little understanding of the anxiety his mum may feel during the morning rush of preparation for work and school (the suggested fixed resource reading should help here). Mum's anxiety will only be important in terms of how it affects James. His desire to be outside playing rather than concentrating on breakfast and packing his school bag is 'normal', even if sometimes difficult for an adult to understand.

If we refer back to the trigger we also have some clues about James's social development. We know that he was co-operative in X-ray. We know that he can communicate effectively. We need to consider these points in with reference to child development theories. Attachment theory may help us to examine the nature of James' co-operation. Bee and Boyd (2004) describe a number of experiments designed to assess the links between a child's behaviour and the strength of attachment with the mother. A child who is securely attached is confident in strange situations and is easily consoled when threatened or frightened. James may be in a strange situation, but he has been co-operative. Does this, therefore, mean that he has a strong attachment with his mother? Can we, therefore, conclude that she is caring and supportive towards her son, and that consequently this is purely an accident where she has simply got confused in the retelling of the story? However, this strange situation is also frightening, and James is in pain, but he does not appear to have asked for comfort from his Mum. We have no indication that she accompanied him to X-ray, and we know that she has spent time outside the department on her mobile phone, presumably trying to keep work and father informed. We also know that she wants father to take over support for James in the department. Do these actions seem typical of a caring and supportive mother? Perhaps we also need to think about behaviours demonstrating no preference for mother when with a stranger. This explanation may fit with certain elements of James's co-operative behaviour, for example we have no evidence that he asked for his Mum and he appears to have been happy to talk to the nurses. We cannot make judgements at this point but it is clear that more information is needed.

Remember that it is his mother's perception of this 'normal' behaviour that we need to discover, but we need to use our own knowledge of children and development if we are to be objective and analytical. If mum recognises that he is not being awkward or difficult, then we might be reassured that this incident was an unfortunate accident. However, if we are not reassured that his is the case and have concerns that mum does not understand 'normal' behaviour, then more questions may have to be asked. Again this will be discussed further in the response to question 4.

3. Parental emotions and responses to stress: Not the easiest thing to assess objectively in an accident and emergency department. Parents are usually anxious at this time. They may be feeling a range of confusing emotions: worry, anxiety, fear, guilt to name but a few. Mum obviously has a lot on her mind, for example James, work, and his father. Maybe thinking about how she appears to have prioritised these elements may help us in assessing her response to this situation and it might be useful to sit down with her to discuss the situation. She is obviously worried about missing work and needs some support from James's Dad, and is maybe finding James a bit of a handful according to the information we have in the trigger.

4. Parental and child interactions and behaviour: These are obviously going to be affected by the alien environment. From the conversation in the trigger it is not clear whether Mum accompanied James to X-ray. Or maybe this was when she was overheard talking to Dad. Again it is important to consider child development theory and whether it would be reasonable to expect the mother of 5 year old to accompany him. Also, is it usual for a 5 year old to be quite so co-operative?

5. Quality of child and parent attachment: Perhaps in one sense this **is** the hardest *judgement* to make, as it appears to be a largely subjective assessment of something almost immeasurable in a very stressful situation. But in another way it is a judgement made after making an assessment of the other four factors and identifying the key issues from each.

It is becoming clear that some objective assessment of this family will have to be made. There is some doubt about the cause of the accident and, therefore, some doubt about Mum's supervision of James. The initial assessment of the above factors will not be decisive in it but will inform any future discussions and decisions.

The most important thing that you and other nursing staff can do is communicate with James and his Mum, and Dad if he arrives, to take over from Mum. You will need to observe their interactions and how they communicate with each other, and then document objectively your observations. You will need to give them all the opportunity to discuss the incident but without making any judgements about their abilities or the situation.

Question 3: Is James's injury consistent with either of the stories told?

During his stay in the accident and emergency department James will undergo a number of investigations to both confirm his injury and assess his physiological status. His treatment will be determined by the results of both.

The most important factors in determining his injury are the account of how it happened and the X-Ray. We have discussed at length the implications of the different stories, which have been told, but have not thought, about the nature of the injury. While an X-Ray cannot either confirm or deny the story it can indicate whether the fracture sustained is consistent with an accident of the kind stated. If it is then the staff are totally reliant on their communications with mum and James to discover the truth. They may never receive what they believe to be the truth.

On the other hand, the radiologist may feel that it is unlikely that the fracture shown on the X-Ray could have been caused by either of the accidents described by James or his Mum. In this situation then further discussion needs to take place with Mum and she has to make aware of the concerns the staff have.

Within the Hospital Trust there will be a nurse with responsibility for Child Protection. It would be appropriate for the two staff nurses to seek her advice.

Question 4: What should the two staff nurses do?

The most important thing is, they have to do something.

Initially one of them should sit down somewhere quiet and private and talk to Mum. Their concerns should be clearly expressed and Mum should be given the opportunity to explain the discrepancies in the two accounts. This conversation should be recorded in James's notes in accordance with recommendations from Lord Laming in the Climbié Enquiry (Laming, 2003). The Department of Health have also published guidelines, which would be useful for the two nurses to follow in this situation. The document is called *What to do if You're Worried a Child is Being Abused*. The guidelines clearly state that practitioners should discuss concerns with parents and the child in language appropriate to their age and understanding (Department of Health 2003). If the nurses are happy with the explanations and the situation at this point then no further action needs to be taken.

If the nurses are not satisfied, then they need to discuss their concerns with either the named nurse for child protection or with their manager. Again, this discussion should be recorded in James's notes. Mum and James should also be informed of the concerns and that this discussion is taking place. Again it might be decided at this point that no further action needs to be taken.

Alternatively the manager may agree that there is cause for concern and it might be decided to check with Social Services as to whether James's name is on the Child Protection Register. If the answer is affirmative then this demonstrates that there have already been concerns for his safety and, therefore, Social Services need to be informed of the current concerns.

If the answer is negative then it does not mean that there is no cause for concern. It could be that there is no previous history. Or there might be a history of concern but which has not been serious enough to require his name to be placed on the Register. Should this be the case then the staff are largely reliant on Mum being honest regarding the history.

If the staff have concerns about James's safety at home then they should make a referral to Social Services. If referred by telephone, confirmation should be made in writing within 48 hours and an acknowledgement should be received from social services within three working days (Department of Health 2003). An investigation will be initiated within seven days of the referral.

It is important that Mum and James are kept informed of everything that is happening and are reassured that all actions taken are the best interest of James, and ultimately the family.

Reflect on your learning

- Recognising child abuse requires excellent observation skills.
- Knowledge and understanding of anatomy and physiology, psychology, sociology and the legal framework is essential to inform and support observations.
- A sensitive approach and response is required by all involved in the process.
- It might be easier 'not to see' something – this is not an option. Children deserve your support and intervention when necessary.

References

Baker, C. D. (2002) *Female Survivors of Sexual Abuse*. Hove: Brunner Routledge.
Bee, H., Boyd, D. (2004) *The Developing Child*, 10th edn. Boston: Allyn and Bacon.
Bowlby, J. (1984) *Attachment and Loss, vol 1*, 2nd edn. Harmondsworth: Penguin.
Bray, M. (1997) *Sexual Abuse: The Child's Perspective: Poppies on the Rubbish Heap*. London: Jessica Kingsley.

Browne, K. (1995) Child abuse: Defining, understanding and intervening, in Wilson, K., James, A. *The Child Protection Handbook*. London, Balliere Tindall. Chapter 3, pp. 43–65.

Dartington Social research Fund (1999) *Child Protection Messages from Research*. London: HMSO.

Dent, R. J. (1991) Support from the educational services, in Balty, D., (ed) *Sexually Abused Children*. London: British Agencies for Adoption and Fostering.

Department of Health (1991) *The Children Act, An Introductory Guide for the NHS*. London: HMSO.

Department of Health (1999) *Working Together to Safeguard Children*. London: The Stationary Office.

Department of Health (2003) *What to Do if You're Worried a Child is Being Abused*. London: The Stationary Office.

Faller, K. C. (2003) *Understanding and Assessing Child Sexual maltreatment*, 2nd edn. London: Sage.

Fitzgerald, J. (1991) Working with children who have been sexually abused, in Balty, D., (ed) *Sexually Abused Children*. London: British Agencies for Adoption and Fostering.

Goldberg, S. (2000) *Attachment and Development*. London: Arnold.

Hendrick, J. (1993) *Child Care Law for Health Professionals*. Oxford: Radcliffe Medical Press.

Hoier, T. S., Shawchuck, C. R., Pallotta, G. M., Freeman, T., Inderbitzen-Pisaruk, H., MacMillan, V. M., Malinosky-Rummell, R., Greene, A. L. (1992) The impact of sexual abuse: A cognitive-behavioral model, in O'Donahue, W. Geer, J. H. (eds) *The Sexual Abuse of Children: Clinical Issues*, vol 2. New Jersey: Lawrence Erlbaum Associates.

Holmes, J. (1993) *John Bowlby and Attachment Theory*. London: Routledge.

Howe, D., Brandon, M., Hinnings, D., Schofield, G. (1999) *Attachment Theory, Child Maltreatment and Family Support, A Practice and Assessment Model*. Basingstoke: Macmillan Press.

Johnson, C. F. (2004) Child Sexual Abuse. *The Lancet* 364, pp. 462–70.

Laming, L. (2003) *The Victoria Climbié Inquiry*. London: HMSO.

Lipovsky, J. A. and Kilpatrick, D. G. (1992) The child sexual abuse victim as an adult, in O'Donahue, W., Geer, J. H. (eds) *The Sexual Abuse of Children: Clinical Issues*. vol 2. New Jersey: Lawrence Erlbaum Associates.

Munro, E. (2002) *Effective Child Protection*. Sage Publications.

NSPCC (2000) *Child Maltreatment in the United Kingdom: A study of the Prevalence of Child Abuse and Neglect*. London: NSPCC.

Nursing and Midwifery Council (2004) *Code of Professional Conduct*. London: NMC.

Parton, N., Wattam, C. (eds) (1999) *Child Sexual Abuse: Responding to the Experiences of Children*. Chichester: John Wiley and Sons Ltd.

Sheridan, M. (1997) From Birth to Five Years: Children's Developmental Progess (revised and updated by Frost, M., Sharma, A.). London: Routledge.

Smith, G. (1995) *The Protectors Handbook*. London: The Women's Press Ltd.

Smith, M. (2004) Parental mental health: Disruptions to parenting and outcomes for children, *Child and Family Social Work*, 9, pp. 3–11.

Smith, P. K., Cowie, H., Blades, M. (2003) *Understanding Children's Development*, 4th edn. Oxford: Blackwell Publishing.

6

Ambulatory Care
Lynda Smith

Learning outcomes

- Discuss the development of ambulatory services within health service provision for children and their families.
- Discuss the management of care within the resuscitation area of an Accident and Emergency department (A&E).
- Discuss the assessment and nursing management of minor injuries within an Accident and Emergency department.
- Discuss with rationale the pre-operative and post operative care of children undergoing day surgery.
- Analyse the role of parents in ambulatory settings.

Introduction

This chapter focuses on the provision of ambulatory care for children and families. The triggers within the chapter will facilitate the development of knowledge and understanding of specific aspects of care management and delivery within a range of ambulatory care settings.

The concept of ambulatory care in the United Kingdom is a growing one as services are developed to meet both healthcare policy and the particular needs of the child and family. Ambulatory care has its roots in the United States in the 1960s and is geared towards the needs of the child who does not require admission to hospital (Heller 1994). This is reflected in the various definitions of ambulatory care:

> Any treatment or nursing intervention that does not take place during an overnight stay. (Turner 1998, p. 12)

> Health services provided on an outpatient basis to those who visit a hospital or clinic and depart after treatment on the same day. (Mosby 1995)

Heller (1994) offers a comprehensive view that not only does ambulatory paediatrics refers to the care of children who do not require admission to hospital as inpatients but includes children seen in primary care and community paediatric settings as well as in hospital, in accident and emergency or in outpatients and those looked after in their own homes.

The relevance of ambulatory care within health care provision can be seen in the recent publication by the Department of Health as part of the NHS Plan (Department of Health 2000). The *National Service Framework for Children* in its standard for 'hospital services; ambulatory care' describes a combination of, a defined acute assessment area or beds, capacity to respond to General Practitioner (G.P.) rapid referral and close collaboration with A&E services (Department of Health 2003).

The focus of this chapter in terms of ambulatory care provision will be the provision of secondary care services with links to primary care to facilitate a seamless approach to care for children and their families.

! Trigger 6.1: Journey through Day Care

The intention of this trigger is to explore the process of safe preparation and recovery of children undergoing surgery.

The Trigger

Hallam Hospital NHS Trust

Child Health Services
Silversmith Road
Steel
S45 5ND

0112 345678

Date as postmark

Dear Mrs Lewis

Re: Daniel Lewis D.O.B. 15/10/01: Consultant Mr Smith Operation: Bilateral myringotomy/Insertion of grommets

Daniel's day surgery has been arranged for Monday 11th November 2004. Please bring Daniel to Disney Day Care Ward on Floor B at 7.30 am in the morning. You will need to bring a sample of Daniel's urine with you. He should not have anything to eat after 12 midnight Sunday. A clear fluid drink can be taken up to 5 a.m.

If you have any queries please contact me on the above telephone number or the staff on Disney ward

Yours sincerely

L Jones
Admissions

Situation

The Day Care Ward at Hallam NHS Trust provides both medical and surgical day care to children. A variety of medical and surgical care management is carried out involving a wide range of staff from within the multidisciplinary team. Nursing care is individualised to each child and family's needs and nursing staff are supported in this by the play therapist and healthcare assistants. Nursing staff on Disney ward are afforded every opportunity to ensure care is evidence based and responsive to ongoing change within healthcare and service provision.

Daniel Lewis is three years old and has had persistent otitis media with effusion. As his referral letter indicates he is to be admitted to the ward for bilateral myringotomy and insertion of grommets. He is accompanied by his mother and his father will arrive later to take them home. Daniel is an only child.

Feedback

As a result of your analysis of Daniel and his family's care needs, select one aspect of care and present the evidence base to practice for it in the form of a summary of the evidence. Guidance and an example of this type of format is included in the feedback section. This could form the basis of a presentation at a journal club or similar meeting where evidence and the implications for practice development are discussed, thus maintaining up to date clinical practice.

The facts

What are the main facts in this trigger? Make a list:

Hypotheses: What may these facts mean?

- Daniel has a recurrent problem that may have implications for his growth and development.
- Day care surgery may be of benefit to children and their families.
- Surgery requires specific care management pre-operatively and post operatively.

Questions developed from the hypotheses

1. Why does Daniel need surgery?
2. What support will Daniel and his family need for planned day-case surgery?
3. What is the rationale for Daniel's pre-operative care?
4. What is the rationale for Daniel's post-operative care?

Trigger 6.1: Fixed resource material

Read the following to help you answer the questions. (You may also wish to search and review other up-to-date research and evidence-based literature, and seek other relevant resources to provide you with the answers to your questions.)

Action for Sick Children (2004) *Meeting the Needs of Children and Young People Undergoing Surgery*. London: Action for Sick Children.
Campbell, S., Glasper, A. E. (1995) *Whaley and Wong's Children's Nursing*. London: Mosby, pp. 529–32.
Huband, S., Trigg, E. (2000) *Practices in Children's Nursing*. Edinburgh: Churchill Livingstone, chapters 27 and 28.
Smith, F. (1995) *Children's Nursing in Practice: The Nottingham Model*. Oxford: Blackwell Science.
www.doh.gov.uk/daysurgery
www.rcn.org.uk

Trigger 6.1: Fixed resource sessions

Otitis Media in children

Otitis media is one of the most common childhood infections. It is defined variously depending on the combination of symptoms experienced. In Daniel's case, otitis media with effusion is inflammation of the middle ear in which a collection of fluid is present. It is commonly referred to as 'glue ear' (Campbell and Glasper 1995). For many children with acute otitis media their recovery is spontaneous. However, for some there are concerns that any accompanying hearing loss may lead to delays in the development of their communication and interpersonal skills and changes in the child's behaviour (Robertson 2001; Rovers et al 2004).

Treatment for recurrent otitis media has been the subject of much debate with regards to its efficacy, both medical and surgical management. Where long term antibiotics have been used there has been concern surrounding side effects such as increased antibiotic resistance (Rovers et al 2004). Short course antibiotics have only a limited effect of a relatively short duration (Campbell and Glasper 1995). In some cases steroids have been utilised in combination with antibiotics but again the effect is only short term (Butler and van der Voort 2004).

Surgical treatment for persistent otitis media with effusion has equally been subjected to scrutiny, this in part, due to the large numbers of children receiving such treatment irrespective of the severity of the problem. Guidance from the Department of Health in the early 1990s, recommended surgery only for those children with severe glue ear. This led to a steady decline in the numbers undergoing surgery (Black and Hutchings 2002).

The impact of surgery on an individual child remains optimum where the right child has the right surgery (Rovers et al 2004). Where surgery is indicated a myringotomy is performed (that is a small incision in the tympanic membrane) and a tympanostomy tube placement called a gromet. This reduces pressure in the middle ear and prevents recurrence of fluid build up. The tube falls out naturally after several months and the hole heals naturally.

Day case surgery

Day surgery has increased significantly in the past 15 years. This can be viewed from two perspectives. First in terms of service provision it is seen as more cost effective and allows healthcare Trusts to maximise their resources. The drive towards value for money and subsequent rationalisation of service provision is evident in Government policy starting with *Working for Patients* (DHSS 1989). Subsequently reports by Thornes (1991) and the Audit Commission (Audit Commission 1993) both encouraged the development of day surgery facilities.

With less inpatient care there is the potential to reduce hospital beds and associated resource costs as the service does not cover a 24 hour period. There is also a reduction in waiting lists which has also featured highly in government targets for health service provision. Most recently the Department of Health in 2002 provided a guideline for hospital Trusts to achieve a 75 per cent target for day case surgery for all elective cases set out in the *NHS Plan* (Department of Health 2000). This guideline reiterated the need to expand day surgery and combat inefficiency to provide faster more efficient services that will decrease waiting times.

Thornes (1991) set out recommendations specifically for the provision of day care services for children which included the need for children's day case units, appropriately trained staff, emphasis on preparation and information and support after discharge with community services a key area for communication. Elements of this have been reinforced in the 2002 guidelines from the Department of Health. Although there is scant reference to children, they are acknowledged as needing to be nursed in paediatric areas with play facilities provided and registered children's nurses available to care for them. The guideline does discuss in detail preparation, support and after care although this is generic to all day case surgery.

The benefits of day care from the child and family's perspective have largely been reduction of trauma in being admitted to hospital as an overnight stay is not required. This minimises any separation of the child from their family. This again is reinforced by the Day Surgery Operational Guide as they highlight that an overnight admission is often the most distressing part of visiting hospital (Department of Health 2002).

While this is seen as reducing any unnecessary stress on the child the impact on the family largely goes unrecognised as the emphasis is on the child. More recently studies have sought to explore parent's experiences of day care and the role they play in it. (Hughes and Callery 2004) in their qualitative study highlighted three specific issues; first the need for in-depth preparation for surgery particularly with regards to the practical, emotional and social impact of caring for their children following surgery. Second, post discharge support is required at different levels for families who were often reluctant to access what had been provided. Telephone follow up was suggested to open up lines of communication to enable parents to more easily ask for support. This is an initiative that is already in place in some hospital Trusts (Higson and Bolland 2000). Follow up arrangements do vary around the country and an awareness of local services is important as you move between different areas of work. To return to the study, the third issue surrounded specific negotiation with regard to care, particularly at what point they felt ready to take their child home and decisions on when their child would be ready to resume their usual activities.

Other studies have focused on the benefits of parental involvement in their child's care. Kristensson-Hallstrom et al in their quantitative study assessed the impact of giving parents information and education about post-operative care on the child's recovery and the time spent in hospital (Kristensson-Hallstrom et al 1997). The study found that parents in the intervention group were well prepared and, therefore, assumed a greater part of their child's care. These children appeared to have less pain; fewer children vomited post-operatively and were able to go home earlier.

This study highlights the importance of preparation in day-care provision, in this instance in terms of post-operative management. The subject of preparation of child and family for day surgery has been a key focus in the delivery of quality care for some time, particularly as there is likely to be a lack of time on the actual day of surgery. This has led to a number of initiatives with variations on pre-admission programmes becoming the norm. Early developments of these (Glasper and Stradling 1989) reported the beneficial use of therapeutic play sessions, presentation of the hospital journey and tours of facilities in preparing children for admission. Subsequent growth in Saturday Clubs, pre-admission clinics and a range of audio-visual material all contribute to reducing the potential anxiety of hospital admission. More recent developments have seen the developing role of the children's nurse in carrying out the pre-operative assessment (Rushforth 2000).

The implications for day surgery children can be seen to be beneficial with preparation and support being major considerations in the delivery of quality care. The shortness of stay, therefore, makes it essential that care pre-operatively, post-operatively including following discharge is planned effectively to maximise the support and care needed to achieve a successful outcome for the child and family.

Pre-operative and Post-operative care

Pre-operative care

Many aspects of pre-operative care are generic to all patients undergoing surgery irrespective of the length of stay. The importance in delivering this care is that it is planned with regards not only to the safe preparation of a child for theatre, but also the particular needs of the child and family and the specific operation they are going to have.

The following includes the main areas that need to be considered when planning care pre-operatively, there may be some variations according to individual hospital Trust policy and you will need to be aware of these.

The emphasis in pre-operative preparation is on the physical and psychological aspects of the child's care and the needs of the parents. As a children's nurse in planning care you need to determine what you already know including what evidence supports your action and what you therefore need to know. These are considerations for you when reading the following outline plan of care and may help you determine your selection of an aspect of care to review its evidence base.

All planned care should be underpinned by a model of nursing appropriate to children incorporating the philosophy of the unit which is usually family-centred care and delivered using a systematic approach to nursing. This provides the framework that will organise the care. The Nottingham model is a good example that is suited to children and families (Smith 1995).

As with all admissions it is necessary to have an initial assessment on admission. Some of these details may be recorded at the pre-assessment clinic and completed on admission. Details selected are pertinent to a child undergoing surgery and, therefore, other details that are collected in the course of an admission have not necessarily been included here, for example immunization status. As you review the list in Table 6.1 consider the rationale underpinning the assessment.

In addition to the initial assessment data, specific areas of consideration for the nurse are:

- *Anxiety of the child and or family*: The nurse needs to consider the type of support needed. This may be determined by the amount of preparation the family have been able to access prior to admission. Information given at the right time and reinforced at different times during the whole of the day case journey, including their information needs and how and when these are these are to be met.

Table 6.1 Pre-operative assessment

- Child's general health prior to admission – important as this will indicate fitness for surgery, particularly with ENT (ear, nose and throat) problems as it can be difficult for the child to be infection free.
- Previous hospital admissions
- Reason for admission
- Child/family's understanding of reason for admission – This is an important part of the preparation process
- Medication/current treatment
- Baseline observations to establish the norm for the child
- Weight to calculate medication and anaesthetic agents
  Sensitivities/allergies
- Screening: varies according to past history and presenting problem
  - Urinalysis – checking for glucose/ketones in the unlikely event the child was an undiagnosed diabetic or proteins which might indicate infection
  - FBC (Full blood count) to check, for example, for anaemia and again any indication from the WBC (white blood cells) of infection

These are the most likely tests for Daniel for other admissions there may be:

  - Blood test for Sickle cell/thalassaemia
  - CXR (chest xray)
  - Swabs for MRSA
  - Nose and throat swabs for signs of infection
  - Other tests will be specific to the type of operation being carried out
- Pain management – It is good practice as part of the preparation to introduce local procedures for pain management early before the child experiences pain, particularly where a tool is involved which needs the child/family to understand its use. It is an opportunity for the family to raise any concerns they may have.

- *Parental involvement*: The involvement of parents in the theatre journey has become the norm over the last 20 years with it being accepted practice for parents, should they wish, to accompany their child to theatre and stay during the induction of anaesthesia. This has also continued into parents sitting with their child in the recovery area or PACU (post anaesthetic care unit) until they are ready to return to the ward. This practice is not as widely accepted as parents in the anaesthetic room. This subject forms the example evidence base to practice in the feedback section at the end of the chapter.

Most hospital Trusts will have documentation specifically designed for use in day care and will include the pre-operative assessment and the preparation needed to transfer a patient safely to theatre. This will include a preoperative checklist that is checked prior to the child leaving the ward and again in the theatre reception. This includes consideration of the following:

Pre-operative fasting: Knowing and recording when the child last had anything to eat or drink. Current recommendations are that infants can be breast fed until four hours before anaesthesia, children a light meal six hours before and clear fluids up to two hours before (Simini 1999). You will need to consult local guidelines as to the minimum fasting times as they vary between Trusts.

It is important that patients are fasted sufficiently to ensure there is no risk of regurgitation during induction of anaesthesia which could lead to pulmonary aspiration of gastric contents. This has been a contentious area of practice with concerns raised over patients being starved for unnecessary lengths of time. There remains variation in practice across hospitals although excessive starving certainly for planned surgery has been reduced significantly. It is an area that nurses need to be aware of particularly in day surgery where the practice of starving their child for theatre is left to the parents. Children who are put to bed early evening and not woken for a drink later can still be starved for a much longer period than is necessary.

Consent: You need to be aware of who legally can consent. This subject is covered in more detail in Chapter 7. In the case of Daniel his parents will have consented as he is not legally old enough to consent on his own behalf and he would not be deemed competent to do so.

Pre-medication: Most commonly this consists of ametop or emla cream. These are local topical anaesthetic agents that are applied to the sites where cannulation will take place. Where a child is particularly anxious then a sedative may be indicated but it is not routine practice. Other drugs given prior to theatre will be indicated by any pre-existing medical condition or the specific surgery being performed.

Theatre checklist: These are completed to ensure essential information is provided to theatre staff to ensure safe care that meets the child's needs. An example of the type of information contained within the documentation is in Table 6.2.

Pre-operative care aims to prepare a child safely for theatre and minimise any distress or anxiety during this process. When transferring a child to theatre this may include them being carried, walking or driving toy motorised cars. Theatre trolleys are often decorated as popular images such as Thomas the tank engine. Distraction of the child during the whole process is beneficial in minimising stress to the child and ultimately to the parent as well.

Table 6.2 Theatre checklist

Documentation: case notes/x rays/drug card
Fasting time
Weight
Pre-medication
Consent form
Identity bracelet
Loose teeth
Jewellery – removed or taped
Nail polish or makeup removed to facilitate monitoring of hypoxia
Marking of limbs
Allergies
Toy/comforter
Empty bladder
Theatre gown – Often the child chooses to stay in his/her own nightclothes.

Post-operative care

Preparing for return of the child: This is often an anxious time for parents who just want to know that their child is safe following the anaesthetic and surgical procedure. It is important that they are encouraged to have something to drink and eat as often parents have starved themselves at the same time as their child. Where parents are able to sit by their child's bedside in recovery this needs to be facilitated according to local policy.

There may be specific preparation at the child's bedside in terms of any equipment required. This is not necessary for Daniel's surgery but it is good practice to check that oxygen and suction are available and working at the bedside.

Return to the ward: The care will depend on the type of surgery that has been carried out. The focus here will be on Daniel but would need to be adapted for other types of surgery. Thus the aspects of care selected are concerned with; post operative observations, pain management, eating and drinking, elimination, observation of operation site, discharge preparation and follow up support. Other aspects of post operative care are detailed in Chapter 7.

- *Observations*: These are usually of temperature, pulse and respiration and will be recorded on his return; the frequency will reflect his condition. Commonly they are carried out half hourly, then hourly, two hourly and four hourly. The length of time is largely determined by the child's recovery and local policy. Time spent in day care is kept to a minimum and this is reflected in the length of time and frequency that observations will be undertaken for.

- *Pain management*: Peri-operatively the anaesthetist often gives analgesia to minimise discomfort post-operatively. Pain management strategies need to take cognisance of Daniel's age; three years, and, therefore, the selection of a pain tool needs to be appropriate to a young child such as Whaley and Wong's smiley faces (Wong 1995). Involvement of the parents is crucial as they know their child best and will be able to recognise when he is in pain. Pain management in children has received a great deal of attention in recent years and there are many guides and tools to choose from. Most clinical areas have adopted one for their use and how this is recorded and acted upon will follow local guidelines. The Royal College of Nursing has produced a comprehensive guideline for clinical practice on the recognition and assessment of acute pain in children, information on the guideline can be accessed from their website: www.rcn.org.uk.

- *Eating and drinking*: To some extent it is necessary to be guided by local policy as with many aspects of pre- and post-operative care there are local variations. With the type of surgery that Daniel has undergone there are no contraindications to eating and drinking, unlike bowel surgery for example. It is necessary to ensure that he is fully awake from his anaesthetic and maintaining his own airway safely. Starting with small amounts of clear fluid if this is tolerated it is possible to progress quickly to free fluid and diet. Nausea and vomiting can be a post-operative complication for some children. This can be linked to the anaesthetic agents, the length of the starvation period and if the child is in pain. For the child experiencing post operative nausea and vomiting (PONV) it can be distressing and prolong the recovery time. These children need a quiet environment, to avoid sudden movement in position and not feel that they must start drinking (Rose and Watcha 1999). It is necessary to deal with the cause in these instances and if it does not resolve administer an anti emetic drug.

- *Elimination*: It is common practice to check that a child has passed urine post-operatively. However in this instance Daniel's surgery did not involve the genital area and his anaesthetic was of a relatively short duration such that it is unlikely that he will develop post-operative urinary retention. Failure to pass urine should not, therefore, preclude him from being discharged.

- *Operation site*: This is usually checked for any signs of oozing. Both ears will have a dressing in place this usually falls out. Parents are advised that after two weeks their child should be able to go swimming but not jump or dive in the water. Gromets may also fall out and this is a common occurrence and not a cause for concern (Huband and Trigg 2000).

- *Discharge*: This is planned for the day unless there is an aspect of post-operative management requiring an overnight stay. Planning for discharge is an integral part of the nursing process and should start at assessment. It is much easier to resolve problems and plan care early rather than find that something has not been identified or planned for when it is time to go home.

The discharge care plan will include assessment criteria that will ensure that discharge is carried out in a timely and appropriate way according to individual need and service provision. The Royal College of Nursing has produced a guide for discharge planning for day surgery that takes account of physical, psychological and social criteria (RCN 2004).

Follow up support varies around the country from the provision of a telephone number for enquiries, to telephone contact to check that there are no concerns, to district nurse or children's community nurse follow up at home. The management and provision of services can, therefore, vary greatly. Research has shown that parents do not necessarily want to be routinely visited at home but want to be able to access reassurance and advice should they need it (Smith and Daughtrey 2000). The provision of paediatric community services remains variable in the UK although it continues to grow and develop as ambulatory care provision becomes a significant part of child health services and services are reconfigured to meet the changing needs of the population.

Parents have a great need for information that will enable them to support their children once they have returned home. This information needs to be both verbal and written and particularly cover the expected progress of their child's care so that they know how and when to respond. Who to contact and in what circumstances is an important aspect of this and can be the cause of stress in parents. When to resume normal activities both at school and home is also essential information for parents.

 # Trigger 6.1: Feedback

Go to Chapter 6 Trigger feedback on p. 171

Trigger 6.2: Child in accident and emergency: Minor injuries

The intention of this trigger is to explore the management of minor injuries in a paediatric Accident and Emergency department.

The Trigger

Luke is seven years old and while playing in the garden fell and bumped his head, he was not unconscious. He is upset, crying and there is a small amount of blood visible from a wound at the back of his head. His mum is not initially concerned but shortly after the accident Luke vomits twice and is drowsy. She telephones NHS direct for advice and is advised to take Luke to the local hospital. Mum and Luke arrive at the accident and emergency department of the local District General Hospital. Luke's father is on his way from work to join them.

Situation

You are a Registered Nurse undertaking a second pre-registration course in children's nursing and have recently started a placement in the accident and emergency department of a District General Hospital that sees several thousand children per year. There is a small separate waiting/play area and treatment room designed for children.

Feedback

Using your experience and knowledge of working with children and their families prepare a guide that outlines the areas of consideration when assessing and treating children of Luke's age in an A&E that is within a District General Hospital. This will be for use in the department by those less familiar with children. The fixed resource material will help you.

The facts

> **What are the main facts in this trigger? Make a list:**

Hypotheses: What may these facts mean?

- There needs to be an assessment of the child's head injury.
- Assessment in A&E may be different.
- Injuries need treatment.
- There is an upset child in a strange environment.
- Children can be seen in largely adult orientated A&E.

Questions developed from the hypotheses

1. How is assessment of minor injuries undertaken?
2. How are head wounds treated?
3. What would be an appropriate environment for children in A&E?
4. What communication strategies are needed to facilitate the care of a seven year old?
5. What discharge support is needed?

Trigger 6.2: Fixed resource material

Read the following to help you answer the questions. (You may also wish to search and review other up-to-date research and evidence-based literature, and seek other relevant resources to provide you with the answers to your questions.)

Huband, S.,Trigg, E. (2000) *Practices in children's nursing*. Edinburgh: Churchill Livingstone.

Department of Health (2003) *Getting the right start: National Service Framework for Children Standard for Hospital Services*, accessible from the Web at: www.doh. gov.uk/nsf/children/gettingtherightstart

Trigger 6.2: Fixed resource sessions

Children and families in accident and emergency

The provision of facilities for children and families in accident and emergency are located either in designated departments within children's hospitals or as an adjunct to the facilities provided for adults in general hospitals. This latter provision varies greatly. In some hospitals this may be an entirely separate area of the accident and emergency department, staffed by specialist staff while in others there may be some provision of facilities for children such as a play area, treatment room for example, employment of children's nurses, but essentially provision is largely within an adult focused department.

Children account for up to a third of all attendees at A&E which has been recognised by government reports from 1991 (Department of Health 1991) and most recently by the *National Service Framework for Children, Young People and Maternity Services* (Department of Health 2004). These reports have focused on the appropriate provision of services to meet the needs of children and families. This includes keeping separate children and adult patients so that children are not exposed to potentially frightening scenes, providing child friendly treatment and ensuring rooms and waiting areas have suitable play facilities.

Triage and assessment

Assessment within the Accident and Emergency Department is designed to be responsive to need. This need is prioritised according to the child's individual condition by a triage nurse.

All children are classified as either having an emergency sign which requires immediate treatment, a priority sign which requires prompt assessment and treatment or non-urgent which can wait for assessment and treatment (Gove et al 1999).

Accident and Emergency departments have triage categories that are then linked to algorithms of the presenting problem based on the patient's history. The system follows a medical model although triage is a nursing activity. These flow charts are used to facilitate consistent decision-making during the assessment process which enables care to be prioritised according to need (Walsh and Kent 2001). Each triage category also indicates the target time for treatment. According to current Department of Health guidelines the maximum wait in A&E is four hours.

The Sheffield Children's Hospital Accident and Emergency department developed triage criteria and categories with associated algorithms. These will be used for the two children presenting at A&E in this chapter:

A	(Red)	Immediate	0 minutes
B	(Orange)	Very urgent	10 minutes
C	(Yellow)	Urgent	60 minutes
D	(Green)	Standard	120 minutes
E	(Blue)	Non-urgent	240 minutes

The algorithm for head injury (Table 6.3)will be used to assess Luke.

Luke presenting with vomiting, drowsiness but no loss of consciousness, is likely to be categorised as D. His neurological status will be assessed by the nurse and if this deteriorates following his initial assessment his triage category may alter.

The assessment by the triage nurse will include observations and in this case neurological observations using a paediatric coma scale, pain assessment, history such as details of the accident, personal details, contact information, particularly if the child is unaccompanied and next of kin need to be contacted, activities of living – the level of detail of which may depend on the presenting problem – any other relevant information that may affect the child and or his treatment (Smith 1995).

Table 6.3 The algorithm for head injury

Head Injury

Airway Compromise
Breathing Inadequate ————————— Y ————————→ A (Red)
Circulation Inadequate
Unresponsive
|
N
↓
Significant History/Mechanism
Severe Pain ————————— Y ————————→ B (Orange)
Altered Conscious Level
(AVP~)
|
N
↓
History LOC
Moderate Pain ————————— Y ————————→ C (Yellow)
Focal Neurological Signs
Persistent Vomiting
|
N
↓
Headache/Haematoma
Mild Pain ————————— Y ————————→ D (Green)
Recent Problem
|
N
↓
Old Injury > 48hrs ————————— Y ————————→ E (Blue)
No Pain

Significant history/mechanism:
   high speed RTA, thrown from vehicle
   fall from height (dependant upon age of a child)
   surface landed on
   penetrating wounds

Focal neurological signs:
   weakness of a limb
   altered sensation
   pupil reactivity/reactions

Persistent vomiting:
   > 3 times

Source: Reproduced with the permission of the A&E Department at the Sheffield Children's Hospital

Head injury assessment and management

You may find it useful to revise your knowledge and understanding of the structures and their function in the brain as this will help you make the links to the symptoms being experienced by a patient with a head injury. There are differences between the adult brain and that of a developing child that may have an impact on the trauma and damage sustained. For example the brain comprises 15 per cent of body weight at birth compared with 3 per cent in adulthood. The paediatric scalp is thinner and more elastic and at greater risk of avulsion (tearing) injuries. A child's undeveloped brain has less cerebral spinal fluid buffer space as the subarachnoid space is smaller. Trauma can, therefore, injure the bony structure resulting in fractures, the vascular system resulting in tearing or bleeding of blood vessels, the brain tissue causing contusion (bruising). This may lead to bleeding, swelling and obstruction of cerebral spinal fluid (Barnes 2003; Thomas and Taylor 1997).

Intervention in head injuries needs to be timely in order to minimise secondary brain injury that occurs as a consequence of the original injury. This reinforces the importance of obtaining a detailed and accurate history of the accident and the child's response following it. A detailed physical examination of the child's level of consciousness and body systems for signs of intracranial pressure will be evaluated and indicate subsequent management (Barnes 2003; Thomas and Taylor 1997).

Luke has sustained an injury to the back of his head, the occiput, and there is bleeding from a laceration to his scalp. Children have increased bleeding from the scalp as there are a large number of blood vessels in the cutaneous layer of the scalp (Barnes 2003). The decision to bring Luke to A&E is due to the nausea and vomiting he is experiencing and the drowsiness. These can be signs of a changing neurological status potentially indicating a rise in intracranial pressure (ICP). Pallor and vomiting are common after minor head injury in young children and result from vagal nerve stimulation. Persistent vomiting is an indication that admission is warranted (Hull and Johnston 1999).

Luke has attended A&E with a minor head injury. This has been defined as a period of unconsciousness lasting no longer than 15 minutes, a Glasgow coma score of 13–15 and a normal neurological examination (Harrison 1991).

The Glagow Coma Score is recognised internationally as an assessment tool and used extensively for coma scoring. Designed for adults it nonetheless has appeal for use with children as it attempts to provide some objective measure of the patient's status. However the differences between adult and child responses limited it use and led to a number of modified versions of the Glasgow Coma Scale (Warren 2000). The modified Glasgow Coma Scale in use in a large number of paediatric centres in the United Kingdom is one that has been benchmarked by the National Paediatric Neuroscience Benchmarking group and can be obtained from the Birmingham Children's Hospital (Barnes, 2003; Warren, 2000).

The Glasgow Coma scale scores three areas; eyes opening, best verbal response, best motor response. Descriptors define the potential scores for each area and after assessment the total score is out of 15. A fall of 2 or more points in GCS is significant and a GCS of less than 8 requires urgent airway management (Hull and Johnston 1999).

The neurological assessment chart also includes assessment of pupil size and reaction, temperature, pulse, respiration, blood pressure and limb movements. Signs of raised intracranial pressure (ICP) can be detected from carrying out these observations and monitoring any changes as follows:

- *Temperature*: Increase in temperature may indicate that a rising ICP is causing pressure on the hypothalamus.
- *Pulse*: Bradycardia can indicate raised ICP caused by excessive pressure on the medulla.
- *Respiration*: Pressure on the medulla and damage to the brain stem can depress respiration.
- *Blood Pressure*: Hypertension again due to pressure on the medulla is a sign of raised ICP. Classic symptoms of ICP are bradycardia and hypertension.
- *Pupil reaction*: If the ICP rises, pressure on the optic nerve affects the eyes' ability to react to light. Pupil size should be checked and whether eyes respond equally and briskly to light. If the response becomes sluggish this may indicate pressure on the optic nerve.
- *Limb movement*: Weakness may indicate damage in certain parts of the brain or in the spinal cord.

The Coma Scale offers some objectivity in the assessment of the child's condition but also the nurse often picks up on less tangible signs indicating deterioration and parents can contribute their knowledge of the child's normal behaviour (Clayton 1999).

Assessment of the child will be ongoing during the time spent in A&E, the frequency of the observations determined by the child's condition and local policy and procedures. It is not routine to X ray the skull for fractures. A CT scan may be considered if there is significant trauma or indicated by clinical findings (Barnes 2003; Warren 2000). A CT or MRI scan will show if raised intracranial pressure is due to oedema, contusion or haemorrhage (Hull and Johnston 1999).

Luke has a scalp laceration which will need cleaning and closure. This is commonly carried out using tissue adhesive which is quick, easy and causes minimum discomfort all factors that are important when caring for children (Mattick et al 2002).

After a period of observation and providing there is no deterioration in his observations Luke will be allowed home. Follow up care is not indicated. His parents will be given verbal and written advice on the signs and symptoms to observe at home that may indicate a need to seek further advice. It may also be appropriate to discuss prevention of future accidents with both Luke and his parents.

→ Trigger 6.2: Feedback

Go to Chapter 6 Trigger Feedback on p. 171

! Trigger 6.3: Child in 'Resusc'

The intention of this trigger is to provide the opportunity to explore the management of children in the resuscitation area of the accident and emergency department. While this trigger does not reflect ambulatory care the A&E setting does and it seems pertinent to include the care of the child requiring resuscitation here rather than in the acute chapter. Nurses working in A&E departments will experience a wide range of care need from minor to major injuries responding to whatever presents at any time.

The Trigger

Staff nurse in A&E talking to ambulance crew.
   Staff Nurse on telephone:

> Yes I can hear you, ten months old you said, Chloe Brown, convulsion at home lasting 3 minutes, temperature 39.5 degrees, heart rate 140/minute . . . (pause in conversation) Just started convulsing again, cyanosed, apnoeic, bring her straight to resusc.

Situation

You are part of the team in the resuscitation room as Chloe Brown is brought in by the ambulance staff. You have been designated to look after her parents and in addition to the emotional support they will also need you to keep them informed about the care Chloe's receiving as they are present with you in the resuscitation room.

Feedback

Prepare an evidence-based fact sheet for parents that you could use to explain Chloe's problems and subsequent care. Use of language is important as you do not want to appear condescending nor do you want to present the information in a way that is inaccessible to the parents. In these days of wide spread Internet use can you include a website that would be suitable for parents wishing to find out more information about this particular medical problem.

The facts

What are the main facts in this trigger? Make a list:

Hypotheses: What may these facts mean?

- The child needs immediate assessment and treatment.
- This is distressing for parents.
- There may be a link between the seizure and the child's temperature.

Questions developed from the hypotheses

1. What immediate assessment and treatment is needed?
2. What is a febrile seizure?
3. How can parents be supported?

Trigger 6.3: Fixed resource material

Read the following to help you answer the questions. (You may also wish to search and review other up-to-date research and evidence-based literature, and seek other relevant resources to provide you with the answers to your questions).

Barnes, K (2003) *Paediatrics A Clinical Guide for Nurse Practitioners*. Edinburgh: Butterworth Heinemann.

Huband, S., Trigg, E. (2000) *Practices in Children's Nursing*. Edinbugh: Churchill Livingstone, pp. 73–81.

Offringa, M., Moyer, V. A. (2001) Evidence based paediatrics: Evidence based management of seizures associated with fever. *British Medical Journal*, 323 (7321), pp. 1111–4.

Walker, W. (1999) Do relatives have the right to witness resuscitation?' *Journal of Clinical Nursing* 8 (6), pp. 625–30.
www.resus.org.uk

Trigger 6.3: Fixed resource sessions

Emergency Management

Emergency management of care in resuscitation

The algorithm used in this instance clearly indicates A (Red) due to Chloe's cyanosis and apnoeic episodes. Emergency management focuses on the ABCs. That is airway, breathing and circulation. National guidelines are produced by the resuscitation council (Resuscitation Council 2000) and followed by all practitioners providing life support. All students and qualified staff are required to attend a yearly update for life support skills within their local Hospital Trust or School of Nursing. You may find it helpful to revise basic life support so that you can apply this knowledge to the management of Chloe. Basic life support (BLS) continues even with the introduction of advanced life support (ALS) and it is important that nurses maintain skills in its delivery as the effectiveness of BLS can affect the outcome of ALS (Huband and Trigg 2000).

Basic life support will already have been commenced in the ambulance and continued on arrival to A&E. If Chloe's breathing remains compromised advanced life support will start in the resuscitation room as the assembled team of nurses and doctors take over her care. Advanced life support is covered in detail in chapter 8.

Important in the management of any child in the resuscitation room is the effective team working of the staff in there. It is important that each knows their role during any emergency or resuscitation procedure. Staff will be allocated roles at the start of each shift so that they are prepared to respond when required.

Management of seizure

A febrile seizure is defined as a 'brief, generalised, clonic or tonic clonic seizure that occurs within the context of a febrile illness' (Barnes 2003 p.183). The seizure involves the sudden loss of consciousness; a tonic phase of 10-20 seconds which involves symmetrical extension of the limbs, arched back and cessation of breathing. The clonic phases involves, generalised jerking. Respiration is usually irregular and the patient may pass urine, open their bowels or salivate (Huband and Trigg 2000).

As observed with Chloe infants in particular are prone to apnoea during the seizure, therefore, observation is an important part of the nurse's role. This will be a frightening and distressing experience for the parents and they will need a lot of support during and after the seizure.

Emergency management of the seizure focuses on ABC as discussed earlier and if the seizure is prolonged administration of anticonvulsant drugs. This is usually rectal

Table 6.4 Algorithm for fits, faints and floppy episodes

Fits, Faints, Floppy Episodes

Airway Compromise
Breathing Inadequate
Circulation Inadequate ————————— Y —————————→ A (Red)
Unresponsive
|
N
↓
Severe Pain
Significant History/Mechanism
Hypoglycaemia BM<2.7mmols
Delayed Capillary Refill ————————— Y —————————→ B (Orange)
Purpura
AVPU
|
N
↓
Moderate Pain
Focal Neurological Signs ————————— Y —————————→ C (Yellow)
Pyrexia > 38.5°C
Bulging Fontanelle
|
N
↓
Mild Pain ————————— Y —————————→ D (Green)
Known Seizure Disorder
|
N
↓
Second Opinion ————————— Y —————————→ E (Blue)
> 24hrs Post Episode

Significant history/mechanism:
    high speed RTA, thrown from vehicle
    fall from height (dependant upon age of child)
    surface landed on
    penetrating wound

Focal neurological signs:
    weakness of a limb
    altered sensation
    pupil reactivity/reactions

Delayed capillary refill:
    > 2 seconds following continuous pressure on a digit for 5 seconds (interpretation
    should be made in light of ambient temperature)

Source: Reproduced with the permission of the A&E Department at the Sheffield Children's Hospital

diazepam or paraldehyde. Table 6.4 details the algorithm for fits, faints and floppy episodes.

Recent guidelines suggest that children under 18 months, those having a complex seizure, and those for whom antibiotics were administered warrant admission (Armon 2003). A simple febrile seizure lasts less than 15 minutes and is not repeated in the same episode and recovery is complete in one hour. A complex seizure is either prolonged, over 15 minutes, focal or with incomplete recovery (Capeworn 1998). In respect of these guidelines Chloe will need to be admitted for inpatient care.

Once emergency care to stabilise the presenting features of Chloe's condition has taken place the emphasis is on clinical assessment to find a focus for the infection and control the temperature. A full infection screen may be carried out to exclude infection in particular meningitis. Where no focus is located a clean catch urine sample needs to be obtained to exclude urinary tract infection. If an infection is identified then antibiotics will be commenced.

Management of temperature

You may wish to review the regulation of body temperature; that is how heat is produced in and lost from the body and the nervous control by the hypothalamus and the vasomotor centre in the brain. To manage pyrexia in children antipyretics such as paracetamol and or ibuprofen are administered. Other measures include the use of a fan to cool ambient temperature in the environment, removing excess clothing and encouraging fluids.

Parents in resuscitation

It is very distressing for a parent to see their child having a seizure particularly as they frequently look cyanosed and have some difficulties breathing. Involvement of the family underpins the practice of children's nursing and over decades this has come to encompass all aspects of their child's care. As with Daniel's care management in Trigger 6.1 it has become the norm of practice for parents to be with their child in the anaesthetic room, this is being extended in many areas to the recovery or PACU (post anaesthetic care unit). Likewise in accident and emergency departments it is becoming more acceptable for parents to be present during resuscitation.

The subject of witness resuscitation creates ethical, practical and professional considerations with as many pros as cons put forward. As you read the following you might want to consider your own personal view about this practice and, in addition to your own experiences and with further reading, analyse the issues it raises and come to some conclusion about whether there should be a blanket policy about witness resuscitation supported with guidelines to ensure safe practice for all involved or whether it remains the decision of individual Trusts and emergency teams. As part of your personal reflection may wish to consider key ethical principles as part of your decision-making process for example beneficence, non maleficence and autonomy. The article by Walker (1999) provides useful commentary on these issues.

Evidence suggests that the majority of people prefer to be there (Williams 1996) although for some healthcare professionals particularly doctors there is a felt need to protect relatives from what is a traumatic event. The Resuscitation Council (1996) recommended that families should be given the opportunity to be present. However there remains a concern that family members may impede the resuscitation. This could involve indirectly affecting the decision-making of the team which might mean prolonging a futile resuscitation attempt, hysterical relatives intervening physically. There may be an increase in the stress level of staff who feel that their actions are being scrutinized which might also lead to errors and resulting litigation. From a practical perspective there is little available space during resuscitation and there would be a need for an additional member of staff to be there supporting the relative (Jarvis 1998; Rosenczweig 1998).

The literature sources are both theory and research based, national and international. Where studies have been undertaken they have either been focused on staff attitudes or relatives' experiences of the event. The latter have concluded that the adjustment to death was easier, that they felt their presence was beneficial to the patient and that in the longer term better coping and grieving processes were reported (Hanson and Strawser 1992) Similar findings were concluded by Robinson (Robinson 1998) who found no adverse psychological effects among relatives interviewed one month after resuscitation. Relatives who were not present at resuscitation have also been found to regret that decision (Ellison 1998). Witness resuscitation enables the relative to see that everything was done and eliminates the not knowing what is happening during the resuscitation (Rattrie 2000).

This sphere of practice will for some remain controversial as we apply our own values and beliefs to the issues it raises. The evidence suggests it is beneficial to those relatives present. However the overwhelming consideration is that this practice is based on informed choice by the family and that the support of family members is constant throughout the resuscitation and counselling is available subsequently should there be a need.

→ Trigger 6.3: Feedback

Go to Chapter 6 Trigger Feedback on p. 171 below

? Chapter 6 Trigger feedback: What do you know?

Trigger 6.1 Daycare

In answer to the questions for this trigger you will be able to utilise the fixed resources and the additional reading given.

1. Why does Daniel need surgery?
2. What support will Daniel and his family need for planned day-case surgery?
3. What is the rationale for Daniel's pre-operative care?
4. What is the rationale for Daniel's post-operative care?

The fixed resources also highlighted the need for you to identity what your current knowledge base is, how you know what you know and identify areas where new knowledge is needed. This is the purpose of selecting an aspect of care and analysing the evidence base to its practice. The following is an example. You will find Chapter 2 useful in guiding your analysis.

Parents in the Post Anaesthetic Care Unit (PACU)

Evidence has been collected following a search of electronic databases and collated using a matrix (see Table 6.5).

Conclusions from the evidence

I have included three examples of evidence into the subject area. There are a number of others that I could have included but the aim is to demonstrate how to collate evidence, the quality of the evidence and its use for informing practice.

The evidence presented shows that it is a subject area that has been researched and it is particularly linked to developing practice protocols for parents being present in recovery areas. Most of the studies have been designed to capture the essence of that experience either as a justification for the practice or to develop the practice. The sample selection and size and data collection approach have limited the generalisability of the findings but nevertheless they do provide collectively a consistent feedback that parents want to be in the recovery room with their child and that they are in a position to help their child. Therefore, allowing parents into PACU/recovery improves the experience for children. However this has not been investigated specifically by the studies and the reduction of stress and anxiety for the child is based on parental and staff perceptions alone. There is an evidence base to practice with regards to parental presence in recovery, however, there is an absence of robust research. Where parental presence in recovery is not the norm of practice children's nurses will need to continue to advocate for children and families and work with individual hospital Trusts to facilitate this practice as much as is practicable within the boundaries of current service provision.

You may also find Peter Callery's article a useful guide on analysing evidence. In this article he uses parents in the anaesthetic room as an example (Callery 1997).

Adopting this approach maintains a questioning and analytical approach to practice.

Table 6.5 Parents in the Post Anaesthetic Care Unit (PACU)

Author/Year	Type of evidence	Methodology	Findings	Limitations	Strengths
Hall et al 1995	Research	Questionnaire to parents pre and post operatively n = 144 pre 132 post operatively Questionnaire to staff after each case n = 132	Parents want to be there Parents feel they can help their child Staff find parents helpful	Questionnaire Design and timing	Includes parents and staff perceptions
Smith and Bassett 1996	Audit of parents and staff	Questionnaire to parents n=22 Staff: Ward n = 13 PACU n = 11	Parents felt they knew their child and could help PACU staff felt children benefited but work load had increased	Small sample size	Includes parents and staff perceptions Identifies area for further practice development
Turner 1997	Research	Questionnaire to parents views of recovery room n = 96	Benefited parent and child Preparation important	Small scale questionnaire mainly closed questions. Findings not generalisable	Highlights beneficial to child and parents

Trigger 6.2 Child in A&E: minor injuries

The answers to the questions can be obtained from the fixed resources and the suggested further reading. Below is an outline answer to the feedback requested for this trigger.

The care of children in adult orientated A&E is an important consideration. The majority of nurses working in these areas are adult trained and while these areas do employ children's nurses it is usually insufficient to provide 24 hour cover (Walsh and Kent 2001). Education is, therefore, important. I have highlighted below the key areas you may have selected as being important in putting together a guide for adult nurses, with the knowledge gained from this book and the additional reading you have undertaken you will be able to expand upon and fill in the detail for these areas.

Children are different: They are not mini adults

Family-centred care:
You may wish to link this specifically to the A&E environment and the potential involvement of parents in their child's care including being present in resuscitation

Environment:
Child-friendly waiting and treatment areas to try to minimise stress and anxiety of an unfamiliar and . . .

Communication:
Use strategies for communicating with children at different ages.
Knowledge of children's cognition, for example, Piaget, will help you approach children in a way that is appropriate to their level of understanding
The use of play and distraction that is age appropriate including examples

Observation monitoring:
Vital Signs will be different and how you go about collecting them will vary according to the age of the child. You may wish to include examples here

Pain assessment and management:
Age-appropriate tools and examples can be included as well as calculation and administration of drugs for children

Trigger 6.3 The child in 'resusc'

The answers to the questions can be obtained from the fixed resources, the suggested further reading and additional material that you have included which may resemble the following.

Question 1. What immediate assessment and treatment is needed?

This can be answered in part from the fixed resource sessions 'Emergency management' and from the additional material included below. In the fixed resource session you were asked to revise BLS in particular as it relates to an infant Chloe's age. In the resuscitation room of an A&E you have the advantage of access to staff and equipment thus it will be easy to monitor vital signs and administer oxygen for example. The review detailed below reiterates the principles of BLS applied within the context of A&E.

The aim of BLS is to maintain ventilation and circulation until any underlying causes for the patients problems can be diagnosed and treated. Using the guidelines from the Resuscitation Council the emphasis for Chloe at this stage is to assess and respond to airway compromise and inadequate breathing:

Airway: Chloe is a ten month old infant,

- To open the airway the head should be placed in a neutral position.
- This can be achieved using the head tilt/chin lift.
- Place one hand on the child's forehead and two fingers of the other hand placed on the chin.
- Gently tilt the head back and lift the chin but do not over extend the neck.

Breathing: Check if Chloe's airway is open by:

- LOOKING for chest movement
- LISTENING for breath sounds at Chloe's nose and mouth
- FEELING for expired breath on your cheek
- Look Listen and Feel for 10 seconds
- If Chloe is breathing turn onto her side and check for continued breathing.
- If Chloe isn't breathing remove any obvious obstruction and start ventilation using self-inflating bag-valve-mask with reservoir and face mask. This should provide a good seal around Chloe's nose and mouth.
- Deliver 5 inhalations slowly: 1–1.5 seconds each.
- The aim is to achieve 2 effective breaths.
- Observe for chest movement with each inflation. If the chest does not rise reposition the airway as before. If this is still unsuccessful there may be airway obstruction.

In Chloe's case we do not suspect aspiration of a foreign body. In other circumstances where there were no other indicating factors in the collapse and this was suspected then the sequence in the BLS guidelines for removal of foreign body would be started. As Chloe has been convulsing and inflation was poor then suction may clear the airway of any secretions that could have collected in the nasopharynx.

Circulation:
- Assess circulation by taking a pulse and observe for other signs of life such as movement.
- In infants the brachial pulse is palpated for 10 seconds.

However, in the resuscitation room a collapsed infant would have been connected to an ECG monitor and it is likely that this will have happened in Chloe's case if she arrived into the resuscitation room apnoeic.

- Chest compression should be commenced if the pulse is less than 60 beats per minute.
- To locate the site for compressions draw an imaginary line between the nipples and place two fingers one finger breadth below in the centre of the sternum.
- Compress by 1/3 of the depth of the chest at a rate of 5 compressions followed by one breath/inflation. This forms one cycle; the aim is to achieve 20 cycles per minute.

Question 2. What is a febrile seizure?

Question 3. How can parents be supported?

Material additional to the fixed resource is presented in the format of the requested feedback. In developing your evidence-based fact sheet you will need to read in detail the subject area. From this you will be able to select key points that parents will want to be informed about. Parents will continue to have some anxiety about febrile seizure as there is chance that it may happen again. They will want to be as prepared as possible. Your approach may take the form of commonly asked questions and answers. This will help the layout as parents will want to be able to access relevant information quickly and easily. It is good practice to develop this type of information sheet. As more clinical problems that require treatment emerge parents will always need to have accessible information. Examples of parent information leaflets can be found in Smith (1995) and at most hospital Trusts. Some are put onto Trust websites as Internet use becomes more widespread.

The following questions and answers are suggestions. You may have included other areas for consideration:

Q   *What is a febrile seizure?*
A   Changes in electrical activity in the brain can lead to a child becoming unconscious with stiffening of the body followed by jerking of arms and legs. Sometimes a seizure is called a fit or convulsion.

Q   *Who is affected?*
A   Seizures are common in children. 3 per cent of all children between 6 months and five years have a febrile seizure. Boys and girls are equally affected.

Q   *Will my child have more seizures?*
A   30 per cent of children will go on to have one more seizure. A small proportion of children have more than two seizures. Children are more likely to have another seizure if there is a family history of febrile seizures or if their first seizure occurred under one year of age.

Q   *Will my child have permanent damage?*
A   There is a lack of evidence to suggest that children who have occasional

febrile seizures have any long term neurological problems. The risk of non febrile seizures in the future is very small.

Q   *Can I prevent my child having a febrile seizure?*
A   You cannot prevent it happening because illnesses that cause high temperatures cause the seizure. If your child has a high temperature it will help to keep them cool and may help prevent a seizure happening. You can do this by:

- removing excess clothing;
- not overheating the room;
- encouraging your child to drink; and
- giving paracetamol or ibruprofen regularly to reduce the temperature.

Q   *What should I do if it happens again?*
A   If your child has a seizure:
- Lay your child on their side with their face turned downwards to prevent choking.
- You do not need to do anything else, the seizure will stop by itself.
- Take note of the time if you can.
- Do not leave your child.
- Wait for the seizure to stop.
- If the seizure lasts longer than 5 minutes and you have been given a drug (diazepam) to insert into your child's bottom give this now.
- The seizure should stop within 10 minutes, if this does not happen dial 999 for an ambulance.
- If you have not been given a drug to administer and the seizure has lasted longer than 5 minutes then ring for an ambulance.
- Most fits stop after a few minutes and in these cases you will need to let your doctor (GP) know what has happened.

Further information and support is available from: www.epilepsy.org.uk

This is a useful website for parents. Although a febrile seizure does not mean a child will develop epilepsy the website contains useful information on the condition and it is relevant to care management in the UK.

It is important that you reference at the end of the information sheet the sources you have used. This will demonstrate that the information is based on current knowledge of the subject area. For the purposes of the questions and answers above the following sources have been used (Armon et al 2003; Barnes, 2003; Offringa and Moyer, 2001).

Reflect on your learning

- Ambulatory care is an important element of healthcare provision for children and their families
- Day case surgery has benefits both for patients and their families in reducing the need for a hospital stay and for the health service in terms of effective utilisation of resources.
- The use of a range of support strategies for the child and family during ambulatory care is paramount to a successful episode of care.
- The care of children within A&E environments should take place in an appropriate environment with care provided by specialist staff.
- Ambulatory care requires the provision of a range of ongoing support measures including telephone follow up/advice line, paediatric community nurses, and prompt and clear lines of communication between primary and secondary care to facilitate a seamless service.

References

Armon, K., Stephenson, T., MacFaul, R., Hemingway, P., Werneke, U., Smith, S. (2003) An evidence and consensus based guideline for the management of a child after a seizure, *Emergency Medicine Journal* 20, pp. 13–20.

Audit Commission (1993) *Children First: A Study of Hospital Services*. London: HMSO.

Barnes, K. (2003) *Paediatrics*. Edinburgh: Butterworth Heinemann.

Black, N. Hutchings, A. (2002) Reduction in the use of surgery for glue ear: Did national guidelines have an impact, *British Medical Journal* 11 (2), pp. 121–4.

Butler, C., van der Voort, J. (2004) Oral or topical nasal steroids for hearing loss associated with otitis media with effusion in children, *The Cochrane Database of Systematic Reviews* 3.

Callery, P. (1997) Using evidence in children's nursing. *Paediatric Nursing* 9 (6), pp. 13–17.

Campbell, S., Glasper E. A. (1995) *Whaley and Wong's Children's Nursing*. London: Mosby.

Capeworn, D., Swain, A., Goldsworthy, L. L. (eds) (1998) Handbook of Paediatric Accident and Emergency Medicine. London: Saunders.

Clayton, M. (1999) Minor head injury: a cause for concern. *Paediatric Nursing* 11 (5), pp. 16–18.

Department of Health (1991) *Welfare of Children and Young People in Hospital*. London: HMSO.

Department of Health (2000) *NHS Plan*. London: Department of Health.

Department of Health (2002) *Day Surgery Operational Guide: Waiting, Choice, Booking*. London: Stationery Office.

Department of Health (2003) *Getting the Right Start: National Service Framework for Children Standard for Hospital Services*. London: Department of Health.

Department of Health (2004) *The National Service Framework for Children, Young People and Maternity Services*. London: The Stationery Office.

DHSS (1989) *Working for Patients*. London: HMSO.

Ellison, G. (1998) Witnessed resuscitation: The relatives' experience. *Emergency Nurse* 58, pp. 27–9.

Glasper, E. A. Stradling, P. (1989) Preparing children for admission. *Paediatric Nursing*, pp. 18–20.

Gove, S.Tamburlini, G., Molyneux, E., Whitesell, P., Campbell, H. (1999) Development and technical basis of simplified guidelines for emergency triage assessment and treatment in developing countries, *Archives of Diseases of Childhood* 81, pp. 473–7.

Hanson, C., Strawser, D. (1992) Family presence during cardiopulmonary resuscitation. Foote hospital emergency departments nine year perspective. *Journal of Emergency Nursing* 18 (2), pp. 104–6.

Harrison, M. (1991) The minor head injury, *Paediatric Nursing* 3 (10), pp. 15–19.

Heller, D. (1994) Ambulatory paediatrics: Stepping out in a new direction. *Archives of Disease in Childhood* 70, pp. 339–42.

Higson, J., Bolland, R. (2000) Telephone follow up after paediatric day surgery, *Paediatric Nursing* 12 (10), pp. 30–2.

Hughes, J., Callery, P. (2004) Parents' experiences of caring for their child following day case surgery. *Journal of Child Health* 8 (1), pp. 47–58.

Hull, D., Johnston, D. (1999) *Essential Paediatrics*. Edinburgh: Churchill Livingstone).

Jarvis, A. (1998) Parental presence during resuscitation: Attitudes of staff on a paediatric intensive care unit. *Intensive and critical care nursing* 4, pp. 3–7.

Kristensson-Hallstrom, I., Gunnel, E., Elander, G., Malmfors, G. (1997) Increased parental participation in a paediatric surgical day-care unit. *Journal of Clinical Nursing* 6 (4), pp. 297–302.

Mattick, A., Clegg, G., Beattie, T., Ahmad, T. (2002) A randomised controlled trial comparing a tissue adhesive with adhesive strips for paediatric laceration repair. *Emergency Medicine Journal* 19, pp. 405–7.

Mosby (1995) *Mosby's Pocket Dictionary of Nursing, Medicine and Professions Allied to Health*. London: Mosby.

Offringa, M., Moyer V.A., (2001) Evidence based paediatrics: Evidence based management of seizures associated with fever. *British Medical Journal* 323 (7321), pp. 1111–14.

Rattrie, E. (2000) Witnessed resuscitation: Good practice or not. *Nursing Standard* 14 (24), pp. 32–5.

Resuscitation Council (1996) *Should Relatives Witness Resuscitation*. London: Resuscitation Council UK.

Resuscitation Council (2000) Resuscitation Guidelines for Use in the United Kingdom. London: Resuscitation Council.

Robertson, J. (2001) Development outcomes do not differ for early or delayed tympanostomy tube insertion in young children with otitis media. *Evidence Based Nursing* 4 (4), p. 108.

Robinson, S., Mackenzie-Ross, S., Campbell Hewson, G. L. Egleston, C. V., Provost, A. T. (1998) Psychological effect of witnessed resuscitation on bereaved relatives. *The Lancet* 352, pp. 614–17.

Rose, J., Watcha, M. (1999) Post operative nausea and vomiting in paediatric patients. *British Journal of Anaesthesia* 83 (1), pp. 104–17.

Rosenczweig, C. (1998) Should relatives witness resuscitation? Ethical issues and practical considerations. *Canadian Medical Association* 158 (5), pp. 617–20.

Rovers, M., Schilder A,, Zielhuis, G., Rosenfeld, R. (2004) Otitis media. *The Lancet* 363, pp. 465–73.

Royal College of Nursing (2004) *Discharge Planning*. London: RCN.

Rushforth, H., Bliss, A., Burge, D., Glasper, A. (2000) Nurse-led pre-operative assessment: A study of appropriateness. *Paediatric Nursing* 4 (2), pp. 15–20.

Simini, B. (1999) Preoperative fasting. *The Lancet* 353 (9156), p. 862.

Smith, F. (1995) *Children's Nursing in Practice: The Nottingham Model*. Oxford: Blackwell Science.

Smith, L., Daughtrey, H. (2000) Weaving the seamless web of care: An analysis of parents' perceptions of their needs following discharge of their child from hospital. *Journal of Advanced Nursing* 31 (4), pp. 812–20.

Thomas, R., Taylor, K. (1997) Assessing head injuries in children. *American Journal of Maternal/Child Nursing* 22 (4), pp. 198–202.

Thornes, R. (1991) *Caring for Children in the Health Services Just for the Day*. London: Action for Sick Children.

Turner, G. (1998) Parents' experiences of ambulatory care. *Paediatric Nursing* 10 (8), pp. 12–16.

Walker, W. (1999) Do relatives have the right to witness resuscitation? *Journal of Clinical Nursing* 8 (6), pp. 625–30.

Walsh, M., Kent, A. (2001) *Accident and Emergency Nursing*. Oxford: Butterworth Heineman.

Warren, A. (2000) Paediatric coma scoring researched and benchmarked. *Paediatric Nursing* 12 (3), pp. 14–18.

Williams, K. (1996) Witnessing resuscitation can help relatives. *Nursing Standard* 11 (3), p. 12.

Wong, D. (1995) *Whaley and Wong's Nursing Care of Infants and Children*, 5th edn. St. Louis: Mosby.

7

Acute Care
Lynda Smith

Learning outcomes

- Analyse current healthcare provision/policy with respect to acute care.
- Discuss the specific healthcare needs of young people.
- Analyse the care of children with acute medical and surgical needs.

Introduction

This chapter explores healthcare provision within secondary care focusing on the nursing management of a range of acute care problems. Concepts that underpin care delivery will be explored such as consent and the specific needs of young people. This is set within the context of a changing healthcare environment. *The National Service Framework Standard for Hospital Services* (Department of Health 2003) aims to ensure that care and services delivered to children is child-centred, appropriate and accessible. The standards it lays out to guide services over the next ten years should be used to inform service provision and delivery as it is integral to the delivery of safe, suitable and quality care for children and families. We know from Chapter 6 'Ambulatory care' that services are being restructured and reconfigured to use available resources most appropriately for the provision of services that meet the needs of today's population. How this is impacting on the provision of acute care needs to be considered as the triggers are worked through.

! Trigger 7.1: Acute appendix

The intention of this trigger is to explore the care of young people within acute care settings as experienced within the context of a young person undergoing surgery.

The Trigger

> The Surgery
> Newbridge Rd
> Newbridge
> NE55 1BL
> 17/01/05
>
> Dear Dr. Jones
> Re Jackie Day DOB 12/01/90 LMP24/12/04
> Thank you for seeing this 15 year old girl with abdominal pain. She presented at the surgery with a 3 day history of central abdominal pain, now locating right lower quadrant. Low grade pyrexia 37.5c. Diagnosis probable appendicitis.
>
> Yours......

Situation

Jackie has been admitted to CSU (Children's Surgical Unit). This is a mixed sex ward admitting children from 0–16 years. The ward layout is three bays of four beds and eight single rooms. There is a playroom for all ages.

Feedback

You have a particular interest in working with young people. With reference to the development of young people and their care needs in hospital prepare a seminar presentation that you have been asked to deliver to the working party of your hospital Trust charged with the implementation of the *National Service Framework for Children, Young People and Maternity Services* (Department of Health 2004).

The facts

What are the main facts in this trigger? Make a list:

Hypotheses: What may these facts mean?

- Jackie is a teenager being nursed with a young age group.
- Jackie has abdominal pain this will need investigation.
- Jackie may need surgery as appendicitis is suspected.

Questions developed from the hypotheses

1. How does appendicitis present?
2. What specific care needs will Jackie have with regards to appendicitis?
3. What are the specific needs of young people in hospital?

Trigger 7.1: Fixed resource material

Read the following to help you answer the questions. (You may also wish to search and review other up-to-date research and evidence-based literature, and seek other relevant resources to provide you with the answers to your questions.)

Barnes, K. (2003) *Paediatrics A Clinical Guide for Practitioners*. Edinburgh: Butterworth Heinemann.
Dimond, B. (1996) *The Legal Aspects of Child Healthcare*. London: Mosby.
Department of Health (1989) *Children Act*. London: The Stationery Office.
www.dh.gov.uk/nsf/children
www.doh.gov.uk/consent
www.clinicalevidence.com

Trigger 7.1: Fixed resource sessions

Appendicitis

Acute appendicitis can occur at any age, additionally there is a genetic predisposition where there is a family history of this problem (Gauderer et al 2003). It is the most common indication for emergency surgery in children ranging from neonates to adolescents. The peak age for occurrence is adolescence and the late teenage years (Rothrock and Pagane 2000).

Acute appendicitis is acute inflammation of the appendix, a narrow sac that is attached to the caecum. It is not known precisely what causes appendicitis although obstruction is seen as the most likely cause, either of faeces or foreign body, if surgery is delayed the appendix perforates leading to peritonitis or abscess formation. The function of the appendix is unknown (Nursing Times 2003) although Rothrock and

Pagane (2000) suggest that it may have a specialised role in the immune system.

Typical presentation is expressed by Barnes in the form of a mnemonic LAMENT (Barnes 2003) However in paediatric patients a large number; 50–70 per cent present atypically and, therefore, for each typical presentation it must be remembered that this may not be the case for a significant number of children who are ultimately diagnosed with appendicitis. Many of the presenting features of appendicitis are age related due to anatomical and developmental differences and understanding these may help in the diagnosis (Rothrock and Pagane 2000).

- Leucocytosis: WBC (White Blood Count) is commonly obtained although the accuracy of the findings in informing the diagnosis is limited.
  Anorexia: Common feature across most age groups.
  Migration of pain: The patient presents with central abdominal pain moving to the right iliac fossa although this sequence does vary, for some patients the pain remains central and for others it starts and remains in the right lower quadrant
  Elevated temperature usually greater than 37.5 degrees Celsius, increasing as symptoms persist to in excess of 39 degrees Celsius.
  Nausea and vomiting: Common feature of appendicitis for all ages, the difficulty is that this can be a feature of a number of problems.
  Tenderness in the right lower quadrant.

The history and examination in Jackie's age group are more reliable, you may wish to explore the presentational differences in a younger age group and the rationale for why they are more likely to present atypically. The order in which symptoms occur varies for different age groups.

One of the recurring challenges is to diagnose appendicitis accurately and thereby prevent perforation, abscess formation and the risk of post-operative complications. In children the presenting features of their illness can be mistaken for gastroenteritis, upper and lower respiratory tract infections, urinary tract infections, gynaecological problems to name but a few of a long list of possible diagnoses. Adolescent girls in particular need to have other pathology checked such as gynaecological or urinary tract problems as they are a group who are at particular risk of misdiagnosis (Barnes 2003).

Diagnosis is based on clinical examination, rectal examination and diagnostic scans such as ultrasound, CT (computed tomography), diagnostic laparoscopy. Rectal examination for tenderness is controversial as there is a lack of evidence to support its value as a diagnostic aid (Rothrock and Pagane 2000). CT scans and ultrasound are valuable aids but still not infallible (Kassutto 2003). Ultrasound is advantageous for female patients in assessing gynaecological causes that can mimic appendicitis as can diagnostic laparoscopy. These reduce the chance of a normal appendix being removed (*Nursing Times* 2003). Plain abdominal X rays have also been used to evaluate the risk of appendicitis but are not reliable in uncomplicated appendicitis (Rothrock and

Barnes 2003; Pagane 2000). Clinical and computer assisted scoring systems (based on clinical and laboratory examination to predict appendicitis) have also been utilised to improve early diagnosis. Studies suggest these are of more value to use with older children (Kassutto 2003; Rothrock and Pagane 2000). In the absence of definitive clinical findings and with limitations with the tests available the diagnosis of appendicitis in children remains extremely difficult.

In females of child-bearing age it is important to ascertain if she is sexually active. With a diagnosis of suspected appendicitis a pregnancy test is usually carried out. This is of course a sensitive area of practice and consideration needs to be given to the individual's right to privacy and confidentiality and consent.

Consent

One of the key messages embodied in the National Service Framework is that services should be child-centred. In particular children and their families should be active partners in decisions about their health care and where possible, be able to exercise choice (Department of Health 2003). The United Nations Convention on Rights of the Child, ratified in this country in 1991, (United Nations 1989) and the Children Act (Department of Health 1989) embody this perspective that children should be consulted and given information and choice regarding their treatment. However the issue of consent in children is a complex area, particularly for teenagers. The question being, can children and specifically in Jackie's case consent for themselves? Consent is required before you examine, treat or care for patients.

Guidance on consent is issued by the Department of Health (Department of Health 2001) underpinned by the law. Legally young people aged 18 have full autonomy to consent or refuse treatment. Aged 16 and 17 they can give valid consent to treatment as they are deemed competent.

Under 16 years consent is legally valid if the person is deemed competent by their doctor. Historically this initially resulted from a court case involving Mrs Gillick who challenged the right of doctors to prescribe the contraceptive pill to her daughter without her knowledge. The landmark ruling deemed consent to be valid in those under 16 if they were considered to be able to make an informed decision (Gillick v Norfolk and Wisbech Area Health Authority and the DHSS 1986). The Children Act also enabled 'competent' children to refuse medical or psychiatric examination.

The issue of consent in children and young people under 16 becomes potentially contentious as there are no criteria in place that define a competent child, leaving it open to interpretation by individual doctors. Additionally as Ross-Trevor points out there is no distinction made between the giving and refusing of consent (Ross-Trevor 1996). In effect this lack of criteria allows for challenges to be made regarding decisions of the 'competent' child resulting in some instances in litigation. This has led to cases where the wishes of the young person have been overridden. It also leads to precedents being set in law that can then be used to influence future cases (Alderson 2000).

The emphasis placed by the NSF (Department of Health 2003, p. 17) is on Trusts to have policies in place that incorporate the guidance from the Department of Health and Professional bodies and also what to do where there is disagreement between the young person and their parent or between the family and the health professional. This should further be underpinned by valid, accurate, up-to-date, accessible and clearly presented information appropriate to their level of understanding so that an informed decision can be made as to whether to consent or refuse treatment.

→ Trigger 7.1: Feedback

Go to Chapter 7 Trigger feedback on p. 198

! Trigger 7.2: Bronchiolitis

The intention of this trigger is to explore the acute care needs of a patient and family with a medical problem.

The Trigger

Hallam Hospital NHS Trust
Day Assessment unit

Hospital No. 03561892   **Date**: 20/01/05   **Time**: 10.30am
Name: Jo Jones   **DOB**: 20/10/04   **Age**: 3 months
Address: 1 Priory Lane   **Next of Kin**: Jane and John Jones
Hallam, S45 1DG
Reason for assessment   **Allergies**
Wheeze and poor feeding   None known
Current Medication   **Contact with infectious illnesses**
None   None
Assessment:
Observations   **Weight**: 7.0Kgs
T 38.0 c
P 140
R 40
BP
Oxygen saturation 95%
History: 2 day history of coryza and snuffles, cough, temperature, not completing feeds (completing half). Worse today now wheezy and struggling to breathe when feeding

---

Examination:
Colour: Pink
Awake and alert
Mild subcostal recession
Diagnosis: Bronchiolitis   **Investigations:** NPA
Plan: Observe during feed and reassess
Paracetamol for pyrexia
Review
Marked recession and drop in oxygen saturation 92% Increased Respiratory rate to 50/minute completed third of feed   Admit Children's Ward

Situation

Jo aged three months has been admitted to the medical ward from the assessment unit. She has a provisional diagnosis of bronchiolitis. Both parents are with Jo and they have been admitted into a single room. Mum is going to be resident on the ward with her. She is their first baby. Jo was a full term baby following a normal delivery and no neonatal problems.

Feedback

Assessment is a key nursing skill and is an ongoing process in a systematic approach to nursing care. Using a head to toe approach identify with rationale your assessment of Jo. When undertaking this type of assessment it is necessary to prioritise depending on the child's presenting problem

The facts

What are the main facts in this trigger? Make a list:

Hypotheses: What may these facts mean?

- Jo may have bronchiolitis.
- Jo is experiencing respiratory distress.
- Feeding is more difficult with this illness.
- Jo's parents will be distressed by her problems.

Questions developed from the hypotheses

1. What is bronchiolitis?
2. What care will Jo need during her admission to hospital?
3. How can Jo's parents be supported during Jo's admission?

Trigger 7.2: Fixed resource material

Read the following to help you answer the questions. (You may also wish to search and review other up-to-date research and evidence-based literature, and seek other relevant resources to provide you with the answers to your questions.)

Barnes, K. (2003) *Paediatrics A Clinical Guide for Nurse Practitioners*. Edinburgh: Butterworth Heinemann.

Huband, S., Trigg, E. (2000) *Practices in Children's Nursing*. Edinburgh: Churchill Livingstone.

Peter, S., Fazakerley, M. (2004) Clinical effectiveness of integrated care pathway for infants with bronchiolitis. *Paediatric Nursing* 16 (1), pp. 30–5.

Smith, L., Coleman, V., Bradshaw, M. (2002) *Family Centred Care: Concept, Theory and Practice*. Basingstoke: Palgrave.

Trigger 7.2: Fixed resource sessions

Bronchiolitis

Bronchiolitis is an acute, highly communicable lower respiratory tract infection that predominantly affects infants and young children. The illness is characterised by cough, coryza, tachypnoea, wheeze, subcostal recession and fever and the infant experiences feeding difficulty. It is a viral illness mainly caused by the Respiratory Syncytial Virus (RSV) and occurs in the winter months. In this country 20 per cent of admissions for lower respiratory tract infections are due to RSV (Handforth 2004). Infants tolerate the illness less well due to their smaller narrower airways. The severity of the illness varies from mild cases that can be managed at home to the most severe requiring admission to hospital and in some cases in need of ventilator support in intensive care. Particular groups of patients are at risk of this being a life-threatening illness including those born prematurely, those with existing disorders such congenital cardiac anomalies and babies in the first few weeks of life (Harrop 2003; Peter 2003).

For those infants and children requiring admission to hospital management of bronchiolitis is based on the presenting clinical problems that are related to respiratory and feeding difficulties. Additionally as a highly communicable disease, infection control procedures will need to be followed. The family will need a great deal of support as it is very distressing to see their baby struggling to breathe and to feed and it is potentially a life-threatening illness. Chapter 3 'Contemporary family-centred care' will help you to consider how and in what practical ways a family-centred approach to care can help Jo's parents at this time.

Breathing: Respiratory support

Ongoing assessment and monitoring of the child's heart rate, respiratory rate and effort and oxygen saturation levels is important as you need to be alert to any deterioration in Jo's condition. Observing her colour and physical state also forms part of your assessment The only approach to management proven to be successful is the administration of oxygen (Handforth 2004). Routine pharmacological treatment of bronchiolitis has proved ineffective. This includes epinephrine, bronchodilators, corticosteroids and ribivirin (Kellner et al 2004; King et al 2004). Antibiotics may be considered where there are other clinical indications such as X ray changes, raised white blood cell count or deterioration (Peter 2003).

Feeding

The effects of symptoms associated with bronchiolitis such as blocked nose, cough, increased respiratory rate and exhaustion result in the baby being unable to feed normally. The degree to which this is affected will determine the management of feeding. It is important, initially, to observe and assess the baby's ability to feed and the amount taken. Fluid requirement is based on 100mls/kg/day to maintain hydration. This is less than the usual requirement of 150mls/kg/day to maintain normal growth and development. Baby's taking less than half their normal feed will need support with their feeding. This may be either by nasogastric feed or if the baby is unable to tolerate gastric feeding and is becoming distressed then fluids will need to be given intravenously to allow the baby to rest. Monitoring the baby's output will also indicate hydration status. It is important that parents are involved and understand the implications of their baby's condition with regards to feeding and the ways in which they can be involved if they wish to. Both verbal and written information is needed to support parents and for those who want to be involved in nasogastric feeding for example then the nurse's role as teacher and facilitator is a key part of family-centred care.

Infection Control

Diagnosis of bronchiolitis is based on clinical signs and from obtaining a nasopharyngeal aspirate (NPA) that detects the presence of RSV. The use of testing to provide a definitive diagnosis enables the cohorting of patients which is essential due to the highly infectious nature of the disease. However evidence suggests it would be more logical to isolate all infants with acute lower respiratory tract infection regardless of cause as knowing that RSV is the cause does not change the clinical course (Bordley et al 2004). Different Trusts will adopt their own infection control procedures in this instance and, therefore, there may be variation in practice in terms of testing for bronchiolitis.

Regardless of whether testing takes place or not infected babies and children are usually cohort nursed or nursed in single cubicles with the aim of preventing the spread of infection. Standard precautions and transmission-based precautions according to local policy will be followed. Hand washing before and after patient contact is essential. RSV is easily transmitted in respiratory secretions and can be passed on through direct and indirect contact. This is vital as the virus can stay on the hands for 30 minutes (Peter 2003). Protective clothing, use of gloves, safe disposal of clinical waste and infected linen, disinfection and cleaning of equipment are all precautions designed to reduce the risk of transmission. This includes not only staff but all family members and visitors.

Bronchiolitis is a self-limiting illness that responds to supportive care as discussed previously. Follow up is not usually required after discharge. A proportion of infants will be prone to recurrent wheezy episodes although most will have grown out of it by 2–3 years of age, although some will go on to be diagnosed with asthma (Peters 2003).

➡ Trigger 7.2: Feedback

Go to Chapter 7 Trigger feedback on p. 198

❗ Trigger 7.3: Fractured Femur

The purpose of this trigger is the specific care needs of children presenting with an acute problem, in this instance a fractured femur that involves a longer stay in hospital than the typical 2.1 days.

The Trigger

Handover from A&E staff to nurse on ward:

This is Luke and his mum. He is 10 years old and was involved in an accident while riding his bike. He arrived in A&E with injuries to his left leg and minor abrasions to left arm. No head injury. He was in a lot of pain and was given entinox and oromorph. X ray confirmed fractured midshaft of femur and splint in place. Neurovascular observations normal. Orthopaedic registrar is on his way.

Situation

Luke has been admitted to the orthopaedic ward at the children's hospital via accident and emergency. It is school holidays and both Luke and his seven year old sister spend time with grandparents while their mother is at work. The children do not have any contact with their father. On admission Luke's mother is with him having arrived at the hospital from work, Lucy has remained with her grandparents at home.

Feedback

As a senior student nurse nearing the end of your course, part of your competency elements in practice on this placement is to teach others. Prepare a teaching session for other students on a specific aspect of Luke's care. You will need to demonstrate underpinning knowledge and rationale to the care selected within the context of Luke's specific needs.

The facts

> What are the main facts in this trigger? Make a list:

Hypotheses: What may these facts mean?

- Luke has a problem that involves a lengthy treatment.
- Luke's mobility is going to be severely affected.

- Luke will be anxious about what the treatment entails.
- Luke's mum may be anxious about implications of any longer term care needs.

Questions developed from the hypotheses

1. What treatment approaches are available to manage a fractured femur?
2. What are the nursing care needs of a patient with a fractured femur?
3. What support will Luke and his family need on, before and after discharge?

Trigger 7.3: Fixed resource material

Read the following to help you answer the questions. (You may also wish to search and review other up-to-date research and evidence-based literature, and seek other relevant resources to provide you with the answers to your questions.)

www.bbc.co.uk/gcsebitesizerevision: This website is useful as a starting point for anatomy and physiology before moving on to more detailed texts
Anatomy and Physiology Made Incredibly Easy (2005) Philadelphia: Lippincott Williams and Wiley.
Beaty, J., Kasse, J. (eds) (2001) Rockwood and Wilkins Fractures in Children, 5th edn. Philadelphia: Lippincott Williams and Wiley.
Ross Wilson, (1996) Anatomy and physiology in health and illness. Edinburgh: Churchill Livingstone.
Tortora, G. Reynolds, S. (2003) Principles of anatomy and physiology. New York: Wiley.

Trigger 7.3: Fixed resource sessions

Fractures

Fractures can occur at any age and are most commonly the result of an accident. In infancy other causes also need to be considered such as non-accidental injury and congenital conditions such as osteogenesis imperfecta.

To understand what happens when a bone fractures it will be useful to have reviewed the structure, development and function of long bones. Key points summarised from the anatomy and physiology text books indicated in the resources are detailed below and can be used as a guide to your further reading.

The development of bone begins before birth and is not complete until adulthood. When fully developed it is one of the hardest connective tissues in the body.

Long bones develop from cartilage. From a primary centre of ossification in the middle of the rod of cartilage enzyme action on osteoblast cells leads to bone formation and mineralization (mainly calcium phosphate). These become osteocytes once they are established in the lacunae. From the primary centre of ossification the diaphysis of the bone is formed and spreads out towards each end. Each end becomes the epiphysis where secondary centres for ossification form usually after birth. Bones grow in length from the epiphyseal cartilage which is between the epiphysis and the diaphysis.

The diaphysis or shaft is composed of mainly compact bone. This bone consists of units called haversian systems. These contain haversian canals (containing blood, nerves and lymphatics), lamellae (concentric plates of bone) and lacunae in the spaces between the lamellae containing lymph and osteocytes (bone cells).

The epiphyses are composed of a thin layer of compact bone inside which is cancellous bone which has a sponge like appearance. Cancellous bone also contains haversian canals and some lamellae. It also contains red bone marrow in which erythrocytes, leucocytes and thrombocytes are formed and mature.

The outer surface of bone has a protective membrane covering; the periosteum which also provides attachment for muscle tendons and ligaments. It also contains osteoblasts.

Fractures are a result of the stress applied to the bone being greater than the resistance of the bone. The fracture is complete when the fragments of bone are separated and incomplete when bone fragments remain attached. Children's bones because they are not fully developed and therefore as hard as adult bones are more flexible. This means they are more prone to certain types of fractures. Following Campbell and Glasper (1995) these are summarised in Table 7.1.

Table 7.1 Childhood fractures

Fracture	Description
Bends	The bone does not break but bends because of the flexibility of a child's bone. The bone does straighten but not completely revealing a deformity. Bends are commonly in the ulna and fibula and may be associated with fractures of the radius and tibia.
Buckle	Occurs more commonly in younger children as a result of compression of the porous bone which buckles. This occurs on the portion of bone shaft next to the epiphysis.
Greenstick	This is an incomplete fracture. The bone angulates beyond the limits of bending but does not break completely. Known as greenstick because it resembles the way a greenstick breaks.
Complete	Bone is completely divided.

Source: Abridged from Campbell and Glasper (1995)

When a child sustains a fracture they may present with a range of clinical signs. These include swelling, pain, tenderness, bruising, deformity and a change in function in the affected limb. These can appear to a greater or lesser extent depending on the individual and the type and location of the fracture.

Managing fractures involves the 3 R's of treatment

- *Reduce*: Regain alignment and length of the bone, this is known as reduction. There are a number of approaches to reduction which will be explored specifically in the context of a fractured femur in the next fixed resource.
- *Retain* realignment and length this is achieved through immobilization. This enables the bone to heal as callus is formed. Callus is the tissue which grows around fractured ends of bone and develops into new bone to repair the injury.
- *Restore* and re-educate for normal function and use

These 3 aspects form the basis of the management of Luke's fractured femur.

Fractured femur

As you read contemporary approaches to the treatment of fractured femurs reflect on your own experiences in clinical practice identifying where you think the strengths and weaknesses of the choice of approach are for the child and family.

There are a number of treatment options for fractured femur and the choice made by the orthopaedic surgeon will be informed by the child's age, weight, concomitant injuries, type of fracture, stability and location (Buechenschuetz et al 2002; Flynn et al 2002).

During the past decade there has been a trend towards surgical treatment of femoral fractures, the two most common procedures being external fixation (EF) and elastic stable intramedullary nails (ESIN). Alternatively children with fractured femurs are placed in traction and depending on their age (usually less than 6 years old) may later be put into a hip spica cast to continue the period of immobilisation while healing takes place.

A number of research papers have evaluated the effectiveness of these approaches in terms of their clinical outcomes (Flynn et al 2002). All of these approaches demonstrate good clinical outcomes for the patient in terms of healing of the fracture. Consideration of wider issues is, therefore, an important part of deciding upon approach such as complications, cost, acceptability to the child and family, impact on the family of lengthy hospitalisation balanced against the support needs that are part of early discharge.

The most challenging age group to manage are the skeletally immature school aged children and adolescents. The younger age group are effectively managed in a hip spica and the much older skeletally mature with the use of the intramedullary nail (Flynn et al 2002).

Traction

Traditionally the school aged group have been managed with a period of traction. Once the limb has been realigned, traction, for example, aThomas splint is applied to keep the bone in position by pulling on it. This can be achieved by using either skin traction where the skin traction kit is applied to the leg and the cord at the end allows a pull to be exerted or for difficult alignments skeletal traction where a pin is inserted in an area of strong bone under general anaesthetic and traction is then applied (Huband and Trigg 2000). It can be balanced (where weights are used) which allows for flexibility in the force exerted or fixed.

The disadvantage is the length of hospital stay, up to two months depending on the age of the child and the injury as this influences the rate of healing. Therefore a long period of immobilization is experienced. Callus formation is regularly monitored radiographically. Nursing care is focused around the activities of living, with particular attention being placed on the following; pain including acute pain associated with the initial injury and management and later muscle spasm, skin care including the traction site and pressure area care Also, performing normal hygiene will be affected and assistance required. Where skeletal traction is used, pin-site care is also needed. Elimination may be more difficult and embarrassing using a bed pan. Decreased mobility may lead to constipation and difficult positioning affecting urination potentially leading to urinary tract infections. Eating and drinking may be affected by loss of appetite. Fluid intake is important to aid elimination and a nutritious diet to aid bone healing. Boredom is a problem and socially and psychologically, play, visitors, schooling are important in providing the child with some routine and normality (Huband and Trigg 2000; Moules and Ramsay 1998). Observations are undertaken for signs of any complications as either the trauma itself or the treatment can cause problems. These are covered in the feedback as a teaching example for a student.

Initiatives to reduce the period of time spent in hospital and for traction to be continued at home have been reported (Clayton 1997; Davies et al 2001) but does require a range of support mechanisms to be in place – in particular a community children's nursing service. Traction is resource intensive. As hospital services are reconfigured there is pressure on acute beds. The need to reduce hospital stay is apparent and this can be seen worldwide not only in this country. Overwhelmingly, if there are ways of managing this problem that reduces the necessity of a prolonged hospital admission for children and their families without compromising outcome then treatment measures that achieve this are to be welcomed.

Surgical intervention

For those children where surgical intervention is indicated the approaches mainly in use include external fixation and flexible intramedullary nail. Studies have evaluated the management and outcome of these procedures including comparative studies of the first two (Buechenschuetz et al 2002; Hedin, 2004; Houshian et al 2004; Mostafa et al 2001).

Each of these methods has advantages and disadvantages and the choice of method will be determined by the clinical presentation of the fracture and any associated injuries and the current practice choice of the surgeon and the hospital.

External fixation: This is a widely available and familiar procedure involving insertion of pins attached to a fixator. The advantage is that mobilization can begin as soon as is tolerated and time spent in hospital significantly reduced. Reintegration back into a normal home and school life can take place with much less disruption than a child who has been hospitalised for up to two months. Reported disadvantages include clinically the risk of pin site infection, delayed union and re-fracture, knee stiffness and from a family's perspective acceptance of the fixator and scarring from the pin sites (Flynn, Skaggs et al 2002; Mostafa et al 2001).

Flexible Intramedullary nail: This also allows rapid mobilization of the patient. It involves the insertion of two flexible nails through the medullary canal up to the fracture site. In effect it provides an internal splint that maintains length and alignment. These nails can later be removed usually 6–12 months after the injury (Flynn et al 2002).

From a nursing perspective there will be many transferable skills associated with a patient undergoing surgery as discussed in previous Triggers in this chapter and Chapter 6 and additional specific considerations because of the particular intervention. Observing for signs of infection because of the invasive nature of the surgery is important. For the child with a fixator pin site care to avoid infection is essential and involves not only the nurse but the child and family who will need to be involved particularly following discharge. Moules and Ramsay (1998) identify that there is no clear consensus regarding the cleaning of pin sites and that local policy and procedure, usually surgeon preference, is followed. Flynn et al (2002) suggest the use of dilute hydrogen peroxide second day post operatively continued until pin entry sites heal. Showering and washing with soap and water are then encouraged. Also there is no consensus whether to cover with woven gauze or leave uncovered and therefore local policy and procedure should be followed.

Restoring function

This will involve physiotherapy to prevent complications of joint stiffness and muscle wasting. Children will be taught exercises to minimise any adverse effects. The physiotherapists will play a crucial role in the mobilisation of children following any of the procedures outlined above. The nurse's role is to support this re-education and to provide ongoing help to the child and family as the child strives to regain normal functioning.

→ Trigger 7.3: Feedback

Go to Chapter 7 Trigger feedback on p. 198 below

? Chapter 7 Trigger feedback: What do you know?

Trigger 7.1: Acute appendix

Question 1: How does appendicitis present?

The presentation of appendicitis can be challenging in children. However, the older child/teenager, that is young people of Jackie's age, more commonly present typically. The detail you should be able to gather from the fixed resource session and additional reading around the subject area

Question 2: What specific care needs will Jackie have?

The nursing care of Jackie undergoing appendicectomy should include the following specific aspects of care. You should be able to use the knowledge gained in Chapter 6 about pre- and post-operative care for the procedures and practices that apply to all patients undergoing surgery.

The surgical approach may be open surgery or laparoscopic. The management of care post-operatively is influenced by the severity of the condition, that is, the degree of inflammation in the appendix and if the appendix perforates.

Jackie has needed open surgery for a severely inflamed appendix, therefore, there are additional areas of nursing care you should have considered.

Pre-operatively: Investigations in support of diagnosis may have included FBC (Full blood count) Urinalysis, radiologic examination.

You will need to have considered your role in support of these investigations as Jackie's advocate and nurse. This may include consent, privacy and confidentiality particularly as sensitive areas of the consultation are undertaken. Consent has been discussed in the second fixed resource session and with further reading you should be aware of the issues and the potential for Jackie to consent herself. Privacy and confidentiality should form part of your answer to question 3.

Jackie will be fasted for theatre, usually outside normal theatre hours this will be on an emergency list, and it is likely that she will have an intravenous infusion sited. In some instances intravenous antibiotics are commenced pre-operatively. Consider the rationale for this approach to care.

Pain assessment and management is important. As Jackie is 15 years old she will be able to articulate clearly the nature and severity of pain experienced and analgesia appropriate to this administered. Protocols for pain management indicate the type of analgesia for the severity of pain indicated. It is also valuable at this stage to discuss the types of pain management available post-operatively so that this can be planned for particularly if PCA (patient controlled analgesia) is required via a morphine infusion.

Body image may be an area that Jackie is anxious about if she is to have open surgery. Location and length of scar for example may be issues that have been discussed with the doctor but need further support from the nurse.

The areas outlined here combined with the relevant information from Chapter 6 on pre-operative care should form a pre-operative care plan designed to meet Jackie's needs.

Post operative Care: In addition to post-operative monitoring to ensure a safe recovery from theatre key areas of care for Jackie include:

- *Pain Management*: Pain levels will continue to be monitored and recorded regularly according to individual hospital Trust policy. Management approaches started pre-operatively will continue. It is likely that Jackie will have received intra operative analgesia to reduce post-operative pain
- *Fluid balance*: Jackie will have an intravenous infusion. The site will need to be checked regularly for signs of extravasation indicated by thrombo phlebitis according to Trust policy. Jackie will initially remain nil by mouth. One of the post-operative complications associated with abdominal surgery is paralytic ileus. Fluids and diet are re-introduced gradually as bowels sounds return. In some instances a naso-gastric tube is passed so that stomach contents, such as gastric juices, that would otherwise collect and cause nausea and vomiting can be drained. Intravenous antibiotic therapy will continue in the immediate post-operative period.
- *Wound care*: With this type of open surgery it is most likely that dissolvable sutures are used. The dressing will be changed the day after surgery and a clear occlusive dressing such as 'opsite' applied. The wound site is observed for signs of infection such as redness. Temperature monitoring will continue for signs of pyrexia indicative of infection.
- *Mobilisation*: This will need encouragement post-operatively and Jackie will need to be supported initially as patients can be reluctant following abdominal surgery for fear of pain particular if they straighten up. Good pain management will also help mobilisation.
- *Discharge*: Timing of discharge will depend on the post-operative recovery of the individual. Management of care in the areas highlighted will indicate when Jackie is ready for discharge. Family support on discharge is important and, therefore, clinically and in conjunction with Jackie and her family discharge will be planned to meet these requirements. Early discharge in uncomplicated

appendectomy like many other surgical procedures is becoming more common. In one reported study this was taking place within 24 hours of surgery provided the patient met strict criteria and were supported by an outreach nurse (Pfeil and Mathur 2004).

Question 3: What are the specific needs of young people?

Seminar: The needs of young people in hospital: In putting together your seminar presentation you should have considered the physical, psychological and social development of adolescents/teenagers. This facilitates links to why young people need to be considered in their own right with regards to service provision. You might briefly refer to some of these in your introduction and highlight how these will be discussed in the context of service provision.

Introduction and Rationale: The needs of adolescents have been referred to specifically in Government reports (Audit Commission 1993; Department of Health 1991; Ministry of Health Central Services Health Council 1959) by professional bodies (Audit Commission 1993; British Paediatric Association 1985; Royal College of Nursing 1994) and have been the subject of research studies (Kari et al 1999; Russell-Johnson 2000). However, it is clear from the most recent publication, the NSF for children, that the experience of young people in hospital still does not meet their needs either they were cared for in an environment suitable for young children or in an adult ward with elderly people, neither of which is appropriate. The NSF identifies that separate adolescent units may be the best solution but acknowledges that this will not always be the case and that many hospitals group young people together in separate bays on a paediatric ward. This indicates that despite much rhetoric on the needs of young people the provision of services is unlikely to include the development of adolescent units. It is important, therefore, that current services are configured to take account of the needs of young people.

Key issues

The following essential areas need to be considered as we review our service provision. These are linked to what earlier writers (Muller, 1992, 1992a) have seen as developmental tasks to be achieved by adolescents as part of their transition to adulthood and centre on their biopsychosocial development. As Muller indicates they would include for example physical and sexual development, developing independence from parents, social skills, academic and vocational skills, norms and values that guide. Hospitalisation can potentially impact on the young person achieving and acquiring these and, therefore, the goal should be to minimise and accommodate the developmental needs of young people in the provision of appropriate facilities and approach to care:

Environment

Location: Adolescent unit or provision of facilities in a general ward environment: There are a small number of adolescent units in the UK. Despite the call for an increase in this type of provision, the care of adolescents has not evolved into a recognised sub speciality unlike in the United States (Shelley 1993). The majority of young people will be nursed in adult or paediatric wards. The difficulty remains that even where the ward has tried to accommodate young people either in single rooms or grouped them into designated bays pressure on beds particularly in the winter months means that this cannot always be guaranteed. This can also be compounded when we consider whether bays should be mixed sex particularly for the older teenager approaching 16 years. Choice is important, providing that choice is available.

Facilities: If part of a young person's transition to adulthood is accommodating their changing body image and their identity formation then the provision of facilities that support this needs to be considered and planned for. More obvious facilities are commonly available such as bathroom door locks, mirrors, full length beds but less consideration has perhaps been given to shaving sockets, sanitary towel disposal. Each area needs to consider a range of facilities they have available and where these can be developed. Asking young people themselves about their experience and any suggestions they may have would be a good start. This could be achieved through Patient satisfaction surveys and involving the PALS (Patient Advisory Liaison Service) representative.

Social and Education

Education is a statutory right. Although provision of a teacher in hospital is available to those children with chronic illnesses requiring recurrent admission to hospital and those whose admission extends beyond two weeks, this can be an anxious time particularly for those undertaking GCSE's. Liaison with school to provide work in their absence is valuable. Provision of a schoolroom or quiet area for study as part of the facilities is needed.

Recreation needs to be considered in the same way, as play is seen as essential to the younger age group. Playrooms are often geared towards the needs of a younger age and a room designed specifically for teenagers would give them an area to socialise in and they would not be sharing with everyone else. In today's technological world of computer games, DVD's would mimic their normal recreational outlet. Maintaining contact with peers would fulfil the social need young people have achieved by encouraging friends as well as family to visit. Part of the ward's policy needs to include ground rules of acceptable behaviour so that there is a balance between freedom and agreed limits, such as being able to leave the ward but ensuring someone knows.

Communication

Privacy and confidentiality: The young person is entitled to have information disclosed kept confidential. This is not to exclude parents but is part of acknowledging that the young person has rights in the same way as adults and, therefore, disclosure would only happen in particular circumstances. This is an important part of a trusting relationship and must be understood by those working with young people. The maintenance of privacy not only in terms of the facilities provided, but also in how practice is conducted. The provision of bed curtains for example does not provide privacy in a bay where it is possible to over hear when often sensitive questions are being asked. Teenagers are easily embarrassed and maintaining their self-esteem is an important part of their identity development. Developing their independence from their parents can be enhanced with clear policies on their involvement in decision-making and seeking their consent.

Conclusion and recommendations

In reviewing the evidence surrounding young people and their needs in hospital the Trust must develop policies and action plans to reflect the key issues presented to this seminar. Particular emphasis must be placed on involving young people in decisions about their care including their preference in the absence of an adolescent unit to be located in either paediatric or adult areas. Respect must be shown for the competent young person to make informed decisions regarding their care and treatment and facilities that meet the physical and social needs of young people should be provided. You might also have considered that much of what has been written about teenagers has tended to be repeated over a number of years and that, while the message remains the same, little has changed. Therefore, what is happening for young people in healthcare and how can we move forward beyond reiterating the same pleas on their behalf is important.

Trigger 7.2: Bronchiolitis

Questions 1 and 2: What is bronchiolitis and what care is needed?

These should have been able to be answered from the fixed resource and the supportive reading.

Question 3: What support would Jo's parents need?

It is important to think about the level of anxiety they will naturally be feeling. Parents are distressed by seeing their child ill in this way. It is frightening, particularly when a child has respiratory distress. As first time parents they are still coming to terms with their role as parents. Parents often feel guilty wondering if it is something they have or have not done. Providing information about bronchiolitis and its treatment will help them understand what is happening, how it is a common problem in babies and how they can be involved in caring for Jo. Using your communication skills, verbal and non-verbal, will help them to come to terms with Jo's problems and feel able to contribute at a level that suits them at different points during their stay in hospital. Chapter 3 'Contemporary family-centred care', focuses on the role of the nurse and family and the involvement of families in negotiated care that empowers them to participate.

Assessment of a baby

When admitting any patient, assessment is the first part of the nursing process. It is an ongoing process as you gather information that enables the development of a plan of care that is holistic to the needs of the individual child and family. While this is a head to toe assessment, in practice you would prioritise your assessment according to the presenting problem, therefore, for Jo, presenting with respiratory distress, your first concern would be to assess this followed by associated areas of concern such as possible dehydration if oral intake had been decreased. For a baby, for example, referred with diarrhoea and vomiting, your first concern might be to assess for signs of dehydration such as checking if the anterior fontanelle is depressed. This is linked to and applied to your knowledge of anatomy, physiology and normal development, thus at what age the fontanelles are open and what the indications of your observations are. I have always found it useful to have a diagram of a baby and add to it key areas of assessment. Having a visual picture then helps you to work systematically through the assessment. Below are some of the areas I would cover including an example of what you would be looking for. You can develop this by working through this outline with regards to Jo, there may have other areas to add:

- Head
  - Conscious level, alert, exhausted
  - Fontanelles: anterior posterior – open/closed, tense/bulging, sunken
  - Hair: clean, head lice
  - Eyes: discharge, dark/hollow/sunken, squint, spectacles
  - Nose: nasal flaring, discharge
  - Ears: discharge, foreign body, hearing
  - Mouth: sore, thrush, furred tongue, mucous membranes
- Chest
  - Sub-costal and intercostals recession
  - Rate, rhythm, depth respiration, noise, e.g., stridor, wheeze, cough, grunting
- Abdomen
  - Distension, rigidity, pain

- Limbs
  - Arms: movement, muscle wasting

- Fingers: nails clean/dirty clubbing
- Legs: movement, gait, muscle wasting
● Skin
  - Clean/ dirty odour, turgor dry/inelastic, bruises/ cuts/ abrasions, rash
  - Colour: perfusion/cyanosis, temperature – hot/ cold clammy sweating
  - Pressure sores
● Genitalia
  - Descended testes
  - Buttocks sore/rash/ thrush urine/faeces
● General
  - Observations: temperature, heart rate/pulse, blood pressure, weight, height/ length, developmental level
● Psychosocial
  - Child/family fears/anxieties, family dynamics, environment

It may read like a list, but as you assess you will be applying your knowledge and understanding of normal growth and development, normal ranges for observations, identifying any deviations and alterations in health status. From working through triggers in this and other chapters you will have also be utilising the underpinning rationale for the significance of your findings.

Trigger 7.3: Fractured femur

Questions 1 and 2: What treatment approaches are available to manage a fractured femur? What are the nursing care needs of a patient with a fractured femur?

These should have been located in the fixed resource sessions and suggested further reading.

Question 3: What support will Luke and his family need on, before and after discharge?

From the fixed resources you will have identified that Luke will need a period in hospital, the length determined by the treatment selected. This will have variable implications for the support need during hospitalisation. The family do have the support of grandparents and this will be valuable in helping Luke's mother who will need to continue working and also provide the support needed to Luke's sister. As it is school holidays the disruption to Luke's education will be minimised which is an important consideration. There is statutory provision for education for sick children. If Luke's period of hospitalisation continues into school time then education will be provided in hospital in consultation with Luke's school. If Luke has a fixator or intramedullary nail, returning to his usual school will need consideration with regards to his safety if access is difficult. Return to school within two to three weeks of surgery have been reported (Buechenschuetz 2002). If suitable arrangements cannot be made for Luke to return to his school, home tuition would need to be offered. It is important that Luke's sister is included and the family unit maintained. Siblings can feel left out if another child's needs seem to be monopolising family time. Luke will need to have follow up over a long period to monitor the healing taking place and long-term sequalae.

Teaching session

This teaching session is based upon developing knowledge and understanding and skill in relation to neurovascular observations.

The fixed resources and your additional reading will help you create an interactive experiential teaching and learning experience for the students. You may choose to present some of the theoretical elements and rationale as a small group teaching session in the clinical area separate from the patient, who probably does not want to hear the potential complications associated with compartment syndrome and the practical element of conducting observations at the bedside with the patient stressing the importance of these observations as part of their recovery.

Neurovascular observations and acute compartment syndrome

Resources used:

Campbell, S., Glapser, E. A. (1995) *Whaley and Wong's Children's Nursing*. London: Mosby.

Edwards, S. (2004) Acute compartment syndrome. *Emergency Nurse* 12 (3), pp. 32–8.

Large, T. (2003) Compartment syndrome of the leg after treatment of a femoral fracture with an early sitting spica cast: A report of two cases. *The Journal of Bone and Joint Surgery* 85 (11), pp. 2207–10.

Middleton, C. (2003) Compartment syndrome: The importance of early diagnosis. *Nursing Times* 99 (21), pp. 30–2.

Acute compartment syndrome

Compartment syndrome is an acute orthopaedic emergency that most commonly follows trauma to the limbs. It results from elevated tissue pressure within an osseofascial compartment caused either by an increase in the contents of the compartment such as blood or other fluids or a decrease in the volume of the compartment such as when a cast or dressing causes constriction. Compartments are areas in the body where muscle, nerves and blood vessels are confined within inelastic boundaries composed of skin fascia (connective tissue) and or bone. As compartment pressure rises above arteriolar pressure, capillary flow decreases while venous outflow is obstructed. This impairs perfusion to compartment structures which results in muscle ischaemia. Necrosis of muscle, nerve and skin tissue may result from this oxygen deprivation

Compartment syndrome following a paediatric femoral fracture can result from a combination of arterial spasm, increased tissue pressures from the injury, direct pressure and elevation of the leg.

Treatment requires relief of pressure. Where a child is in a cast there should be a low threshold for splitting the cast. It may be necessary to undergo surgery; fasciotomy, which involves making an incision and cutting away the fascia to relieve the tension or pressure.

Signs and symptoms

- *Pain*: This appears disproportionate to the injury. Diagnosis of compartment syndrome in children can be difficult as classic signs are often unreliable in children and that increasing analgesia need may be a reliable indicator (Large 2003).
- *Pallor*: This is caused by poor capillary return. The obstructed circulation may make digits appear pale, mottled or bluish in colour.
- *Parathesis*: Altered sensation such as tingling or pins and needles.
- *Paralysis*: A later sign will be that the patient will eventually be unable to move the digits on the affected limb.
- *Pulselessness*: Distal pulses – radial or pedal may be present intermittent, weak or absent. The presence of a pulse does not exclude the diagnosis of compartment syndrome.

A diagnosis of acute compartment syndrome does not need all five signs to be present. Early detection and treatment are essential to avoid irreversible damage. Nerve tissue is capable of regeneration but muscle tissue once infarcted can never recover. Prevention is, therefore, the goal and this can be achieved by careful observation.

Neurovascular observations

These observations should be carried out frequently for a minimum of 12 hours after the injury and usually for a longer period. Huband and Trigg (2000) suggest 24 to 48 hours. This may be determined by the child's condition and local policy and procedure.

From the signs, and signs already identified, the following observations are undertaken to assess their presence and recorded on the patient's chart. Usually this is hourly unless the patient's condition indicates a more frequent observation. Gradually the frequency is reduced until being stopped as indicated above:

- *Colour*: Look at the colour of digits and record what you see. Are they pink or pale bluish or mottled?
- *Temperature*: Touch the digits and record what you feel. Are they warm/hot, cool/cold/clammy?
- *Movement*: Ask the patient to move the digits. Is the movement good, limited, painful? Can they extend them? If patients are asleep this action is carried out by the nurse, noting the reaction to the extension.

- *Sensation*: You need to check all digits, asking the patient about any numbness or tingling or pins and needles.
- *Pulse*: This is checked pre-operatively. Subsequent checking of the pulse of the affected limb identifies, if it is present, strong, faint or intermittent.
- *Pain*: As highlighted previously disproportionate pain is a good indicator of acute compartment syndrome, particularly in children and should be reported as soon as any concerns are felt.

These observations need also to take cognisance of what is the norm for an individual child, if for example they have neurovascular deficits by virtue of pre-existing conditions. This reiterates the importance of holistic assessment of individual patients.

This is a serious potential complication and the significance of undertaking and accurately recording neurovascular observations cannot be overstated. Prompt action on any untoward signs is key to averting or limiting any damage to muscle nerve or skin tissue.

Reflect on your learning

- Acute care provision needs to respond to current changes and developments in healthcare provision.
- Young people have specific healthcare needs which, are acknowledged and now need to be acted upon.
- Hospital admissions are becoming shorter as technology increases and patterns of care change.
- Support in the community from children's nurses needs to continue to be expanded to meet the increased need resulting from shorter hospital admissions.
- The involvement of children young people and their families in the care process is increasing and this needs to be accompanied by effective expansive support mechanisms.

References

Alderson, P. (2000) The rise and fall of children's consent to surgery. *Paediatric Nursing* 12 (2), pp. 6–8.

Audit Commission (1993) *Children First – A Study of Hospital Services*. London: HMSO.

Barnes, K. (ed) (2003) *Paediatrics A Clinical Guide for Nurse Practitioners*. Edinburgh: Butterworth Heinemann.

British Paediatric Association (1985) *Needs and Care of Adolescents*. London: British Paediatric Association.

Buechenschuetz, K. E., Mehlman, C., Shaw, K. J., Crawford, A. H., Immerman, E. B. (2002) Femoral shaft fractures in children: Traction and casting versus Elastic Stable Intramedullary Nailing. *The Journal of Trauma Injury Infection and Critical Care* 53 (5), pp. 914–21.

Campbell, S., Glasper, E. A. (1995) *Whaley and Wong's Children's Nursing*. London: Mosby.

Clayton, M. (1997) Traction at home: The Doncaster approach. *Paediatric Nursing* 9 (2), pp. 21–3.

Clayton, M., Bordley, W., Viswanathan, M., King, V. J., Sutton, S. F., Jackman, A. M., Sterling, L., Lohr, K. N. (2004) Diagnosis and testing in bronchiolitis. *Archives of Pediatrics and Adolescent Medicine* 158 (2), pp. 119–26.

Davies, R. A., Stanislas, M. J. C., Walsh, H. P. J. (2001) A retrospective review of a hospital at home scheme for non-operative treatment of paediatric femoral shaft injuries. *Journal of orthopaedic Nursing* 5 (3), pp. 136–41.

Department of Health (1989) *Children Act*. London: The Stationery Office.

Department of Health (1991) *Welfare of Children and Young People in Hospital*. London: HMSO.

Department of Health (2001) *Reference Guide to Consent for Examination or Treatment*. London: Department of Health.

Department of Health (2003) *Getting the Right Start: National Service Framework for Children: Standard for Hospital Services*. London: Department of Health.

Department of Health (2004) *National Service Framework for Children, Young People and Maternity Services*. London: Department of Health.

Flynn, J. M., Skaggs, D., Sponseller, P. D., Ganley, T. J., Kay, R. M., Leitch, K., Kellie, M. D. (2002) The operative management of pediatric fractures of the lower extremity. *The Journal of Bone and Joint Surgery* 84 (12), pp. 2288–300.

Gauderer, M. W., Green, J. A., DeCou, J. M., Abrams, R. S. (2003) Acute appendicitis in children: The importance of family history. *Annals of Emergency Medicine* 41 (2) p. 289.

Gillick v Norfolk and Wisbech Area Health Authority and the DHSS (1986). Appeal Cases (England), *1AC112*.

Handforth, J. (2004) Prevention of respiratory syncytial virus infection in infants. *British Medical Journal* 328, pp. 1026–7.

Harrop, M. (2003) Respiratory and cardiovascular problems, in Barnes, K. (ed.) *Paediatrics A Clinical Guide for Practitioners*. Edinburgh: Butterworth Heinemann, Chapter 11, pp. 116–24.

Hedin, H. (2004) Surgical treatment of femoral fractures in children: Comparison between external fixation and elastic intramedullary nails: A review. *Acta Orthopaedica Scandinavica* 75 (3), pp. 231–40.

Houshian, S., Gothgen, C. B., Pedersen, N. W., Harving, S. (2004) Femoral shaft fractures in children: Elastic intramedullary nailing in 31 cases. *Acta Orthopaedica Scandinavica* 75 (3), pp. 249–51.

Huband, S. Trigg, E. (2000) *Practices in Children's Nursing*. Edinburgh: Churchill Livingstone.

Kari J. A., Donovan, C., Li, J., Taylor, B. (1999) Teenagers in hospital: What do they want. *Nursing Standard*, 13 (23), pp. 49–51.

Kassutto, Z. (2003) Paediatric appendicitis score. *Annals of Emergency Medicine* 41 (2) p. 288.

Kellner, J. D., Ohlsson, A., Gadomski, A. M., Wang, E. E. L. (2004) Bronchodilators for bronchiolitis. *The Cochrane Database of Systematic Reviews* 4, pp. 1–22.

King, V., Viswanathan, M., Bordley, W., Clayton, M., Jackman, A. M., Sutton, S. F., Lohr, K. N., Carey, T. S. (2004) Pharmacologic treatment of bronchiolitis in infants and children: A systematic review. *Archives of pediatrics and adolescent medicine* 158 (2), pp. 127–37.

Ministry of Health Central Services Health Council (1959) *The Welfare of Children in Hospital*. London: HMSO.

Mostafa, M., Hassan, M. G., Gaballa, M. (2001) Treatment of femoral shaft fractures in children and adolescents. *The Journal of Trauma Injury Infection and Critical Care* 51 (6), pp. 1182–88.

Moules, T., Ramsay, J. (1998) *The Textbook of Children's Nursing*. London: Stanley Thornes.

Muller, D. (1992) *Nursing Children: Psychology, Research and Practice*. London: Chapman and Hall.

Muller, D. (1992a) *Nursing Children: Psychology, Research and Practice*. London: Chapman and Hall.

Nursing Times (2003) Acute appendicitis. *Nursing Times* 99 (3), p. 28.

Peter, S. (2003) *Bronchiolitis*, in Barnes, K. (ed.) *Paediatrics A Clinical Guide for Practitioners*. Edinburgh: Butterworth Heinemann, Chapter 11, pp. 121–4.

Pfeil, M., Mathur, A. (2004) Early discharge following uncomplicated appendicectomy. *Paediatric Nursing* 16 (7), pp. 15–18.

Ross-Trevor, J. (1996) Informed consent and the treatment of children. *Nursing Standard* 10 (50), pp. 46–8.

Rothrock, S., Pagane, J. (2000) Acute appendicitis in children: Emergency Department Diagnosis and Management. *Annals of Emergency Medicine* 36 (1), pp. 39–51.

Royal College of Nursing (1994) *Caring for Adolescents*. London, Royal College of Nursing.

Russell-Johnson, H. (2000) Adolescent Survey. *Paediatric Nursing* 12 (6), pp. 15–19.

Shelley, H. (1993) Adolescent needs in hospital. *Paediatric Nursing* 5 (9), pp. 16–18.

United Nations (1989) *Conventions for the Rights of the Child*. Geneva: UN.

8 Paediatric Critical Care Practice

Helen Bailey

Learning outcomes

- Recognise the clinical signs and symptoms of a deteriorating child.
- Identify the different types of respiratory support available and discuss methods of delivery.
- Demonstrate an understanding of how cardiovascular support is provided.
- Explore the reasons for retrieving children to regional paediatric intensive care units.
- Discuss methods of supporting the family of a critically ill child.
- Differentiate between the levels of nursing care and support available

---

Introduction

Within this chapter the focus will be on children and families experiencing life threatening illness or injury necessitating a need to receive critical care. The term critical care is used to denote a greater dependency on nursing and medical interventions than is usually available within the paediatric ward setting. Primarily the focus examines aspects of the intensive care environment but high dependency care will also be considered.

Critical care

There are four triggers within this chapter, which are all related to the same situation. Each trigger is presented as a transcript of a conversation referring to the same child at different stages throughout his hospital experience. Although these triggers all relate to a child with one specific condition it is important to recognise that the key concepts identified and discussed are transferable to the majority of children requiring intensive care nursing, regardless off illness, injury or reason for admission.

! Trigger 8.1: Recognition of the deteriorating child

The intention of this trigger is to recognise the signs that a child's condition may be deteriorating.

The Trigger

Transcript of Conversation on Paediatric Ward

Student Nurse: Could you please take a look at Charlie for me? He seems less active than before and I can't get a blood pressure to record.

Staff Nurse: Have you checked his other vital signs?

Student Nurse: Yes. His temperature has gone up to 39.2 degrees centigrade. His pulse rate was 180 beats per minute and his respiratory rate was 40 breaths per minute.

Staff Nurse: Did you check his capillary refill time?

Student Nurse: No, I'm not sure how to.

Staff Nurse: Okay. I'm going to take a look at him. Find me a doctor and send him over to me. Come back to Charlie's cot. After that I'll show you how to check the capillary refill time.

Situation

Charlie is ten months old and was admitted to the paediatric ward in a District General Hospital three hours ago. His parents described him as being generally unwell, having a raised temperature and being off his feeds.

Feedback

This trigger requires you to make brief notes in answer to the questions that are raised.

The facts

> **What are the main facts in this trigger? Make a list:**

Hypotheses: What may these facts mean?

- It is a fairly recent onset of illness.
- Charlie may have an infection causing his pyrexia.
- Charlie's pulse rate, respiratory rate and blood pressure are not normal for his age.
- Charlie's capillary refill time may be abnormal.
- Charlie may be developing shock.

Questions developed from the hypotheses

1. What are the normal ranges for pulse rate, respiratory rate and blood pressure in a ten month old child?
2. How do you check capillary refill time?
3. What is the significance of capillary refill time?
4. What causes shock to occur?

Trigger 8.1: Fixed resource material

Read the following to help you answer the questions. (You may also wish to search and review other up-to-date research and evidence-based literature, and seek other relevant resources to provide you with the answers to your questions.)

ALSG (2005) *Advanced Paediatric Life Support: The Practical Approach*, 4th edn. London: BMJ, Chapter 3, pp. 13–18.

Davies, J., Hassell, L. (2001) *Children in Intensive Care. A Nurse's Survival Guide.* Edinburgh: Churchill Livingstone, pp. 2–5.

Jevon, P. (2004) *Paediatric Advanced Life Support: A Practical Guide.* Edinburgh: Butterworth Heinemann, Chapter 3, pp. 21–9.

Trigger 8.1: Fixed resource sessions

Recognition of the deteriorating child

Early recognition of a child who is developing respiratory, circulatory or neurological failure is essential to reduce the risk of mortality or associated morbidity (ALSG 2005). Untreated any of these primary system failures are likely to lead to cardiac arrest. Even with intervention there is a risk of hypoxic damage occurring if there is a delay in initiating appropriate treatment. This may affect all tissues within the body but the brain and kidneys are particularly at risk due to their sensitivity. As a direct result of hypoxic damage, even children who are initially successfully resuscitated, are at risk of dying from multi organ failure or neurological damage days after the initial event occurs (Zideman 1994). Consequently the need for quick and accurate recognition of the child's condition with appropriate intervention is paramount. In order to achieve this a structured approach is required. ALSG (2005) identifies two components to achieving this. First they describe their model for assessing the child as having three key stages.

1. Primary assessment incorporating resuscitation;
2. Secondary survey; and
3. Definitive treatment.

Within each of these stages the actual order of assessment is identified using the ABC approach.

- Airway
- Breathing
- Circulation

Jevon (2004) uses different words and phrases to describe his approach but the fundamental aspects remain the same. He outlines the key components of a rapid assessment of the respiratory, cardiovascular and neurological functions in conjunction with an overall assessment of the child's general appearance.

Having a differential diagnosis is not necessary at this stage of treating a critically ill child. It is more important to ensure that the child has a patent airway, is breathing and has adequate circulation to oxygenate the tissues. Each alphabetical stage is continually being reassessed to ensure that no further deterioration has occurred. Once this has been confirmed it is possible to move on to the next system although it should be remembered that it may not be possible to stabilise all systems without recognising and treating underlying problems. An example of this is that a child presenting with seizures secondary to hypoglycaemia will need to have this treated but identification of the definitive cause of the hypoglycaemia can wait.

Many practitioners will advocate continuing to use the alphabetical system to remain structured. Beyond ABC this continues:

- D – Disability: an assessment of the neurological system.
- E – Exposure: an opportunity to check for rashes, bruises, lacerations, burns and other marks.
- F – Family: keeping them constantly updated about their child's condition and obtaining an accurate history of events leading up to admission.
- G – Glucose: children who are critically ill rapidly consume their energy reserves, increasing the risk of hypoglycaemia occurring. Although this would usually be checked as part of the disability assessment it is useful to have a further reminder to ensure that an easily reversible problem has not been missed.

Essentially, however it is described, recognition of the seriously ill or deteriorating child needs to be quick, accurate and structured with interventions being made in order of priority and importance. Once emergency interventions have been made and the child has been stabilised it is possible to investigate and definitively treat the specific underlying cause.

Circulatory Shock

Shock occurs when there is an acute failure of circulatory function (ALSG 2005). This leads to inadequate provision of oxygen and nutrients to the cells and a build up of waste products such as carbon dioxide within the body. This may occur secondary to a number of underlying causes and this dictates which of five classifications of shock is said to have occurred.

1. *Hypovolaemic shock*: there is an imbalance in the type or volume of fluid available within the circulatory system. Primarily this is due to fluid loss. The mechanism of fluid loss varies but includes haemorrhage following trauma and burns. Infants are also susceptible to developing hypovolaemic shock secondary to gastroenteritis due to the relatively large quantity of fluid that may be lost with diarrhoea and vomiting (ALSG 2005).
2. *Cardiogenic shock*: occurs when the heart fails to pump blood adequately around the body. In infants less than one month of age this is likely to be secondary to an underlying congenital heart defect. In the older child this is more likely to be secondary to a cardiomyopathy or cardiac arrhythmia. There are numerous reasons why these abnormalities may occur.
3. *Distributive shock*: this results secondary to an abnormality within the vessels of the circulatory system. Vasomotor tone becomes altered or may be lost completely leading to inappropriate vasodilation and pooling of blood. Common causes of this in children include septicaemia and anaphylaxis. Less commonly, it may also occur following spinal cord injury doe to loss of autonomic control.
4. *Obstructive shock*: there is an obstruction to normal blood flow around the body. This is most likely to be seen in children who have a tension pneumothorax, haemopneumothorax or cardiac tamponade. Consequently it is most likely to be seen following trauma, surgery or when a child is being mechanically ventilated.
5. Dissociative shock: occurs when there is an inability to release oxygen adequately to the tissues. This may be seen in children with profound anaemia such as that seen in sickle cell disease or following carbon monoxide poisoning.

Irrespective of the underlying cause of shock and the classification, three distinct phases have been identified by ALSG (2005) and are supported by Stack and Dobbs (2004).

Phase one is known as compensated shock. The heart and brain are protected by sympathetic reflexes, which increase systemic arterial resistance (and, therefore, increase blood pressure), divert blood away from non-essential areas and increase the heart rate (to maintain cardiac output). During this stage the systolic blood pressure remains normal because of the compensatory mechanisms but the diastolic pressure may be elevated because of the increased systemic pressure. The kidneys and digestive tract also play a part by conserving as much water as possible. Clinical signs during this phase may include increased heart rate, cool peripheries, decreased capillary return, pallor, agitation or confusion.

Phase two occurs when the untreated child progresses into uncompensated shock. The compensatory mechanisms begin to fail and the circulatory system becomes inefficient. Reduced perfusion means that some tissues receive no oxygen and metabolism in these areas becomes anaerobic. This is a very inefficient system that uses large quantities of glucose with very little energy being produced. It also causes an increase in waste products, most notably carbonic acid (from excess production of carbon dioxide) and lactate (which causes a lactic acidosis). The presence of these two acids in the body alters the chemical balance and the child progresses to develop signs of metabolic acidosis with an associated reduction in myocardial contractility and a reduced response to catecholamines, which are naturally occurring stimulant hormones and neurotransmitters. This reduced response then causes a further decrease in myocardial contractility. Continuing chemical changes and the advancing reduction in blood flow lead to a deterioration in a number of body processes, most notably the coagulation system, which becomes ineffective. Finally the capillary system becomes more porous, allowing fluid to leak out of the circulatory system and into the cells resulting in a further reduction in the circulating volume. Clinically the child who has uncompensated shock will have a falling blood pressure, very slow capillary return, cold peripheries, tachycardia, acidotic breathing, reduced level of consciousness and no urine output.

Phase three is irreversible shock. This diagnosis is made after death, as the child's body is unable to recover once this stage has been reached despite restoration of an adequate circulation. This is because of the massive amount of damage that occurred to the tissues and organs within the body during the uncompensated stage of shock.

Appropriate intervention during either of the first two phases will prevent progression to the next phase. This intervention should follow the structured approach already identified (ALSG 2005). Once airway and breathing have been stabilised it is possible to concentrate on the circulatory system. In almost all cases of a child presenting with shock rapid fluid administration will be required to help restore the circulatory volume. The exception to this is the child demonstrating signs of cardiac failure who will benefit more from drugs to improve myocardial contractility and who may actually deteriorate if given additional fluid.

While fluid is being administered, an underlying cause for the shock should be identified. Clinical signs and symptoms demonstrated by the child, an accurate account of the onset of illness and knowledge of the previous medical history will all help in identifying the diagnosis. Definitive treatment can be instigated at this stage.

→ Trigger 8.1: Feedback

Go to Chapter 8 Trigger feedback on p. 233

! Trigger 8.2: Referral and Retrieval to a Paediatric Intensive Care Unit (PICU)

The intention of this trigger is to examine the reasons why children are referred to paediatric intensive care units for retrieval and to learn more about Charlie's underlying condition.

The Trigger

Transcript of telephone conversation

Ward Doctor: We have a child requiring intensive care. Do you have a bed available?

Intensivist: We have a bed available but I need to know a bit more about the child.

Ward Doctor: Charlie is ten months old, pyrexial, shocked and showing signs of respiratory failure. His capillary refill time is six seconds and he has a purpuric rash developing.

Intensivist: He certainly sounds like he needs intensive care. We will send the retrieval team out to get him. They should be with you within the hour. While you're waiting give him some fluid and see if that improves his capillary refill time. I would also suggest you get an anaesthetist to review him in case he needs intubating.

Situation

The doctor has decided that Charlie is too unwell to remain on the ward and requires intensive care. He is currently on the telephone to a paediatric intensivist in a local hospital.

Feedback

This trigger requires you to design a poster that could be displayed for parents in District General Hospitals giving them information about what to expect if their child needs to be transferred to a paediatric intensive care unit in a different hospital. Brief notes should also be made to answer the questions raised.

The facts

What are the main facts in this trigger? Make a list:

Hypotheses: What may these facts mean?

- Charlie's respiratory failure and purpuric rash are symptoms of his underlying illness.
- Children requiring intensive care need to be retrieved.
- Fluid will help to treat shock.
- Charlie's respiratory function may deteriorate further.

Questions developed from the hypotheses

1. What illness is Charlie likely to be suffering from?
2. Why do intensive care units retrieve critically ill children?
3. What fluid will help Charlie?
4. How will intubation help Charlie's respiratory function?

Trigger 8.2: Fixed resource material

Read the following to help you answer the questions. (You may also wish to search and review other up to date research and evidence-based literature, and seek other relevant resources to provide you with the answers to your questions.)

ALSG (2005) *Advanced Paediatric Life Support: The Practical Approach*, 4th edn. London: BMJ. Fluid resuscitation, pp. 114–16.

Department of Health (1997) *Paediatric Intensive Care 'A Framework for the Future'. Report from the National Co-ordinating Group on Paediatric Intensive care to the Chief Executive of the NHS Executive.* London: Department of Health. Retrieval services, pp. 44–7 (sections 95–102 inclusive).

How to guides: Meningococcal disease – early management (1998) *Care of the Critically Ill*, 14 (8).

Hubband, S., Trigg, E. (2000) *Practices in Children's Nursing. Guidelines for Hospital and community*. Edinburgh: Churchill Livingstone, Endotracheal intubation, p. 79.

Morrison, G. (2000) Transportation of the critically ill child, in Williams, C., Asquith, J. *Paediatric Intensive Care Nursing*. Edinburgh: Churchill Livingstone, Chapter 5, pp. 51–8.

National Meningitis Trust (1996) *Hospital Information Pack*.

Paediatric Intensive Care Society (2001) *Standards for Paediatric Intensive Care*. Sheffield: PICS, Standards for retrieval of critically ill children, Chapter 12, pp. 24–26.

Trigger 8.2: Fixed resource sessions

Retrieval of Critically Ill Children

It has been widely recognised that children requiring intensive care should be cared for in regional lead centres (Britto et al 1995; Department of Health 1997; Pollack et al, 1991). This, therefore, means that critically ill children have to be transported, often over significant distances, to be cared for in a lead centre. This is a potentially hazardous event for the child and numerous studies from both within the United Kingdom and abroad have highlighted the risks involved. In order to minimise these risks it is recommended that children are collected and transferred to the paediatric intensive care unit (PICU) by a team from the lead centre that will be undertaking the definitive care (British Paediatric Association 1993; Department of Health 1997a; Paediatric Intensive Care Society 2001). This would appear to be a reasonable solution given that the child is considered sick enough to require care from medical and nursing staff trained in intensive care. It can, therefore, be concluded that they will require these same staff even more urgently when removed from the relative safety of the hospital environment. This concept is supported by a number of studies that have examined the impact on patient safety of inter-hospital transfer by non-specialist paediatric retrieval teams (Barry and Ralston 1994; Britto et al 1995; Edge et al 1994; MacNab 1991). Dangers highlighted in these studies include the development of life-threatening complications, increased incidence of avoidable secondary insults, and deterioration related to the underlying illness, treatment or the transfer itself. Edge et al (1994) conclude that using a specialised paediatric retrieval team reduces the number of adverse events associated with the transfer of critically ill children.

Even with the identified risks involved in transportation it is still felt that the most appropriate treatment for a critically ill child is to transfer them to a regional centre (Davies 2001). It is, therefore, important to identify standards to be maintained during retrieval. The Paediatric Intensive Care Society have published such standards although these concentrate primarily on clinical guidelines and issues relating to staff qualifications, training and listing necessary equipment (Paediatric Intensive Care Society 2001). A number of other authors since have attempted to build upon this with the production of further evidence and guidelines (Davies 2001; Stack 1997).

Although retrieval to a referral centre is described as best practice there are a number of disadvantages, apart from the potential risks, that have to be considered.

The paediatric intensive care network in the UK is divided into geographical regions that vary in size depending upon population levels. Consequently hospitals within the London area cover relatively small geographical retrieval areas although they serve a large population. In other parts of the country distances can be considerable although in comparison to some other countries such as Australia the United Kingdom has a very compact surface area to cover. This obviously has an impact on the PICU as the retrieval team may be away from the base for some time but equally importantly it can have a significant effect on families.

Having a child admitted to hospital and requiring intensive care is stressful enough. To then be told that your child needs to be transferred to a different part of the country may compound that stress. First parents tend to be separated from their children for the duration of the transfer as most teams feel it is safer not to have parents in the ambulance. Stack and Dobbs (2004) list reasons for this including a lack of space, increased stress on parents and staff and the possible diversion of the staff's attention away from the child. They do however acknowledge that in situations where the child is awake or anxious there are benefits to having a parental presence. Second, upon arrival and for the duration of the stay in the tertiary centre the parents are removed from their home environment. This leads to one of three situations developing.

1. This is the most common scenario. The parents choose to be resident at the hospital and all PICU's should offer adequate accommodation for parents (Paediatric Intensive Care Society 2001). This provides the reassurance of being close to their sick child but may lead to a number of other problems. Being away from home means that the parents may be separated from their normal support structures such as extended family and friends. Even more worryingly they may be apart from their other children. As well as being separated from them they also need to ensure that the siblings are being cared for adequately and need the reassurance that their homes and possibly pets are all receiving the necessary care. In addition to this is the pressure of financing a stay in hospital. Parents need to pay for all of their meals, or buy food if cooking facilities are available, they may need to pay for car parking, laundry facilities and regular telephone calls to relatives. This is combined with the fact that they are unable to go to work and may not be receiving any income. Obviously not all families are going to struggle with this scenario but for a significant number it creates enormous problems.

2. Some parents may choose to stay at home and stay in contact with the unit by telephone. This is an uncommon situation but does occur, particularly in situations where families have no support available to care for other children, have transportation problems or are having difficulties financing trips to the hospital. Nurses are able to keep parents updated of their child's condition over the telephone but should make enquiries about the family circumstances to ascertain if any help can be offered to allow the family to spend time with their critically ill child.

3. Many families use a combination of the above two approaches. It may be that one parent stays resident in hospital while the other parent remains at home or both parents may opt to commute between the hospital and home. Both of these options have their own associated problems but it should be acknowledged that all families are individual with specific needs and should be respected and treated accordingly.

In conclusion it is generally accepted that critically ill children need to be cared for in regional PICU's and in order to optimise their care prior to admission they should be retrieved by a specialist paediatric retrieval team. The team should include a doctor and nurse who are both trained in the provision of paediatric intensive care and have received additional training in the field of transporting critically ill children (Department of Health 1997a). These staff should receive regular updates to ensure their practice remains up to date and in keeping with emerging evidence, as this is a rapidly evolving speciality.

Appropriate equipment needs to be available for staff to use when necessary during the transfer. Some units find that this is best achieved by designing and using a dedicated 'mobile intensive care unit' that is used exclusively for paediatric transfers however this is not compulsory.

Communication with families is vital to minimise anxiety and stress. Prior to transfer a member of the retrieval team should speak to the family. Information imparted at this point should include the reason why transfer is necessary, details of treatments that have already been initiated and practical information about the unit and hospital to which their child is being transferred (Stack and Dobbs 2004). Staff should also ascertain how parents plan to travel to the new hospital and instigate arrangements to provide safe transportation if necessary.

A final key component to communication is that between health professionals in the two hospitals. Establishing strong links between the PICU and the District General Hospitals (DGH) they serve is essential to enhance the care that children receive. Many regions support this through the role of nurse retrieval co-ordinator based within PICU and retrieval link nurses based within each DGH. This enables the PICU to cascade training, information and feedback to each individual area and provides a two-way communication route for staff.

When a retrieval is required it should be initiated by direct consultant to consultant contact. The PICU should remain available to provide advice to the DGH over the telephone if necessary but responsibility for the care delivered to the child remains with the referring hospital until the retrieval team arrives.

Meningococcal Septicaemia

The most common cause of shock in children is septicaemia (ALSG 2005). This is supported by a pyrexia indicating an infective process and the presence of a purpuric rash is indicative of meningococcal septicaemia. Care should be taken when examining a child for a purpuric rash. ALSG (2005) identifies that 7 per cent of children with meningococcal septicaemia do not develop a rash while a further 13 per cent present with an atypical blanching erythematous rash. More importantly, a rash may not be evident when the child first presents or there may be only one or two spots appearing necessitating a thorough examination.

Meningococcal septicaemia or meningococcaemia is caused by the gram negative diplococcus *neisseria meningitidis*. The pathogen can be further divided into strains A, B, C, Y and W135. Vaccines are available for most of these although the vaccine for type B – the most common strain – is still at the testing stage (Nadel and Brownlie 2000). The bacteria are found harmlessly in the nose and throat of about 10 per cent of the population but occasionally, for unknown reasons, cross into the bloodstream causing septicaemia. In some cases the bacteria also penetrates the blood brain barrier resulting in a concurrent meningococcal meningitis.

Meningococcal sepsis often begins with a flu like illness but progresses rapidly, often within the space of just a few hours. The progress may include petechial or purpuric lesions, shock, hypotension, pyrexia, drowsiness, seizures, disseminated intravascular coagulation, multisystem organ failure and coma. Scoring systems are often used to predict the likely severity of the disease process, most commonly the Glasgow Meningococcal Septicaemia Prognostic Score (GMSPS) with a high score indicating a poor prognosis. Advances in technology, greater awareness of the disease and more aggressive pharmacological treatments have significantly improved survival rates in recent years but Stack and Dobbs (2004) still link the disease to a potential 50 per cent mortality rate.

Initial treatment requires intravenous antibiotics – usually cefotaxime or ceftriaxone. All other treatments are supportive and depend upon the degree of organ involvement but will usually include airway management and artificial ventilation, fluid resuscitation, blood products, cardiovascular support and renal replacement therapy.

➡ Trigger 8.2: Feedback

Go to Chapter 8 Trigger feedback on p. 233

! Trigger 8.3: Care of the child in intensive care

The intention of this trigger is to gain an overview of the nursing care required by critically ill children within the paediatric intensive care unit.

The trigger

Transcript of conversation on intensive care unit

Mother: There is so much equipment here it's difficult to see Charlie in the bed. What does it all do?

Staff Nurse: The machine at the top of the bed is a ventilator. That is helping Charlie to breathe. It is connected to the tube in his nose.

Mother: Does it hurt him?

Staff Nurse: No. We are giving him painkillers and sedatives into his bloodstream through these tubes so that he will not feel any pain or be upset.

Mother: What about all those numbers on the monitor?

Staff Nurse: They give us continuous information about what is going on inside Charlie. They tell us about his heart rate, blood pressure and oxygen requirements.

Mother: Why does the red number on the monitor keep flashing?

Staff Nurse: That is telling us his blood pressure is a bit low. We are giving Charlie some drugs called inotropes and they will help to increase his blood pressure.

Mother: Is he going to die?

Staff Nurse: Charlie is very sick and we can't promise you that he is going to survive. He does seem to be responding well to treatment though and we are hoping he is going to recover.

Mother: I feel completely useless. Is there anything I can do?

Situation

Soon after arrival in the intensive care unit the nurse caring for Charlie sits down at the bedside with Charlie's mother to talk to her.

Feedback

This trigger requires you to make brief notes in answer to the questions that are raised.

The Facts

What are the main facts in this trigger? Make a list:

Hypotheses: What may these facts mean?

- A ventilator is a way of providing respiratory support.
- Ventilated children require painkillers and sedation.
- Critically ill children require continuous monitoring.
- Staff must be honest about the possibility of death.
- Mum would like to be involved in Charlie's care.

Questions developed from the hypotheses

1. How do ventilators support the respiratory system?
2. How do inotropes work?
3. How do you talk to families about the possibility of death?
4. How can parent's of critically ill children be involved in their care?

Trigger 8.3: Fixed resource material

Read the following to help you answer the questions. (You may also wish to search and review other up to date research and evidence-based literature, and seek other relevant resources to provide you with the answers to your questions.)

Cook, M. (2000) Care of the dying child, In Williams, C., Asquith, J. *Paediatric Intensive Care Nursing*. Edinburgh: Churchill Livingstone, Chapter 18, pp. 319–28.

Davies, J., Hassell, L. (2001) *Children in Intensive Care. A Nurse's Survival Guide*. Edinburgh: Churchill Livingstone. Drugs – inotropes and infusions, Chapter 9, pp. 153–69.

Haines, C., Wolstenholme, M. (2000) Family support in paediatric intensive care, in

Williams, C., Asquith, J. *Paediatric Intensive Care Nursing*. Edinburgh: Churchill Livingstone. Chapter 17, pp. 307–17.

Paediatric Intensive Care Society (2002) *Standards for Bereavement Care*. Sheffield: PICS, pp. 17–26.

Trigger 8.3: Fixed resource sessions

Respiratory support

Respiratory failure occurs when the respiratory system is unable to provide enough oxygen for cell respiration or is ineffective at removing waste carbon dioxide. It develops either directly because of problems with the respiratory system or indirectly because of problems with the neurological system. Early recognition of respiratory failure is essential to prevent it from progressing into respiratory arrest.

The degree of effort required to breathe gives an indication of the extent of respiratory failure the child is suffering from. Signs include tachypnoea (increased respiratory rate), recession (intercostal, subcostal or sternal), inspiratory noise (stridor), expiratory noise (wheeze), grunting, use of accessory muscles (head bobbing) and nasal flaring.

Not all children with respiratory failure will show the above signs. There are three main exceptions. Children with neurological dysfunction may have a reduced respiratory drive. They, therefore, do not show signs of increased respiratory effort. Similarly children with an underlying neuromuscular disorder such as muscular dystrophy or spinal muscular atrophy may present without signs of increased effort. In this situation the neurological system is sending messages telling the respiratory system to respond but due to the weakened muscle state the response is inadequate. The third group of children who do not demonstrate signs of increased respiratory effort are tiring children. If respiratory failure has been present for some time the child may have insufficient energy to sustain an increased effort and may, therefore, not present with an increased effort.

In these cases the diagnosis is reached by assessing the efficacy of breathing, that is assessing how effective the effort is. This is achieved by listening to air entry, observing chest expansion and recording oxygen saturations. This is supported by observing for signs of respiratory inadequacy affecting other systems. To achieve this checks should be made of heart rate, skin colour and mental status.

The underlying cause of respiratory failure will need to be identified in order to treat it appropriately but simultaneously some method of supporting the respiratory system may be necessary. Support refers to any intervention to reduce the effort required to breathe or increase the efficiency. It may be undertaken electively to prevent a deterioration in the child's condition or as an emergency if the child's respiratory effort is ineffective. In its simplest form respiratory support may refer to the administration of supplementary oxygen but more commonly it is described as a method of providing artificial ventilation.

All people breathe through a process of negative pressure ventilation. Early ventilators such as the 'iron lung' imitated this. Since the 1950s this has been reversed and most ventilation these days is performed using a positive pressure technique.

Artificial or assisted positive pressure ventilation is a way of supporting or controlling a child's breathing by providing the effort to move a mixture of oxygen and air (gas) into the lungs. This can be achieved invasively via an endotracheal tube or tracheostomy tube or non-invasively through the use of a tight fitting facemask. Although non-invasive ventilation has less side effects and potential problems than conventional invasive ventilation, it in not suitable for sicker children, especially those with an underlying respiratory or cardiovascular disease or those with a dramatically increased oxygen requirement (Stack and Dobbs 2004).

It is also possible to categorise ventilation dependent upon the level of support required – the machinery may be responsible for all of the breathing, the child and ventilator may be sharing the work of breathing or the child may be breathing spontaneously through the ventilator circuit while receiving some support.

Controlled ventilation

There are three variables involved in gas exchange – pressure, volume and lung compliance. As it is not possible to control the child's lung compliance it is the remaining two factors that are manipulated to provide optimal ventilation. Although both pressure and volume can be controlled this cannot be done simultaneously. A choice therefore needs to be made either to provide pressure controlled ventilation or volume controlled ventilation.

ALSG (2005) describes pressure controlled ventilation as being preferable in smaller children. This involves the delivery of a flow of gas until a pre-determined peak inspiratory pressure is reached. If lung compliance decreases (lungs become stiffer), the volume of gas delivered will decrease. This will lead to a decrease in oxygenation and gas exchange and should, therefore, be carefully monitored. The advantage of using this ventilation strategy is that the lungs do not become damaged by over stretching (barotrauma).

Volume controlled ventilation delivers a pre-set volume of gas to the lungs with each breath. This is calculated dependant upon the child's weight. If the lung compliance deteriorated significantly the same volume of gas would be delivered but the increased pressure now created raises the possibility of barotrauma occurring. As this is more likely to occur in younger infants this mode of ventilation is not advocated in children under 10kg and its use within the wider paediatric population is diminishing.

Weaning modes

Children cannot go from being fully ventilated to self-ventilating without a transition period. This is known as weaning the child from the ventilator. There are a range of ventilatory modes that are designed for this purpose. All of them involve a gradual reduction in the amount of work being done by the ventilator and a steadily increasing effort being made by the child.

Support

Continuous Positive Airway Pressure (CPAP) requires the child to breathe for him/herself but less effort is required to do so. A continuous flow of gas is delivered to the child so that at the end of expiration a set amount of gas remains within the lungs. This prevents the alveoli from collapsing down completely and, therefore, makes it easier to initiate the next breath. CPAP can be delivered via a number of delivery systems including face masks, nasal prongs, tracheostomies and endotracheal tubes. The amount of gas (and therefore pressure) left in the lungs is measured in cm H_2O.

CPAP is used either as a preventative measure to stop the child requiring full ventilation or as a step down after the child no longer requires full ventilation.

There are delivery systems available specifically for administering CPAP known as CPAP drivers. These involve placing a 'bung' into each nostril, which seals the nostrils but allows the gas to flow in through an opening. This is secured in place using ties and a bonnet. It can be very effective but only works if the child keeps their mouth closed otherwise the pressure escapes. Consequently the use of dummies is advocated for these children with the parents permission. This system has been designed for use with neonates and, therefore, the manufacturers only produce small nasal pieces in a range of three sizes. As this is a completely non-invasive technique it should be possible to use this system within any paediatric setting providing that adequate training and staff numbers are provided. It should be remembered though that the airway remains unprotected.

Drugs

If intubation is undertaken in an emergency, for example during a cardiac arrest, no drugs are required but if this is an elective procedure on an awake child certain drugs need to be administered for the comfort of the child.

The actual choice of specific drugs will vary depending upon local policy and individual practitioner's preference but the types of drugs used are fairly standard.

An intravenous anaesthetic or barbiturate is used to anaesthetise the child. Examples of these include ketamine and thiopentone. A short acting muscle relaxant (paralysing agent) will prevent any muscles within the airway from going into spasm and stop the child from moving. Suxemethonium is commonly used for this purpose. Atropine is always available although not usually administered in case the process of tube insertion causes vagal stimulation leading to bradycardia.

The anaesthetic and muscle relaxant drugs tend to be fairly short acting and if the child is to remain ventilated for a prolonged period further drugs are required as continuous infusions.

Analgesia is given to all intubated children, most commonly morphine. This is to ensure that the child remains free of pain and to minimise any attempts the child may make to fight against the required interventions. Sedation is generally given in conjunction with pain relief for the same reason. Sedation is usually started with intravenous midazolam but is often weaned to oral sedatives such as chloral hydrate or alimemazine within a few days.

Muscle relaxants block messages from the brain to the muscles and, therefore, prevent movement. There is a range of drugs available for this purpose, an example is pancuronium. It is essential when starting muscle relaxants to ensure that respiratory function has been replaced and that adequate analgesia and sedation has already been given to prevent distress and discomfort.

Most practitioners would advocate the minimal amount of drugs being administered to achieve safe and effective ventilation. In reality this means that muscle relaxants, if used at all after the initial intubation, tend to be weaned rapidly. Intravenous analgesia and sedation is significantly reduced once oral medication is being tolerated and absorbed. This reduces the incidence of associated drug withdrawal problems.

Nursing care

It is of paramount importance when caring for a ventilated child to ensure that the airway remains patent and secure at all times. To achieve this the nurse needs to maintain endotracheal tube security, assess the effectiveness of and maintain adequate ventilation, ensure all ventilatory settings and alarms are appropriate, assess the need for suction, performing it as required and respond quickly and appropriately to emergencies.

Involving families in care on a PICU

It is acknowledged that when a child is critically ill the parent may become disempowered as the primary care giver and this role is taken on by nursing staff. Haines and Wolstenholme (2000) identify that parents feel great stress, grief and helplessness when their child is admitted to intensive care. It is reasonable to accept that the nurse will need to undertake many of the technical aspects of the child's care during the critical illness phase but consideration should also be given to preservation of the parenting role wherever possible. This needs to be approached sensitively as many parents faced with the shocking reality of a child in the PICU feel unable to participate, touch or occasionally even visit their child. This may be further compounded by the condition of the child who may be too unstable to be physically handled or by the barrier created by equipment, monitors, tubes and wires. The nurse needs to be able to empower the parent in such a situation in a non-judgemental manner to allow them to re-establish their parenting role in an appropriate manner.

In its simplest form the first intervention the nurse can make is to encourage the family to spend time with their child and talk to him/her. Families may also wish to be involved in creating a more 'normal' environment for their child. This may include displaying photographs of family members and pets, providing favourite toys or comforters such as blankets, playing familiar music or favourite films and for older children in particular, allowing friends to visit as well as family.

Touch is another important aspect of parenting and families should be supported to do so. This may involve simple hand holding or stroking but if the child is stable enough parents should be enabled to hold and cuddle their child if they wish to. With sufficient staff to ensure the security of attachment to vital medical equipment, critical illness and mechanical ventilation should not inhibit this action although it is important that the safety of the child is not compromised.

Families may also wish to be involved in other aspects of their child's care. Commonly this starts with roles that they undertake for their child at home such as washing, dressing, hair brushing and nappy changing. Parents should be supported to fulfil these roles with appropriate help and advice from staff to accommodate the altered circumstances such as how to dress a child with multiple intravenous lines or cleaning the teeth of a child with an oral endotracheal tube in place.

It is important, however, to ensure that the child's needs are met and not just those of the parents. Haines and Wolstenholme (2000) identify that adolescents in particular may be embarrassed at parental involvement in meeting their personal hygiene needs and the nurse may need to act as an advocate for what is thought to be best for the individual child. Care should be taken to try to maintain a balanced level of involvement that is beneficial to all parties without increasing stress for any individual.

Parents may wish to be involved in some of the more traditional medical tasks and the appropriateness of this will need to be assessed on an individual basis. Parents of children with a chronic medical condition may have already adapted their parenting role to include certain medical and nursing skills and they should be encouraged to continue to do so if they wish to. Examples of this include administration of medicines via subcutaneous or nebulised routes, feeding via gastrostomy or nasogastric tubes and tracheostomy care.

Similarly, there is a growing population of technology dependent children within the United Kingdom who tend to spend a prolonged period of time resident in an intensive care unit prior to discharge home with ventilatory support. These families need to undertake extensive training in all aspects of their child's care before safe discharge into the community can occur.

For the majority of children admitted to paediatric intensive care however, the technical interventions required remain the remit of health professionals. Most families are content to know that the 'experts' are caring for their child but the key to ensuring this is effective communication that should be clear, understandable and honest. Families should be spoken to before any intervention to explain what is about to be done, why it is being done and what the aim is. This explanation should include the child so that they are prepared for what is about to occur. By giving this explanation the health professional is giving the family the opportunity to clarify their understanding of the situation and ask any questions. It also enables them to give implied consent for any necessary procedure, which is an area receiving considerable attention within paediatric intensive care units currently.

Trigger 8.3: Feedback

Go to Chapter 8 Trigger feedback on p. 233

! Trigger 8.4: High dependency care

The intention of this trigger is to highlight the differences between paediatric intensive care and high dependency care and to identify how the nurse can ensure a smooth transition between units.

The Trigger

Transcript of Conversation in the Paediatric Intensive Care Unit waiting room

Mother: He's being transferred to the high dependency unit.

Grandmother: That's brilliant. You must be really relieved.

Mother: Well I'm happy that he doesn't need the ventilator any more but I'm worried that he won't get as much attention. They don't have one to one nursing in high dependency.

Grandmother: But surely that's because he doesn't need it anymore?

Mother: I know but you can't help but worry. What if he gets worse again?

Grandmother: I think you should talk to the nurses again and get some more information.

Situation

Charlie was successfully extubated after five days and his mother has just been told he is well enough to be transferred to the high dependency unit. She is telephoning Charlie's grandmother to tell her the news.

Feedback

This trigger requires you to design a simple information leaflet for parents of children who are recovering and being transferred out of intensive care, either to a high dependency unit or a paediatric ward. Brief notes should also be made to answer the questions raised.

The facts

What are the main facts in this trigger? Make a list:

Hypotheses: What may these facts mean?

- High dependency care is a step down from intensive care.
- Parents may still be worried even when their child is being discharged from the PICU.
- Information about the transfer may alleviate anxiety.

Questions are developed from the hypotheses

1. What are the differences between intensive care and high dependency care?
2. How can nurses alleviate family anxiety?
3. What information does the family need to know about the transfer?

Trigger 8.4: Fixed resource material

Read the following to help you answer the questions. (You may also wish to search and review other up to date research and evidence-based literature, and seek other relevant resources to provide you with the answers to your questions.)

Department of Health (2001) *High Dependency Care for Children – Report of an Expert Advisory Group for Department of Health*. London: Department of Health.

Keogh, S. (2001) Parents' experience of the transfer of their child from the PICU to the ward: A phenomenological study. *Nursing in Critical Care*, (6) 1, pp. 7–13.

Paediatric Intensive Care Society (2001) *Standards for Paediatric Intensive Care*. Sheffield: PICS), Standards for paediatric high dependency units, Chapter 10, pp. 19–21.

Trigger 8.4: Fixed resource sessions

Paediatric Intensive Care and High Dependency Care: A History of the Service Development

Paediatric intensive care is a relatively new speciality that was first established in Gothenburg in 1955 (Bennett 1997). Developments did not appear internationally until the 1960's and within the United Kingdom the service remained fragmented and poorly structured until the early 1990s. A significant development was the publication of *Standards for Paediatric Intensive Care* (Paediatric Intensive Care Society 1996). This document, which is updated every five years, offered guidelines for standards of medical and nurse training within the speciality and promoted the concept of having fewer, larger paediatric intensive care units in order to concentrate resources, knowledge and expertise. The publication of this report, at a time when the national press were reporting a significant shortfall in the number of available paediatric intensive care beds prompted the government to establish a National Co-ordinating Group to examine the provision of paediatric intensive care within the United Kingdom. They also provided money for the further development of the speciality.

The co-ordinating group's report *Paediatric Intensive Care 'A Framework for the Future* (Deartment of Health 1997) underpins many of the key principles seen within paediatric critical care settings in recent years. In conjunction with this the Chief Nursing Officer's Taskforce produced a complementary document *A Bridge to the Future* (Deartment of Health 1997a), which has also been hugely influential within the speciality.

Paediatric intensive care can be defined as 'A service for patients with potentially recoverable diseases who can benefit from more detailed observation, treatment and technological support than is available in standard wards and departments' (Paediatric Intensive care Society 2001, p. 5). This definition can be further sub-divided depending upon the degree of support and care required.

Paediatric high dependency care is more difficult to define. It has been described as 'Care provided to a child who may require closer observation and monitoring than is usually available on an ordinary children's ward. For example the child may need continuous monitoring of the heart rate, non-invasive blood pressure monitoring, or single organ support (but not respiratory support)' (Department of Health 1997, p. 7). This report also identifies however that at the time of writing, much of this care was being delivered within general ward areas with increased staffing levels to accommodate this. High dependency is also sometimes provided as a step down from intensive care. It became apparent that there was a significant amount of confusion around the issue of high dependency care with a great deal of disparity in the service being provided throughout the United Kingdom.

To address this specific issue a further report was compiled to examine high dependency care for children (Department of Health 2001). A method of categorising dependency was required to enable monitoring of workloads of different units and to support effective audit initiatives. This was done by examining compromised organ function to identify a core set of high dependency categories.

While the development of core categories for high dependency care is beneficial it should be remembered that this is a medically driven model. Many children are classed as no longer requiring intensive care and being suitable for high dependency care due to a decreased requirement for medical interventions. They may however still have a significantly high nursing dependency requirement. Examples of children who this may apply to include medically stable children requiring long-term ventilation, children requiring rehabilitation following head injury and children with complex psychological needs. Further development in the area of nursing dependency tools may assist in this area.

Preparing parents for transfer out of the PICU

Initial parental responses to the news that their child is to be transferred out of the PICU tend to be favourable as parents recognise that this is a positive step and signifies considerable progress. However, in a study by Keogh (2001) it was highlighted that parents may also respond negatively describing anxieties such as fear of the unknown, new staff and environment and different approaches to care. The reduction in monitoring was also noted to reduce reassurance for the family.

A key theme to emerge from Keogh's study was the impact parental dependency on the PICU nurse has upon parental stress. Studies by Cagan (1988) and Saarmann (1993) have also identified similar issues. When the intensity of this support mechanism is reduced because the child is moving to a different environment the family feel they have lost a significant carer of the child and may feel unable or ill equipped to resume this role themselves. In order to promote a positive experience for children and their families it is important in critical care areas for nurses to redress this balance prior to transfer.

The transition through intensive care, high dependency care, paediatric ward and finally back home needs to be seen as a smooth journey with changes in levels of care being introduced gradually and appropriately. Nurses within higher dependency areas, therefore, have a responsibility to ensure parents and children are adequately prepared for new environments and altered levels and methods of care delivery. Examples of this include withdrawing the intensity of monitoring and frequency of recording of nursing observations prior to transfer to a lower dependency area.

Nurses should also be gradually reducing the amount of direct care being administered to the child and encouraging parents to regain responsibility for this role. This will help parents adjust to the lower staffing ratios found within high dependency units and even more crucially on paediatric wards.

In conjunction with these practical measures, the single most effective tool nurses can use to alleviate child/family stress is communication. By providing children and their families with clear, accurate information prior to the transfer, many anxieties can be minimised or even prevented. This information should be given verbally but the provision of supplementary written information may enhance understanding, prompt questions and is available for parents and children to refer to. The possibility of pre-transfer visits to the unit or ward that the child will be moving to should also be considered. It is recognised that this is not always possible due to workload constraints, parents not being present or urgent transfers due to emergency admissions but nurses should aim to achieve this whenever possible. This becomes a particularly useful technique when children have spent a considerable period of time in the PICU. If this is to be accompanied by a lengthy rehabilitation period on a ward it is advisable to facilitate a number of meetings between the child, family and ward staff to aid a smooth transition to the new environment.

 # Trigger 8.4: Feedback

Go to Chapter 8 Trigger feedback.

Chapter 8 Trigger feedback: What do you know?

Trigger 8.1: Recognition of the deteriorating child

Question 1: What are the normal ranges for pulse rate, respiratory rate and blood pressure in a ten month old child?

The younger a child is the greater their metabolic rate and level of oxygen consumption. This means that the younger a child is, the faster the respiratory rate is going to be. A ten month old child will typically have a respiratory rate between 30–40 breaths per minute. This will increase during illness or following any injury to the child.

The higher metabolic rate also accounts for a higher resting heart rate. A child of ten months will have a resting heart rate of between 110–150 beats per minute. This will also increase with any illness or injury, as the younger child is unable to increase the volume ejected with each beat of the heart significantly. Consequently the only way to increase the cardiac output is to become tachycardic.

Younger children have less systemic vascular resistance than adults and therefore their blood pressure is lower. This steadily increases with age and by adolescence blood pressure parameters are similar to an adults. A ten month old child is likely to have a systolic blood pressure of 70–90 mmHg with a diastolic pressure of 50–55 mmHg.

Question 2: How do you check capillary refill time?

Capillary refill time is calculated by applying pressure (usually with the pad of the fingertip) to the child's skin. This may be done peripherally by squeezing the child's fingertip but is more accurate if performed centrally by applying gentle pressure in the sternal area. A central recording is a more accurate assessment method as cool peripheries may adversely affect the results. This pressure should be maintained for a count of 5 seconds and then released. The nurse should then count how long it takes for blanching to disappear and normal perfusion to return. This should normally occur in less than two seconds. An increase in the amount of time taken for normal perfusion to occur may be an indicator of inadequate tissue perfusion secondary to shock but it is important to ascertain that the prolonged capillary refill time is not being influenced by external factors such as the environmental temperature. As with all nursing assessments capillary refill time should not be considered in isolation but in conjunction with other related observations. The presence of a prolonged capillary refill time in conjunction with tachycardia, hypotension and cool peripheries is highly suggestive of shock.

Question 3: What is the significance of capillary refill time?

The presence of a prolonged capillary refill time of greater than two seconds indicates that the child may have inadequate perfusion. The most common cause of this is hypovolaemia. This would normally indicate that a fluid bolus is required.

Question 4: What causes shock to occur?

You should have found the information to answer this question within the fixed resource session entitled 'Circulatory shock'.

Trigger 8.2: Referral and retrieval to PICU

Question 1: What illness is Charlie likely to be suffering from?

The fixed resource session entitled 'Meningococcal septicaemia' and additional reading materials should have helped you to answer this question. Charlie is suffering from shock, which is probably secondary to sepsis. Statistically, and in the presence of a purpuric rash, this is most likely to be meningococcal septicaemia and consequently appropriate antibiotics should be commenced at the earliest opportunity. It is important, however, to remain vigilant for the possibility of a differential diagnosis as it is not possible to confirm the diagnosis until blood cultures have been tested and this may take a couple of days.

Question 2: Why do intensive care units retrieve critically ill children?

Reading the fixed resource session entitled 'Retrieval of critically ill children' should have identified the answer to this question.

The trigger also asks you to design a poster for parents. You may have chosen to do this fictitiously or related to your local paediatric intensive care unit. The information provided should help to prepare parents for any impending transfer. Detailed below is a summary of some of the information you may have chosen to include on your poster:

- What is meant by 'intensive care'.
- Why the child needs to go to a different hospital.
- Who will be collecting the child.
- How parents will travel to the intensive care unit.
- Details of the hospital and unit location.
- Brief details of facilities for parents on intensive care.
- What to expect in the first hour after arrival.
- Contact details for the unit.
- Contact details of someone to talk to in the referring hospital.

This list is not meant to be exhaustive and may contain very different information to your own poster. Essentially you should try to ascertain what information a family is likely to require once they know their child is to be transferred to an intensive care unit and aim to provide this in a simple, easily understood format.

Question 3: What fluid will help Charlie?

Fluids administered to children can either be identified as maintenance fluid or resuscitation fluid. In this situation the fluid requirement is for resuscitation. As a result of the underlying disease process and the body's compensatory mechanisms in response to this, Charlie has inadequate fluid in his circulatory system to adequately perfuse all of the cells and, therefore, requires fluid for volume replacement.

Fluid for resuscitation should be given as a bolus over a short period of time (5–10 minutes) and then assessed for effectiveness. ALSG (2005) recommend 20 mls per kilogram for this initial bolus and this is supported by numerous paediatric texts. If the child remains fluid depleted at the end of the bolus this should be repeated in the same quantity. If a third fluid bolus is required this provides a good indication that more intensive support is necessary and if PICU staff are not already involved in the resuscitation they should be informed of the child's condition.

The type of fluid used is controversial and may become more significant when large volumes are required. Primarily fluids are classified into two groups – crystalloids and colloids.

Crystalloids can be described as a solution containing ionic or non-ionic solutes that can be diffused through a semipermeable membrane. Most commonly they are a combination of sodium or glucose molecules in water. Crystalloids do not have osmotic properties and, therefore, they are distributed between both the intracellular and extracellular spaces. Fluids which contain no sodium are distributed evenly between all areas whilst 0.9% Saline is confined to the extracellular areas.

The advantages of using crystalloids is that they are simple to make, cheap to buy and do not provoke an adverse reaction in the patient. However a greater volume of crystalloid rather than colloid may be required due to crystalloids dispersing into the cells.

Colloids are naturally occurring fluids which diffuse less readily into the interstitial space and, therefore, are more effective at expanding the intravascular volume. This is because these fluids exert an oncotic pressure, which causes big molecules to remain in the intravascular space. If the oncotic pressure is greater than that of the plasma, they also draw fluid into the intravascular space from the surrounding tissues (known as plasma expanders).

Blood, which can be classed as a colloid, has the additional advantage of raising the haemoglobin and thereby improving oxygen delivery. The main disadvantages are time (as it takes an hour to fully cross match blood), risk of adverse reactions, error and expense.

Human Albumin Solution (HAS) is pasteurised human plasma. It is available in two strengths: 4.5 per cent and 20 per cent, identified by the sodium content. The most commonly used strength of albumin, 4.5 per cent, has a similar electrolyte composition to plasma. The Cochrane Injuries Group Albumin Reviews (1998) identified a significantly higher risk of mortality associated with albumin use in the adult population. The investigators advised that the results be interpreted cautiously but an accompanying editorial recommended a cessation of albumin use in critically ill patients. This report allegedly led to a 40 per cent decrease in albumin use in the United Kingdom (Roberts et al 1999). In the critically ill child, albumin is often thought to be the most effective method of rapid, sustained volume expansion and its use continues to be recommended (Allison and Lobo 2000).

A large randomised trial was conducted in Australia to compare the effectiveness of albumin and saline for fluid resuscitation in the intensive care setting (SAFE study investigators, 2004). Although based within the adult population again the results still have relevance to children. Their conclusions showed no difference in outcome 28 days after administration of either albumin or saline. This is, therefore, not supportive of the earlier Cochrane study.

Waikar and Chertow (2000) identify that the debate about which fluid is most appropriate continues. Literature identifies that local policies primarily direct the choice of fluid at present. It is reasonable to expect that future studies will examine the appropriateness of different fluid types in relation to the underlying diagnosis rather than relying on the existing heterogenous studies. It is also to be hoped that studies specifically relating to the specific needs of children will be forthcoming.

One possible solution to the problem may be the use of artificial colloids. These are made by chemical hydrolysis of collagens to form bigger molecules suspended in an ionic solution. This results in man-made products that possess many of the properties of colloids. Advantages of these include being cheap and readily available, they have a long storage life and do not have the risks of infection associated with blood products due to being man-made. However, there remains a possibility of allergic reaction and they have a short half life within the body once administered when compared to albumin.

Specific nursing care of a child receiving fluid resuscitation includes maintenance and care of the intravenous cannula and line, ensuring that the cannula remains patent and observing for signs of tissue damage or infection. Intravenous lines should be carefully secured to ensure they do not become dislodged or disconnected. The child should be closely observed to monitor for the effect the fluid is having. Signs of fluid overload such as increased respiratory rate and heart rate should be reported to medical staff immediately.

Question 4: How will intubation help Charlie's respiratory function?

You should already have established that with a structured approach it is essential to ensure an adequate airway prior to undertaking any definitive treatment. Intubation involves the placement of an endotracheal tube either nasally or orally into the trachea. This is the easiest way of securing an airway to instigate artificial ventilation.

Stack and Dobbs (2004) identify a number of reasons why this may be necessary in the child suffering from meningococcal septicaemia. It will reduce the effort of breathing and, therefore, reduce the oxygen demand on the myocardium. It will also enable nursing staff to clear secretions quickly and easily, which is necessary for two reasons. First the underlying disease process will be causing fluid to leak out of the cardiovascular system and into the tissues and second large quantities of fluids will be being administered to Charlie simultaneously to maintain adequate perfusion and circulation. Both of these factors significantly increase the risk of pulmonary oedema occurring.

It should also be remembered that Charlie's neurological function may be affected. If the bacteria have crossed the blood-brain barrier, Charlie may have a concurrent meningitis. His neurological function may also have been affected by his multiorgan failure leading to hypoxia and a shortage of oxygen being delivered to his brain. All of these factors may prevent Charlie from adequately protecting his airway and maintaining sufficient respiratory effort, necessitating elective intubation.

Trigger 8.3: Care of the child in intensive care

Question 1: How do ventilators support the respiratory system?

You should have found the information to answer this question within the fixed resource session 'Respiratory support'.

Question 2: How do inotropes work?

Inotropes are drugs that work on specific receptors within the body. Primarily they increase contractility of the cardiac muscle but other actions include increasing the heart rate and producing peripheral vasoconstriction. All of these actions will have the effect of increasing cardiac output, which will help the body to respond to traumatic events such as illness or injury. Inotropes may be naturally occurring within the body or man-made. Naturally occurring inotropes include adrenaline (epinephirine), noradrenaline (norepinephirine) and dopamine. Synthetic inotropes include dobutamine, isoprenaline and enoximone.

Inotropes can have a dramatic effect on the cardiovascular system and consequently should only be administered in situations where the child can be closely monitored. Generally they are not used outside intensive care units, cardiac units or operating theatres. Children receiving inotropic therapy should have electrocardiograph and saturation monitoring and ideally invasive (arterial) blood pressure monitoring. Accurate fluid management is essential and catheterisation is preferable to allow hourly urine output measurements to be obtained. It is essential that there is no obstruction to the administration of the intravenous infusion of the inotropic drugs due to their short half life. To support this inotropes should ideally be administered directly into a central vein, using modern, accurate syringe pump infusion devices, on a dedicated line and all infusions changed at least one hour before the syringe empties. A sudden decrease in the infusion rate or disconnection of the infusion may lead to significant hypotension with associated arrhythmia's and in extreme or prolonged cases, cardiac arrest.

Question 3: How do you talk to families about the possibility of death?

The document *Standards for Bereavement Care* (Paediatric Intensive Care Society 2002) was written to provide guidelines for health professionals working within paediatric intensive care units within the United Kingdom. It was felt to be of particular benefit following recent inquiries into paediatric death and organ retention affecting a number of hospitals. It has become evident however that that this is a valuable document for all staff caring for children who may potentially die, regardless of their clinical setting.

The document summarises guidance for best practice and deals with a number of psychological, practical and legal issues. Chapter 4 'Care of the family of the dying child' was highlighted as a useful resource to help you answer the questions raised within this trigger as this is an area many nurses feel uncomfortable with and inadequately prepared for.

Although within this trigger Charlie was expected to live, this could certainly not be guaranteed. It is important never to lie to families, to ensure they are fully aware of possible outcomes and to address any questions they may have about the potential death of their child openly and honestly. This will help to build a trusting relationship between the family and the health care workers. If an individual feels unable to do this they should gain support and help from a more experienced colleague to ensure that the needs of families are met.

Question 4: How can parents of critically ill children be involved in their care?

You should have found the information to answer this question within the fixed resource session 'Involving families in care on PICU'.

Trigger 8.4: High Dependency Care

Question 1: What are the differences between intensive care and high dependency care?

You should have found the information to answer this question within the fixed resource session 'Paediatric intensive care and high dependency care: A history of the service development'.

Question 2: How can nurses alleviate family anxiety?

You should have found the information to answer this question within the fixed resource session 'Preparing parents for transfer out of PICU'.

Question 3: What information does the family need to know about the transfer?

When designing an information leaflet for families it is important to use simple language and avoid medical jargon and abbreviations. The information should be clearly presented and not overcrowded. Leaflets should be available in other languages for the benefit of families who have little or no understanding of written English.

The exact content of your leaflet will depend on your own perceptions of what is important from the research that has been published and from the information provided in the fixed resource 'Preparing parents for transfer out of the PICU'. It is likely to address some of the key points outlined below.

1. Factual information about the unit the child is being transferred to, for example, layout, parental accommodation, ward routines, telephone numbers.
2. Information about the staffing ratio's within the new ward area so that parents realise that their child will no longer be receiving one-to-one care.
3. Information about their child's decreased need for monitoring and technical information so that they are prepared for this reduction and are able to see this as a positive step.
4. Ideas for how they can start to increase their role in the care of their child.

Reflect on your learning

By working through the triggers and following Charlie's case a number of areas have been considered. Although these have been linked to a particular scenario, the key principles of paediatric critical care nursing can be applied to any child and are outlined below.

- Early recognition of a sick or deteriorating child is vital. A child's condition can deteriorate rapidly and they may be unable to communicate specific details. The use of a structured, systematic approach (airway, breathing, circulation, disability) will assist the assessment process. By utilising such a system it is possible to assess and treat a child appropriately before a definitive diagnosis has been confirmed. Crucially, at this stage, it is the treatment of the symptoms that the child is displaying that is more important than identifying the causative factor although this will obviously become important once the child is stabilised.

- Children requiring intensive care should be cared for in a specialist regional referral centre. If this is in a different location to the referring hospital an experienced paediatric retrieval team should undertake the transfer. Staff within referring hospitals need to establish close communication links with the lead centre in order to ensure that optimal care is given to the child at all times. This will also help to enable families to receive accurate and appropriate information about what to expect for their child during and following transfer.

- Most children who require intensive care are suffering from one or more primary organ/system failures. The affected organ/system will require a replacement strategy or support until the underlying problem has been resolved. Most commonly the affected system will be the respiratory system requiring ventilatory support. Other regularly affected systems include circulatory, renal, hepatic and neurological.

- Constant advances in technology and therapeutic interventions mean that children in intensive care are often surrounded by a plethora of cables, monitors and electrical equipment. While often providing parents with reassurance that their child is receiving the best treatments available, this can all add to the stress, fear and confusion being experienced by families. This if further compounded by the uncertain future of their child and a lack of understanding of what is happening. Communication is vital to allay these fears. Families need regular, accurate and honest information about their child's condition, treatment and progress. This can be further enhanced by ensuring that families are involved in their child's care to the extent that they feel comfortable.

- Although probably not equivalent to admission to intensive care, it is recognised that transfer to a lower dependency setting may be a stressful experience for the child and family. The nurse can help to ease this transition with effective preparation, good communication and by instigating a gradual reduction in the intensity of interventions.

- Simultaneous negotiation of families to be further involved in their child's care will also be beneficial.

In conclusion at all stages of a child's journey through critical care areas the key concepts to be remembered are:

- Structured approach to assessment and treatment.
- Appropriately trained staff available at all times.
- Involvement of the child and family in decision-making.
- Effective communication.

References

Allison, S., Lobo, D. (2000) Debate: Albumin administration should not be avoided. *Critical Care* 4 (3), pp. 147–50.

ALSG (2005) *Advanced Paediatric Life Support: The Practical Approach*, 4th edn. London: BMJ.

Barry, P. W., Ralston, C. (1994) Adverse events occurring during inter hospital transfer of the critically ill. *Archive of Diseases of Childhood* 7 (1), pp. 8–11.

Bennett, N. (1997) Paediatric intensive care: A developing speciality. *Paediatric Anaesthesia* 7, pp. 495–500.

British Paediatric Association (1993) *The Care of Critically Ill Children. Report of the multidisciplinary working party on paediatric intensive care*. London: British Paediatric Association.

Britto, J., Nadel, S., Levin, M., Habibi, P. (1995) Mobile paediatric intensive care: The ethos of transferring critically ill children. *Care of the Critically Ill* 11 (6), pp. 235–8.

Cagan, J. (1988) Weaning patients from intensive unit care. *Maternal and Child Nursing* 13, pp. 275–7.

Cochrane Injuries Group Albumin Reviews (1998) 'Human albumin administration in critically ill patients: A systematic review of randomised controlled trials. *British Medical Journal*, 317, pp. 235–40.

Davies, J. (2001) 'Paediatric retrieval – aiming for the gold standard, *Care of the Critically Ill* 17 (3), pp. 94–8.

Davies, J., Hassell, L. (2001) *Children in Intensive Care. A Nurse's Survival Guide*. Edinburgh: Churchill Livingstone.

Department of Health (1997) *Paediatric Intensive Care 'A Framework for the Future'. Report from the National Co-ordinating Group on Paediatric Intensive care to the Chief Executive of the NHS Executive*. London: Department of Health.

Department of Health, NHS Executive (1997a) *A Bridge to the Future. Nursing Standards, Education and Workforce Planning in Paediatric Intensive Care*. London: Department of Health.

Department of Health (2001) *High Dependency Care for Children – Report of an Expert Advisory Group for Department of Health*. London: Department of Health.

Edge, W. E., Kanter, R. K., Weigle, C. G. M., Walsh, R. F. (1994) Reduction of morbidity in inter hospital transport by specialized pediatric staff. *Critical Care Medicine* 22 (7), pp. 1186–91.

Haines, C., Wolstenholme, M. (2000) Family support in paediatric intensive care, in Williams C, Asquith J. *Paediatric Intensive Care Nursing*. Edinburgh: Churchill Livingstone.

How to guides (1998) Meningococcal disease – Early management. *Care of the Critically Ill* 14 (8).

Hubband, S., Trigg, E. (2000) *Practices in Children's Nursing. Guidelines for Hospital and community*. Edinburgh: Churchill Livingstone.

Jevon, P. (2004) *Paediatric Advanced Life Support: A Practical Guide*. Edinburgh: Butterworth Heinemann.

Keogh, S. (2001) Parents' experience of the transfer of their child from the PICU to the ward: A phenomenological study. *Nursing in Critical Care* 6, pp. 17–13.

MacNab, A. J. (1991) Optimal escort for inter hospital transport of pediatric emergencies. *Journal of Trauma* (31) 2, pp. 205–9.

Morrison, G. (2000) Transportation of the critically ill child in Williams, C., Asquith, J. *Paediatric Intensive Care Nursing*. Edinburgh: Churchill Livingstone.

Nadel, S., Brownlie, R. (2000) Care of the critically ill child with infectious disease, in Williams C, Asquith J. *Paediatric Intensive Care Nursing*. Edinburgh: Churchill Livingstone, pp. 199–227.

National Meningitis Trust (1996) *Hospital Information Pack*.

Paediatric Intensive Care Society (1996) *Standards for Paediatric Intensive Care*. Sheffield: PICS.

Paediatric Intensive Care Society. (2001) *Standards for Paediatric Intensive Care*. 2nd edn. Sheffield: PICS.

Paediatric Intensive Care Society. (2002) *Standards for Bereavement Care*. Sheffield: PICS.

Pollack, M. M., Ruttimann, U. E., Tesselaar, H. M., Bachulis, A. C. (1991) Improved outcomes from tertiary centre paediatric intensive care: A state-wide comparison of tertiary and non tertiary care facilities. *Critical Care Medicine* 19, pp. 150–9.

Roberts, I., Edwards, P., McLelland, B. (1999) More on albumin. Use of human albumin in UK fell substantially when systematic review was published. *British Medical Journal* 318, pp. 1214–15.

Saarmann, L. (1993) Transfer out of critical care: Freedom or fear?' *Critical Care Nursing Quarterly* 16, pp. 78–85.

SAFE Study Investigators (2004) A comparison of albumin and saline for fluid resuscitation in the intensive care unit. *New England Journal of Medicine* 350, pp. 2247–56.

Stack, C. G. (1997) Stabilisation and transport of the critically ill child. *Current Anaesthesia and Critical Care* 8, pp. 25–30.

Stack, C., Dobbs, P. (2004) *Essentials of Paediatric Intensive Care*. London: GMM.

Waikar, S., Chertow, G. (2000) Crystalloids versus colloids for resuscitation in shock, *Current Opinion in Nephrology and Hypertension* 9, pp. 501–4.

Williams, C., Asquith, J. (2000) *Paediatric Intensive Care Nursing*. Edinburgh: Churchill Livingstone.

Zideman, D. (1994) Resuscitation in infants and children, in Colquhoun, M. (ed.) *ABC of Resuscitation*. London: BMJ.

9 Neonatal Intensive Care

Angela Thurlby

Learning outcomes

- Describe the contexts of the Neonatal Intensive Care Unit (NICU) and the Special Care Baby Unit (SCBU).
- Understand the physiology of the newborn with reference to maintaining homeostasis for a baby requiring specialised care at birth.
- Explain interventions to maintain optimum physical development for babies being cared for within these contexts.
- Explore the needs of the families within the NICU.

Introduction

This chapter introduces you to the Neonatal Intensive Care Unit (NICU). It will focus on defining which babies are cared for in this context, identifying the characteristics, causes and problems of premature and small for date (SFD) babies. Along with being able to provide expert nursing care for these babies it is necessary to understand the effects that admission of a baby to the NICU has on the parents and other family members. It is also important to identify the support mechanisms and facilities available to parents. The long-term consequences, for some of these babies, are such that they may require extensive follow-up and support for a number of years. Facilitation of effective communication between the multi-disciplinary team, the parents and external agencies are crucial throughout their care. Also, maintaining a constant stream of explanations and information has been identified as a source of reassurance and empowerment for parents struggling to come to terms with the unexpected events of a baby born at the limits of viability or with the prospect of bringing up a child who will need special support for a long period.

The triggers will provide a 'snapshot' to help you to gain an overview of the care required by the babies and their families within this context. Nursing these babies is complex and very demanding, therefore, nurses working in the NICU have undertaken further specialist post-basic training. The opportunity to observe care in this situation is a unique and challenging experience.

! Trigger 9.1: The Neonatal Intensive Care Baby Unit

The intention of this trigger is to introduce you to the context of neonatal intensive care nursing and to highlight some of the problems which necessitate a baby being admitted to the NICU.

The Trigger

Joanne is a 28 year old primigravida who is married and living with her husband. She is a teacher and he is a dentist. She experiences a normal uneventful pregnancy until 28 weeks gestation when she suddenly develops abdominal pain and spontaneous rupture of her membranes. She is taken into the local maternity unit and her baby boy is born 30 minutes later. The mother has no history of medical problems.

At birth the baby weighed 1.450 Kg, was active and making some respiratory effort, but needed assistance with oxygen and Continuous Positive Airway Pressure (CPAP). He was also given a dose of surfactant. Following his resuscitation he was taken to the Special Care Baby Unit (SCBU) to be stabilized before being transferred to the Neonatal Intensive Care Unit (NICU) in another maternity hospital 20 miles away. A chest X ray at 4 hours old revealed that he had developed respiratory distress syndrome (RDS) and he received a further dose of surfactant. His respiratory support continued until he was weaned from CPAP, eventually managing to breathe unaided.

His mother was transferred to the other hospital to be near to him and was discharged home after a few days, managing to visit daily, with his father visiting in the evenings. The baby was fed continuously via a nasogastric tube using expressed breast milk. His mother was encouraged to express breast milk and to bring it with her when visiting.

The baby remained in the NICU for three weeks before he was well enough to be transferred back to the referring unit to complete his care. He was finally discharged home at 3 months old with follow-up clinic appointments to monitor his progress.

The situation

You are about to commence on a placement within the Neonatal Intensive Care Unit (NICU) where you will be faced with similar scenarios in practice. Think about how the experience of this baby and his family differs to that of a baby born at term with no problems.

Feedback

Plan and present an information booklet for parents explaining why their baby has

RDS, how it will be treated and how they can become involved in the care of their baby in the NICU. Make notes from the fixed resources and references to help provide some of the information.

The facts

What are the main facts in this trigger? Make a list:

Hypotheses: What may these facts mean?

- A baby can be born and survive earlier than expected.
- A baby who is premature will need help with breathing.
- CPAP and surfactant will help a premature baby with its breathing.
- The baby will need transfer to the Neonatal Intensive Care Unit.
- His parents will find this situation distressing and difficult.
- The baby will benefit from the mother's breast milk.

Questions developed from the hypotheses

1. Why are babies born prematurely, how is it defined, where should they be nursed?
2. What are the problems and complications and what care is needed?
3. What is Respiratory Distress Syndrome, how is it managed?
4. Why is breast milk needed?
5. How will the parents be supported?

Trigger 9.1: Fixed resource material

Read the following to help you answer the questions. (You may also wish to search and review other up-to-date research and evidence-based literature, and seek other relevant resources to provide you with the answers to your questions.)

Boxwell, G. (ed.) (2001) *Neonatal Intensive Care Nursing*, 2nd edn. London: Routledge.

Fraser, D. M., Cooper, M. A. (eds) (2003) *Mayes' Midwifery: A Textbook for Midwives*, 14th edn. London: Churchill Livingstone.

Johnston, P. J. B. (1998) *The Newborn Child*, 8th edn. London: Churchill Livingstone.

Rennie, J. M., Roberton, N.R.C. (2002). *A Manual of Neonatal Intensive Care*, 4th edn. London: Edward Arnold.

Rennie, J. M., Roberton, N. R. C. (eds) (1999) *Text Book of Neonatology*, 3rd edn. London: Churchill Livingstone.

Roberton, N. R. C. (2005) *Roberton's Textbook of Neonatology*, edited by Janet M. Rennie, 4th edn. Edingburgh: Elsevier Churchill Livingstone.

Smith, L., Coleman, V., Bradshaw, M. (eds) (2002) *Family-centred Care*: Concept, Theory and Practice. Basingstoke: Palgrave.

Sparshott, M. (1997) *Pain, Distress and the Newborn Baby*. Oxford: Blackwell Science.

Wong, D. L. (1995) *Whaley and Wong's Nursing Care of Infants and Children*, 5th edn. St Louis: Mosby.

Yeo, H. (ed.) (2000) *Nursing the Neonate*, 2nd edn. Oxford: Blackwell Science.

Infant. www.infantgrapevine.co.uk

Midirs Midwifery Digest. www.midirs.org

BLISS The Premature Baby Charity. www.bliss.org.uk

Kangaroo Care. www.prematurity.org/baby/kangaroo.html

UNICEF Baby Friendly Initiative. www.babyfriendly.org.uk

Trigger 9.1: Fixed resource sessions

The Contexts of the NICU and SCBU

The baby in the case history was born in a maternity hospital where the mother was receiving her antenatal care and where she was planning to have her baby after a normal pregnancy. However, these plans were interrupted when the she went into spontaneous premature labour resulting in the birth of her baby at 28 weeks gestation. Following his birth he required transfer to another hospital for intensive care due to his premature arrival and respiratory difficulties.

This is not an unusual event as not all maternity hospitals are equipped to deal with premature babies who require ventilation or other forms of intensive nursing care. All maternity units will have a special care baby unit (SCBU) where they can provide supportive care prior to the baby's transfer to an NICU. This involves a team of medical and nursing staff from the NICU retrieving the baby from the referring unit bringing with them a range of specialised equipment in an especially equipped ambulance. They will assess and stabilize the baby prior to transfer. This will also involve separation of the baby from its parents for a short period of time until the mother can be transferred to be near to her baby. The nursing staff will ensure that the parents are given a chance to see and touch their baby prior to the transfer and the medical staff will give them an explanation of why their baby needs to be transferred. The nurses will also take pictures of the baby for the parents to keep especially if the mother has had a surgical delivery requiring an anaesthetic rendering her unable to have contact with her baby for a few days. In these circumstances the father has a key role in that he will follow the baby to the regional unit to see his baby settled there and to talk to the staff. He will also be able to keep the mother informed of events. He will need support from other family members during this time especially if he has other children to care for. You will find more information about supporting parents in the fixed resource material.

Therefore the current structure for neonatal care is:

- Regional neonatal intensive care units where expert intensive care is provided for premature babies and babies of any gestation who are ill at birth. Mothers will be referred to these centres for delivery or retrieval teams will collect the baby following delivery and stabilisation. The baby will be returned to the referring unit when their condition stabilizes. These units also provide specialist neonatal surgery.
- Sub-regional neonatal intensive care units are a subsidiary to the regional unit. They will retrieve babies and provide intensive care. They will transfer any baby requiring surgery to the nearest surgical unit.
- Special Care baby units are based in all maternity hospitals. They care for babies from 32 weeks gestation. They also provide emergency treatment for smaller babies until transfer to a regional unit can be arranged. There are usually one or two intensive cots and the baby will stay if it can be managed in that context.
- Transitional Care units are usually based in a maternity ward and care for babies who, for example, require treatment for jaundice or infection but are otherwise well. This keeps the baby with or near to its mother and cared for by midwives or neonatal nurses, thus preventing unnecessary transfer of the baby into an intensive care unit.

Therefore, babies admitted to the NICU will fall into the following criteria:

- Any baby weighing less than 1.700 kg from 23–34 weeks gestation.
- Any baby who is ill at birth, for example, extremely premature or small for date babies.
- Term babies who have suffered birth asphyxia or meconium aspiration requiring extensive resuscitation at birth.

- Any baby with severe congenital abnormalities requiring emergency treatment or surgery. Babies with congenital abnormalities who are not seriously ill usually stay with their parents on the maternity ward in order to help the parents to bond with their baby, for example a baby with Downs Syndrome who is otherwise well.

The definition and causes of premature babies

The definition of a premature baby is one born before 37 completed weeks of gestation (World Health Organisation 1992). A normal pregnancy usually lasts for about 38 to 42 weeks. At these gestations the baby is classed as term. It will weigh about 3.5 kg and is usually able to survive under normal circumstances with its parents and without the need for specialised Intensive care (Johnston 1998). According to the above definitions the baby described in the case history will be classed as premature because his gestation was only 28 weeks. A premature baby will have differences in its appearance and needs to those of a term baby.   The Human Fertilisation and Embryology Act (1990) stated that a baby is capable of surviving from the 24th week of pregnancy. Therefore, viable gestational age is by law considered to be 24 weeks and over whatever the weight of the baby. These two definitions give an indication of the gestational range that premature babies can be classed in, for example, any baby between 24 and 37 weeks gestation. With this in mind there will be a vast difference in the size, appearance and needs of babies at the different gestations. At birth regardless of its size and gestation the nursing and medical staff will record the weight, length and head circumference. These measurements are recorded on centile charts which show the average weight, head circumference and length for the different gestations (Johnston 1998 pp. 45, 108).The baby's actual measurements when recorded on this chart can then be compared with the normal measurements for its gestation. These measurements are reassessed regularly. Weight is also used to determine the baby's daily nutritional, fluid needs and medication doses in the NICU (Johnston 1998; Rennie and Roberton 1999; Yeo, 2000).

The developing foetus is dependent on the mother for its respiration and nutrition. It will be influenced by the mother's metabolic and cardiovascular state and environmental factors. The foetus has a limited ability to adapt to stress or to modify its surroundings. This creates a situation in which the prenatal environment exerts an influence on the foetal development which will affect its wellbeing and outcomes in the immediate and long-term future. Of all babies 3 to 4 per cent are premature and almost all of them weigh less than 2.500 kg. It is from this group that 60 per cent of all neonatal deaths occur (Johnston 1998; Rennie and Roberton 1999). There are many factors that can adversely affect the growth and development of the foetus and increase the risk during the pregnancy, labour and delivery or in the neonatal period. Some of these factors are summarised as follows:

- Where there is a previous obstetric history of mid-trimester miscarriage or where the mother has had an abortion.
- Where the maternal age is outside of the optimum childbearing ages of 18–40.
- An increased risk has been identified in groups with poor socio-economic status these risks have been linked to poor diet, unemployment, smoking, alcohol and drug abuse (Wilcox 1995).
- Congenital abnormalities can be associated with premature birth.
- Maternal infection during pregnancy can affect the baby in utero and lead to premature delivery.
- Multiple pregnancies can result in premature deliveries. This is due to the number and size of the foetuses.
- Pregnancy induced hypertension (PIH) can lead on to pre-eclampsia. This is a condition peculiar to pregnancy characterised by hypertension, proteinuria and systemic dysfunction resulting in the need to deliver the baby early because of the risks to the mother and the baby (Fraser and Cooper 2003).
- Antepartum haemorrhage (APH) is defined as bleeding from the maternal genital tract after the 24th week of pregnancy. The bleeding is from the placenta and can lead to placental insufficiency and a smaller baby who may be delivered prematurely (Fraser and Cooper 2003).
- Placenta praevia is a condition in which the placenta is attached to the lower segment of the uterus which can lead to placental bleeding and early delivery of the baby by caesarean section (Fraser and Cooper 2003).
- Placental abruption is premature separation of the placenta from the uterine wall which can occur any time from 24 weeks to term (Fraser and Cooper 2003). It is an obstetric emergency which results in the need to deliver the baby immediately and can lead to foetal death.
- Maternal diabetes can be associated with premature delivery and immature lung development in the baby.

However 40 per cent of premature deliveries are spontaneous with no apparent cause (Rennie and Roberton 1999, Wilcox et al 1995) as with the baby in the case history.

In practice midwives and obstetricians will identify possible risk factors from the history when a pregnant woman presents for the booking visit and on subsequent visits to the antenatal clinic. Some of the risks can be minimised by advising the woman on healthy diet, to stop smoking and drinking alcohol or by referring her for help if she has a problem with drug addiction. Regular blood pressure, health checks and, where necessary, ultrasound scanning, are used to monitor the progress of the pregnancy and provide early recognition of potential problems, which can be treated before they become too serious.

The characteristics of premature babies

Premature babies will differ in their appearance to their term counterparts and often the parents are shocked by this as they will be unprepared for what to expect and will need time to come to terms with what has happened. One of the biggest concerns expressed is that the baby is very small and they worry about causing the baby harm it they touch it.

- The head of a premature baby will appear to be large compared to the body however the proportional head size is usually normal. This is because the brain will be growing faster than the body during the early stages of development. By the time the baby reaches term the head will appear to be more in proportion (Yeo 2000).
- The skin will appear red, oedematous (because of retained fluid) and transparent depending on the gestation. A very premature baby of 26 weeks gestation will have a very thin skin with the epidermis being only two or three cells thick. As the baby develops the skin will show increasing levels of maturity and by 34 weeks epidermal development is complete. It can take two to four weeks for the stratum corneum to form giving the skin the same maturity as a term baby (Boxwell 2001; Johnston 1998; Yeo 2000). Premature babies also have little or no subcutaneous fat and the blood vessels can be seen through the thin layer of skin on the abdomen which will appear large and prominent when compared to the chest which appears small (Johnson 1998; Rennie and Roberton 1999; Yeo 2000).
- Their tone is poor and movement is limited because of their under developed muscles and skeleton.
- Their cry is weak and they would sleep for long periods if left to rest.
- The heart rate is normally about 120 – 150 beats per minute at rest.
- The respiration rate is about 40 – 60 breaths pre minute at rest.
- The blood pressure range is about 60/30.
- The genitalia may be under developed. In girls the labia minora is prominent and in boys the testes may not have descended.
- The ears are also very soft due to an absence of cartilage.
- Their urinary output is poor at first but will gradually increase over first 48 hours. This is due to a combination of the immaturity of the kidneys and the reduced levels of fluid given to premature babies with respiratory difficulties (Johnston 1998).

The problems and complications

Premature babies can experience many problems until they are well enough to go home with their families. Most of these occur due to their premature status and can be managed within the contexts of the NICU and SCBU.

- The management of fluids and nutrition can be difficult due to an inability to coordinate sucking and swallowing.

When attempting to feed, a premature baby will become easily tired out. Initially they may require a combination of intravenous feeding with ten per cent dextrose or total parenteral nutrition (TPN) and continuous nasogastric feeding with breast or formula milk until full breast or bottle feeds can be slowly introduced.

On admission to the NICU the baby will be weighed and the amount of fluid that the baby can be given will be worked out according to this weight and the regime, which dictates the hourly amount to be given. In practice they usually start at 60 ml per kg per hour for the first 24 to 48 hours. The amounts on the regime can then be increased by 30 ml increments as the baby's condition improves. As the urinary output increases the oedema will begin to diminish. They are usually weighed weekly and once the weight increases beyond the birth weight the amounts of milk can be increased. The initial weight gain will be slow because of their problems and the demands made on their metabolism. Weight is a significant measure for the parents as it is often seen as one of the signs of progress and they easily become discouraged if the baby loses weight following any setbacks.

- Physiological jaundice can be prolonged because the liver functions are immature. This inhibits their ability to conjugate and excrete bilirubin efficiently (Day et al 1997).
- Hypoglycaemia occurs due to the baby being born before enough glycogen can be stored in the liver (Rennie and Roberton 1999).
- The temperature is difficult to maintain due to immaturity of the temperature regulating system in the hypothalamus (Fellows 2001).
- Infection is a risk due to immaturity of the immune system.

The early recognition of the symptoms and treatment with antibiotics is important. Infection screening will be carried out if the baby develops any signs of infection and a 10 day course of broad spectrum antibiotics will be commenced following collection of all samples. Scrupulous hand washing and drying by staff and visitors has been proved to be the most effective way of reducing the risk of infection (Yeo 2000). All equipment used is sterilised and only used for one baby. Visiting policies are in place to protect the babies from too many visitors. Parents are encouraged to visit and stay near their baby at all times, other visitors are allowed at the discretion of the parents and staff caring for the baby. Special arrangements are also considered for siblings to visit with parental support.

- Respiratory Distress Syndrome (RDS) occurs due to a lack of surfactant in their lungs (Cameron 2001).

RDS is one of the main causes of morbidity and mortality in premature infants which usually affects babies born before 32 weeks gestation as they have few alveoli resulting in reduced surfactant production. Production usually begins from 20 weeks gestation and there is a small amount present at 24 weeks steadily increasing up to 34 weeks when there is a surge in production to prepare for birth. Surfactant stabilizes the size of the alveoli and equalises the surface tension preventing their collapse when breathing out (Gibson 1997; Rennie and Roberton 1999). Therefore, a lack of surfactant leads to alveolar collapse on expiration and impaired gas exchange because of the thickness of the alveolar walls thus decreasing the amount of oxygen able to diffuse into the blood. Also the baby's diaphragm and intercostal muscles are still developing, which may mean that the respiratory efforts will be inadequate to sustain life. The lungs are described as being 'stiff' and difficult to expand. The associated hypoxia can cause right-to-left shunting through the foramen ovale between the atria in the heart and left-to-right shunting through the ductus arteriosus between the pulmonary artery and aorta, which leads to a failure of the transition from intrauterine to extrauterine life. This leads to pulmonary ischemia and damage to the developing lungs (Cameron 2001).

RDS can also be associated with:

- Perinatal asphyxia due to hypoxia and acidosis.
- Hypothermia, a temperature of less than 35°C causes a decrease in the production and efficiency of surfactant.
- RDS can also occur in infants of diabetic mothers where surfactant production can be reduced due to the maternal diabetes even in term babies. There is also a higher incidence of asphyxia due to the larger size of baby (Cameron 2001; Rennie and Roberton 1999).

The onset of RDS usually occurs within 4 hours of birth. The baby becomes increasingly tired with the effort of breathing and develops signs of distress. The diagnosis of RDS is confirmed with a chest x-ray at 4 hours old.

The signs of RDS include:

- Diminished breath sounds because of poor air entry.
- Grunting on expiration. This is caused by the baby trying to force air past its partially closed glottis in an effort to keep air in the alveoli at the end of each breath to prevent atelectasis (collapse of the alveoli when breathing out).
- As the baby becomes more exhausted nasal flaring, apnoea, increased respiratory rate and cyanosis become apparent.

The treatments for RDS include the administration of maternal steroids prior to the baby being delivered. This is only possible with prior warning and was not an option for the mother in the case history who delivered soon after the onset of labour. Giving the steroids to the mother initiates a stress response in the foetus, which will increase surfactant production and mature the lungs. Once born ventilation may be required if the baby is less then 30 weeks and surfactant replacement if the baby is less than 28 weeks gestation (Cameron, 2001).

Surfactant replacement has been shown to reduce the severity of RDS. The OSARIS trial (OSARIS Collaborative Group 1992) demonstrated that early administration was the most effective (Ainsworth and McCormack 2004; Cameron 2001; Soll 1999). The dose of surfactant is injected directly down an endotracheal tube into the lower trachea. The baby will be ventilated to disperse the surfactant as far as possible into the lungs. Further doses can be given in the same manner. The baby needs to be lying supine and flat. Suction should be avoided for at least four hours. After administration pulmonary compliance can improve rapidly, requiring prompt adjustment of ventilator settings and the inspired oxygen concentrations to avoid too high levels of oxygen.

If the baby is deemed suitable the surfactant is given immediately and an X ray is obtained as soon as possible within the first 30 minutes if the baby is less than 26 weeks (Cameron 2001). Following this the baby will be transferred to the NICU to continue with its treatment and care.

Long term problems and complications following premature birth

There is also a risk that premature babies may develop complications which can delay their progress and lead to long-term problems.

> Bronchopulmonary Dysplasia (BPD) becomes apparent when it is difficult to wean the baby from the ventilator usually after 28 days from birth.

BPD occurs as a result of barotrauma from ventilator pressures, oxygen toxicity, surfactant deficiency and pulmonary immaturity (Yeo 2000). The baby will become ventilator and oxygen dependant for several months eventually being discharged home needing low flow oxygen and steroids until the lungs have recovered. Some never fully recover and hospital admissions are frequent with repeated chest infections and difficulties maintaining nutrition. They are also at risk of developing cor pulmonale because of pulmonary oedema, hypoxia and fibrosis in the lungs. These complications can lead to death during this time. Once they start to gain weight the damaged lung tissue can regenerate and their lung function can improve. However they may have some developmental delay and neurological impairments (Mc Cormick et al 1996).

> Necrotising enterocolitis (NEC) is a condition that is characterised by ischaemic changes and necrosis of the gastrointestinal tract (Parker 1995).

The specific cause remains enigmatic, but several risk factors have been identified suggesting that the pathophysiology is multifactorial. Most of the aetiological factors describe events in a population of physically stressed high-risk neonates (Boyd 2001; Parker 1995). There appears to be a complex relationship between mucosal injury, infection and the use of hyperosmolar enteral feeds, that is, those associated either preterm formulas (Boyd 2001). It is the most common surgical emergency in the neonate, which can lead to perforation of the bowel that can be lethal carrying a 30–50 per cent mortality rate (Boyd 2001). It usually affects babies weighing below 1.5 kg, occurring during the between the third and tenth day of life following the initiation of milk feeding. It can be treated medically by stopping enteral feeding and commencing the baby onto total parenteral nutrition with intravenous antibiotics for 14 days slowly introducing milk feeds as their condition improves. However if there is a perforation of the bowel the baby will need surgical intervention to remove the affected area and may need a temporary colostomy or ileostomy until the condition has been treated and milk feeding has been re-established (Boyd 2001; Yeo 2000).

> Retinopathy of prematurity (ROP) is a condition which affects the retinal blood vessels which can lead to blindness if not monitored and treated in its early stages.

It is more common in very premature babies below 28 weeks. The exact cause is not known but it is thought to relate to high concentrations of oxygen causing the developing vessels in the retina to proliferate rapidly leading to haemorrhages and peripheral separation of the retina (Johnston 1998; Yeo 2000). In cases where it does not progress beyond this stage there is little effect on the child's eyesight. In more severe cases it can lead to fibrosis and opacity behind the lens which can be treated with cryotherapy to halt the progression of the disease (Johnston 1998). In practice all babies below 32 weeks are monitored for signs of ROP. Inspired oxygen concentrations are kept below 40 per cent unless a higher concentration is needed. Oxygen levels are continuously monitored by the use of pulse oximetry and regular blood gas analysis to ensure that the baby receives the right level of oxygen (Johnston 1998).

> Peri-intraventricular haemorrhage (PIVH) can occur in the brain of babies below 32 weeks gestation. It is associated with repeated episodes of hypoxia and hypotension leading to intracranial bleeding.

The greatest time of risk occurs in the first 72 hours after birth (Johnston 1998). The risk can be diminished by preventing wide variations in blood pressure and hypoxia. The bleeding starts in the fragile vessels in the germinal matrix in the ventricles of the brain. At these stages the baby will be asymptomatic and the haemorrhages can resolve without causing any problems. However if the haemorrhages continue to develop the ventricles become distended. Bleeding can also extend into the brain tissue which can lead to peri-ventricular leukomalacia (PVL) where cysts form within the damaged brain tissue. This may result in the baby's death or lead to long-term developmental problems and cerebral palsy (Johnston 1998; Yeo 2000).This problem is very difficult to predict and prevent but careful nursing, minimal handling and management of the baby's blood pressure and oxygen especially during the first 72 hours can help to prevent the occurrence (Yeo 2000). In practice regular ultrasound scans of the brain are carried out using a portable scanning machine which means that the progress of the bleeding and the healing process can be monitored without too much disturbance to the baby. Images of the scans are taken at each stage and kept in the baby's notes. The parents are kept informed of the prognosis especially if the bleeding has been severe and the outcome for the baby is in doubt.

The care of premature babies

So far this chapter has concentrated on the care and treatments of some of the medical problems experienced by premature babies in the NICU. Recently, there have been rapid advances in the technology as well as an increased understanding of the preterm baby's development and behaviours. These advances have modified and influenced the practice of neonatal nurses leading to a medically focused management of care. However over the past decade it has been recognised that the environment in the NICU can be over-stimulating, unpredictable and too complex for the newborn to cope with and that this can have an adverse effect on the short-term and long-term outcomes of the babies (Als 1994; 1996 Becker 1995; D'Appolito 1991; Peters 1996). Despite this awareness, the babies are often exposed to loud noise, bright light, painful procedures and excessive handling. As a result efforts are made to reduce the impact of these factors and to make the nursery environment more conducive. Blackburn (1998) stated that the NICU has grown in both intensity and challenge – he describes it as technology-filled, somewhat chaotic, yet with a warm and caring environment.

It is now becoming apparent that medical knowledge with the use of technology is insufficient in guiding the whole of neonatal nursing care, but that integration of other patterns and concepts is essential to expert nursing practice for high risk babies and their families (Phillips 1994).

It must be remembered that although premature babies are small, vulnerable and immature in terms of their development they are still complete and competent human beings who need the support of specialised care in order to grow and develop normally. It is in recognition of the need to nurture the babies through these early stages of development that the concept of developmentally sensitive care was developed and is now practiced where the baby receives care based on its own need and the cues which it gives to carers and not on routine events which may come at a time when the baby is trying to sleep (Als et al 1994, 1996; Als 1998).

The concept of developmentally sensitive care requires rethinking the relationships between babies, families and health care providers. It is a nursing-focused model of care, which will work in partnership with the medical model and in collaboration with other specialists such as physiotherapists, speech therapists, nutritionists and the family.

Developmentally sensitive care includes activities designed to manage the environment and individualize the care of premature babies based on behavioural observations. The goal is to promote a stable, well-organised and competent baby who can conserve energy for growth and development.

A well-known formal approach to developmental care is the Neonatal Individualized Developmental Care and Assessment Programme (NIDCAP) first developed by Dr Als in 1986. In this model, interventions are designed to simulate the environment in utero and to promote normal development. Care is based on the baby's behavioural and physiological cues, and on the nurse's knowledge of normal development and functional ability. In developing her theory Dr Als describes the premature infant as 'the extrauterine foetal neonate' who is in a mismatch situation by virtue of having irreversibly left the support of the intrauterine environment but their nervous system is geared to many more weeks in that environment. Rapid brain growth and differentiation between 26 and 40 weeks renders the premature baby vulnerable to neurological and developmental delays (Als et al 1994, 1996).

NIDCAP provides a framework for understanding the behaviour of premature babies where their behaviours are grouped according to five subsystems of functioning. Each subsystem can be described independently, yet functions in relation to the other subsystems. The process of subsystem interaction – how the five subsystems work together and influence each other – is what is meant by the term 'synaction'. This synaction is combined with the infant's continuous interaction with the environment to formulate the synactive theory of infant development (Als et al 1986).

The five subsystems are described as:

1. *Autonomic*: the basic physiological functioning necessary for survival. The observable indicators are skin colour, tremors/startles, heart and respiratory rate.
2. *Motor*: tone, movement, activity and posture.
3. *States*: the level of central nervous system arousal – sleepy/drowsy, awake, alert and fussing, crying.
4. *Attention/Interaction*: the availability of the baby for interacting in terms of alertness and the robustness of the interaction.
5. *Self-regulatory*: the presence and success of the baby's efforts to achieve and maintain a balance of the other four subsystems.

The basic concept underlying this approach is that the baby will defend itself against stimulation if it is inappropriately timed or is inappropriate in its complexity or intensity. If an inappropriate stimuli persists the baby will no longer be able to maintain a stable balance of subsystems, for example, it will decrease or increase its heart or respirations, skin colour may change, and muscle tone decrease. If properly timed and appropriate in complexity and intensity, stimulation will cause the baby to search and move toward the stimuli, while maintaining a stable balance for example good colour, regular heart and respiratory rate and good muscle tone (Als et al 1994, 1996).

The pre-term infant's systems are not fully developed and ready to function and its behaviour is generally characterized by disorganization and signs of stress. They are very dependent on their environment to help maintain a balance between the subsystems. Technology, which focuses care on the autonomic system, comes at the expense of the other systems which are dependent on an adaptive environment (Als et al 1994, 1996).

Some of the following strategies are used in practice to help the baby to maintain a balance between the subsystems:

- Clustering of care activities enables the baby to have longer periods of quiet and rest. Increased rest will save energy needed for optimal growth and development.

- Quiet times are also arranged during the day in an attempt to cut down on handling and disturbance. This is a multidisciplinary approach meaning that during these times the babies are not handled unless necessary in an emergency. Lights are dimmed and noise levels are reduced. Visiting parents are given the choice to stay with their baby during these times with many choosing to sit quietly by the incubator or to take time out for a rest themselves. Only essential staff will remain in the area to deal with any problems and they can use the time to quietly catch up with any paperwork.

- Pacifiers are used for non-nutritive sucking during tube feeds. Non nutritive sucking helps the baby to develop a sucking reflex and to associate a feeling of fullness with sucking. Pacifiers are used with the parents consent as many who wish to eventually breast feed are concerned that the use of a pacifier may interfere with the baby's ability to suck from the breast. The parents are reassured that this will not happen, and are advised of the benefits of pacifier use to help the baby to associate the action of sucking with the feeling of a full stomach which can encourage sucking at the breast or bottle later (Barros et al 1995; Vibhuti and Ohlsson 2000; Webster 1999; Yeo 2000).

- Supported positioning is used for premature babies who tend to lie in a 'frog like' flattened posture with the limbs extended and their hips abducted as they do not have the strength to resist gravity (Turrill 1992; Young 1994). This can lead to long-term muscular skeletal and developmental problems if left lying for long periods of time in fixed, extended positions without a change (Downs 1991; Fay 1988; Turrill 1992; Young 1994). The use of supported prone, supine or side lying positions helps the baby to achieve state control. The aims are to encourage a balance between flexion and extension and to provide support for the extremities towards the midline in order to maintain body symmetry (Young 1994). This can be managed using rolled up sheets and blankets to provide support and boundaries for the baby to flex against, other methods of support, such as soft gel-filled wedgies and prone pillows, help to keep the baby in a comfortable flexed position. The baby is supported in such a way as to encourage the flexion that would have occurred naturally in the uterus if they had reached term gestation and grown enough to make contact with the walls of the uterus. This is referred to as 'physiological flexion' (Fay 1988) which prepares the baby for birth and gives a normal newborn its ability to balance against gravity and to lie in a flexed foetal position. This also helps with the later developments of normal hand eye co-ordination, hip positions and scapula alignment all of which lead to the ability to sit up and bring the hands to the midline and mouth when exploring new objects during the first two years (Downs 1991; Fay 1988; Turrill 1992; Young 1994). In practice the neonatal physiotherapists advise nursing staff and parents of the best techniques to use. The babies will also be placed on soft quilted sheets to prevent them from being flattened against a hard mattress. The prone position has been shown to be the best position for very premature babies who are being monitored constantly in the NICU as it helps with oxygenation and energy conservation (Heimler et al 1992). As the baby's condition improves it is advised that the supine (back) lying position only is used as advocated by the Department of Health (1991) 'Back to Sleep' campaign for the prevention of cot death. Recently this advice to parents has been reinforced by the Department of Health (2004) in Reduce the Risks: an Easy Guide. Parents are advised about all of these issues before discharge (Lynch 1997).

Other useful strategies such as holding the baby's hand by gently placing a finger in the baby's palm which stimulates the grasp reflex can help with the self regulatory responses. Also slow the pace or give the baby a break if signs of stress are noted (Als et al 1994, 1996).

● Parental education about how to support the baby's developmental agenda is also essential to developmentally focused care (Als et al 1994, 1996; Reid 2001).

Parents can be taught how to understand their premature baby's behaviour and observe more closely their baby's individual behaviour. It is also suggested that this will help them to 'reset' their expectations and thus offer more infant-led support. Facilitating parent teaching by helping the parents to understand the individuality of their baby and how they can offer support promotes stability and development making parental teaching and learning opportunities that are more specific and responsive to their baby' needs with improved skills for handling and care (Reid 2001).

● The use of Kangaroo care has many benefits for both the baby and the parents. Involving the patents with this type of interaction can promote bonding and family centred care.
● The management of pain and distress can be a problem because the babies experience repeated exposure to invasive procedures and the need for ventilation.

Assessment of pain is difficult in a small baby who cannot verbalise its feelings. Concerns are expressed whether enough is currently done to relieve this suffering and to provide comfort for the babies (East 2001). Despite vast amounts of research into the subject there is still uncertainty about how to assess pain and how to differentiate pain cues from other cues indicating distress and illness. Over the past decade a number of pain assessment tools have been researched and developed which are currently being trailed or are in use in some NICU's (Bildner and Krechel 1996; Lawrence et al 1993; Horgan et al 1996; Sparshott 1996; Stevens and Frank 1995). These assessment tools are based on observations of various physiological and behavioural cues that have been observed during painful events. Charts have been devised that enable these cues to be recorded and scored to provide a more objective assessment of the baby's pain in order to initiate the prescription of pain relief. However, there are concerns over the use of pharmacological agents such as opiates unless the baby is already on ventilation as these can depress respiration and there is also a fear of addiction. Opiates are used for babies who are post-op or who are distressed and on ventilation. Paracetamol may be used for mild pain but long-term usage is not advised as there is uncertainty about its effects on the developing liver (East 2001).

Non-pharmacological pain relief using baby massage and appropriate touching techniques, which can also involve the parents, is now becoming an important part care.

Premature babies have a poor tolerance to excessive handling which is often associated with painful procedures. Unfortunately they experience very little comforting touch. Techniques of touch and handling have been developed which allow for loving touch and massage to be modified for use with premature babies (Acolet 1993; Feldman and Eiderman 1998; Field et al 1990; Vickers and Ohlsson 2000).

It has been observed that the parents offer the best form of loving touch, which does not appear to disturb the baby (Appleton 1997).

Pacifiers are also used during stressful and painful events to provide some comfort to help to keep the baby calm.

The pacifier can also be used in conjunction with sucrose. The action of the sweet tasting solution is thought to stimulate the endogenous pain control mechanism and sucking helps the baby to regulate itself to gain control over the pain and to experience comfort (Engerbretson and Wardell 1997; Pinelli and Symington 2000; Vibhuti and Ohlsson 2000; Yeo 2000).

The use of swaddling, facilitated tucking and containment holding, where the carer or parent will place hands gently around the baby's head and body, also provides feelings of comfort and security especially during and following painful events (Hill et al 2005; Ward-Larson et al 2004).

Family care

The family will find this a difficult and distressing time during which they will require constant support, information and reassurance (Turrill, 1999).

Some are parents for the first time and have no idea of how to undertake this role for their baby, who may have a life threatening condition that casts doubt on its survival.

In some cases the parents experience the birth and death of their baby within hours. Supporting parents during this time is a very special but demanding aspect of neonatal nursing. Much has been written about the problems associated with separation of the parents from their baby at birth, bonding and attachment, and the feelings experienced by the parents within this context (Affonso and Hurst 1992; Henson 2001; Klaus and Kennell 1982; Pederson et al 1987; Redshaw 1997;). All agree that when a baby is born early or sick the whole family is thrown into crisis and that parents experience a grieving process of giving up the blueprint infant they had imagined in order to be able to accept the infant they have. (Henson 2001).

Lau and Morse (1998) identify that this can evoke strong negative feelings such as:

- Grief;
- Anxiety;
- Fear;
- Sense of failure;
- Helplessness;
- Shame;
- Denial;
- Shock; and
- Disappointment.

Most neonatal units will have systems in place designed to support the parents. However for the nursing staff the needs of the family can be eclipsed by the need to provide the highly technological care required by the baby especially in the early stages of the admission and assessment of the baby's immediate medical needs. Although parents are able to be with their baby throughout this time they are often left dazed and confused by the rapid turn of events whereby they find themselves thrust into an alien technological world along with their newborn baby who they have yet to get to know. Henson (2001) uses the term 'family support' when referring to the needs of the parents which involves enabling the parents to care for, to take responsibility for and to gain knowledge about their sick and premature infant. She also suggests that the work of supporting the families can be very demanding which can leave the nurses feeling exhausted and dispirited. Others use the term 'family-centred care' (FCC) (Beresford 1997; Derbyshire 1995; Lau and Morse 1998; Nethercott 1993; Smith et al 2002; Taylor 1996). The focus of Chapter 3 is family-centred care as a concept for children's nursing and while it is not specifically applied to the neonatal context many of the principles contained in it are directly transferable.

FCC when defined and analysed has many different components. Ultimately in the context of the NICU it concerns:

- The relationship of the parents with their infant.
- Their participation in the infant's care and any decisions, which are made.

It seeks to help the parents to develop a relationship with the nursing and medical staff that is equal, whereby they can become active rather than passive recipients, which can elevate their position on the neonatal unit to that of equal partners with the health care professionals (Henson 2001).

It is not about whether appropriate resources and facilities are available or about whether they are allowed to perform parenting tasks. It is about the ability of nurses to provide family nursing, simply to care and support the family of a sick or premature infant (Henson 2001). Although much has been written about the application of FCC there is still some uncertainty of how to apply this concept within the neonatal setting.

The original focus for FCC comes from paediatric nursing where the child is an established member of the family but as Turrill (1999) points out intensive care of the newborn is unique in that it involves a new person who the parents need to get to know. Turrill (1999) explains that although as yet no model of FCC is generally accepted in neonatal nursing, the principles of FCC are central to the care of babies and families within this context.

As well as recognising the complex psychological needs of the parents there is also a need to provide practical support for their physical well being especially for a visiting mother, who may still be experiencing pain and discomfort from the delivery. While the mothers are inpatients on the maternity ward they will still be cared for by the midwives and are usually escorted between the maternity unit and the neonatal unit. The midwives have the opportunity to visit with the mother to find out what is happening in order to be able to give support.

Midwives normally have the responsibility for the care of the mother and the baby for as long as necessary post-delivery either in hospital or within the community once the mother has been discharged. After this time they come under the care of the health visitor. Because the babies in the NICU may be in hospital for a long period a liaison health visitor working in the neonatal unit will keep the parent's GP practice informed of the baby's progress and inform them when the baby is due to be discharged.

Most neonatal units will have various facilities for the parents to use such as quiet rooms for parents to rest in and to be able to make drinks and meals. Rooms are also available for the parents to stay should their circumstances require them to stay near to the baby especially if the baby has been transferred from another hospital. Some units also provide family rooms for parents and other siblings to stay together. They will have access to other health care workers such as social workers to provide practical advice and support especially if the family is experiencing difficulties with finance, travelling and visiting or if the family have social problems that need to be sorted out before the baby can go home. There is usually a direct phone line to the room where their baby is being cared for and they are encouraged to phone at any time and speak directly to the nurse caring for their baby. They can visit at any time and to stay as long as they want. It is during these times that they will get to know the nurses and medical staff as well as their baby and the gradual process of building the bridges necessary to help them to begin to take on their parental role begins. The nurses will help the parents to join in with the care by doing nappy changing and mouth care. As their confidence improves they will to do more for the baby and make more decisions. A skilled nurse will enable the parents to do this giving them back a sense of control.

It also needs to be recognised that families will come from different social and cultural backgrounds, which may influence their understanding and acceptance of the situation and that each family should be treated as individual when assessing their need for support. All who have carried out the research or been studied agree that the most important aspects for supporting the family are good communication and a constant exchange of information between the carers and the parents. Having a good understanding of the baby's condition and day-to-day progress helps to empower the parents to feel able to make decisions in partnership with the nursing and medical staff (Lau and Morse 1998; Redshaw 1997; Smith et al 2002; Turrill 1999).

Breast feeding

The benefits of human milk for term and pre-term infants has long been established and documented. As a result it is now common practice to help and encourage mothers of premature babies in the NICU to express their breast milk so that it can be given to the baby via a nasogastric tube until the baby is strong enough to suck and take breast feeds. Human milk is easily digested and contains anti-infective properties, which are especially good for a premature infant who has an immature immune system. The IgA from the mother will afford the baby some protection from infection for the first few weeks. One of the most compelling reasons to give a premature baby breast milk is the protection it gives them against developing necrotising enterocolitis (NEC). Infants weighing less than 1.850 kg at birth and receiving formula feeds are six to ten times more likely to develop NEC than those fed with breast milk. Breast feeding can also enhance bonding between the mother and her baby (Parker 1995; Wheeler and Chapman 2000). There are longer-term benefits in that children who have been breast fed score higher at psychomotor and mental development skills than those fed on formula milk. This link between improved intelligence and breast-feeding is due to the long chain polyunsaturated fatty acids found in breast milk, which give improved vision, brain growth and cognitive development (Lucas and Morley 1992; Lucas et al 1994).

In practice mothers who wish to breast-feed their baby will be helped with expressing and storage of their milk, which is given to the baby as soon as possible. If the mother is expressing large amounts of milk it is stored in the fridge for up to 24 hours and can be frozen for up to three months and given to the baby as needed (Jones 1996). As the baby grows stronger breast-feeding will be gradually introduced. Although all mothers are informed of the benefits of breast milk for their premature baby some chose not to breast feed or express milk, this decision is usually respected and those babies will be fed with formula milk. Special low-birth weight formula feeds have been developed which may be used where growth is slow. Although human milk is important some supplementation may also be necessary due to the varying amounts of milk produced by the mother and the varied nutritional requirements of very ill premature babies. This can be done either with formula milk or with a breast milk fortifier such as Eoprotein (Wheeler and Chapman 2000; Yeo 2000).

→ Trigger 9.1: Feedback

Go to Chapter 9 Trigger feedback on p. 281

! Trigger 9.2: Admission to the Special Care Baby Unit (SCBU)

The intention of this trigger is to introduce you to some of the problems that small babies experience which necessitate admission to the Special Care Baby Unit (SCBU)

The Trigger

Alice was delivered by elective caesarean section (ECS) under epidural anaesthetic at 38 weeks gestation weighing 2.250 kg at birth. Her mother has a history of antepartum haemorrhages. She smokes and is a social drinker. She is a 19 year old single mother and has no contact with the baby's father but is supported by her parents.

At birth Alice was crying loudly and active. As soon as she was separated from the cord and dried she was wrapped in warm towels and shown her mother who was able to hold her for a few minutes before she was put into a warmed cot, under a heater ready for an examination by the midwife.

On examination she was active, jittery and anxious. Her blood glucose was 1.8 mmols/l and her temperature was 36.2°C. She was otherwise normal. She was offered a feed at 90mls/kg and the post feed blood glucose was 2.0 mmols. Following this she was put into an incubator and admitted to the SCBU. An intravenous infusion with 10 per cent dextrose was commenced and feeding was changed to intermittent hourly tube feeds. After a few hours her temperature was 36.8°C and her blood glucose 2.6 mmols/l. Her mother visited later and had contact with her daughter and an explanation of what was happening.

The mother was asked if she wanted to express breast milk but she declined stating a wish to bottle feed when her daughter was well. By the third day Alice was stable and feeding well, taking three hourly bottle feeds of formula milk. She had also developed physiological Jaundice which was treated with phototherapy for four days.

During subsequent visits the mother was able to give Alice her care. She was also enabled to carry out kangaroo care (KC). Alice responded well to being close to her mother and her mother said it helped her to develop a feeling of closeness with her daughter. After ten days Alice was discharged home.

The situation

You will be working in a Special Care Bay Unit where you will care for babies with similar histories to the one discussed above. This baby appears well at birth but will need admission to the SCBU.

Feedback

Using the fixed resources and referenced material develop an evidence-based information package for new staff explaining the definition, characteristics and causes of small-for-date babies. Include the reasons why hypothermia, hypoglycaemia and jaundice occur and how these are managed.

Develop a leaflet for parents explaining what Kangaroo care is, its advantages and how they can undertake KC with their baby.

The facts

> **What are the main facts in this trigger? Make a list:**

Hypotheses: What may these facts mean?

- Babies can be born by caesarean section for different reasons.
- Mothers who experience antepartum haemorrhage or who smoke and drink alcohol during pregnancy will have small babies.

- A term baby should be able to maintain its temperature and blood glucose within the normal limits if not it may be admitted to the SCBU.
- Physiological jaundice is a problem for newborn babies.
- Kangaroo care can help with bonding.

Questions developed from the hypotheses

1. What is the definition of small-for-date babies?
2. What are the characteristics and causes of small-for-date babies?
3. Why do small babies have a problem with maintaining their temperature? How will it be managed?
4. Why do small babies have a problem maintaining their blood sugar? How is it managed?
5. Why do newborn babies develop physiological jaundice, how is it managed?
6. What is Kangaroo care?

Trigger 9.2: Fixed resource material

Refer to those for Trigger 9.1.

Trigger 9.2: Fixed resource sessions

The definition of a small-for-date baby

A small-for-date baby is a one whose weight falls below the 10th centile for its gestational age (World Health Organisation 1992). Centile charts can be viewed by referring to Johnston (1998, pp. 45, 108). This definition indicates that a baby can be both premature and small-for-date or term and small-for-date, for example:

- A baby at 28 weeks gestation who weighs 900 grams or less.
- A term baby who weighs 2.5 kg or less.

From this definition and the previous definition of the premature baby you should be able to decide that Alice is a term baby who is small for date.

About 6.7 per cent of babies born in the UK will weigh less than 2.5 kg. One third will be small for date, 70 per cent will weigh between 2 kg and 2.5 kg, about 50 per cent of those weighing 1.5 kg to 2 kg will have minimal or no illness in the neonatal period (Johnston 1998; Rennie and Roberton 1999).

Gestational age can be calculated by using ultrasound scanning where the parameters of the baby's skull and femur will be measured and compared. From this, the age in days, the size and weight can be determined. It can also be determined if the baby is the correct size for gestational age of if it is growth restricted or larger than expected (Johnston 1998; Proud 1994; Yeo 2000).

Poor foetal growth may indicate placental failure and without intervention the baby may die. A growth-restricted baby will have been deprived of nutrients in utero due to placental insufficiency causing a lack of nourishment from the placenta. As a result it will not have been able to lay down any spare stores of glycogen or fat and once born the baby will have problems maintaining its blood glucose and body temperature. A Caesarean section may be carried out when the baby reaches a viable age (Yeo 2000). This is discussed later in the chapter.

The characteristics of small-for-date babies

As with the premature baby a small-for-date baby will look different to a term baby even though in some cases the baby may be near to term gestation. Again this is a difficult time for the parents who need time to adjust to the baby's appearance and the fact that the baby may need to be admitted to the SCBU. A small-for-date baby will also appear different to a premature baby but may experience similar problems.

Therefore, a small for date baby can appear:

- Active and wide-awake at birth depending on its gestation. If the baby is also premature it may be sleepy and less active.
- Wizened in appearance with a dry, lax and cracked skin and very little subcutaneous fat due to poor nourishment.
- They will look anxious and their cry will be loud possibly fuelled by hunger.
- The abdomen appears flat or scaphoid due to the diminished storage of glycogen in the liver.
- The cord will appear dull, yellow, thin and stretchy.
- May be irritable and 'jittery' due to low blood glucose.
- The head size can be asymmetrical or symmetrical.

Asymmetrical babies have a normal size head and brain for gestational age but their abdominal circumference is small in comparison because they have depleted fat and glycogen stores in the liver. However the brain has received sufficient nourishment to develop normally (Yeo 2000).

Symmetrically small babies will have a head and abdominal circumference which are decreased but in proportion. This is often diagnosed early in the pregnancy from the first scan. It is more serious as it indicates a longer period of time without adequate nutrition to the brain and organs and the baby will be slow to make up the deficiency after birth. The long-term prognosis is guarded as to their future intellectual development because the baby will have missed out on vital periods of brain growth and development (Wood et al 2000; Yeo, 2000). The origins of developmental difficulties have been attributed to:

- Delay in neurological maturation;
- Early cerebral injury;
- Social factors; and
- Poor early growth. (Wood et al 2000).

The causes of small-for-date babies

The socio-economic, medical and maternal factors are the same as those for a premature baby in particular:

- Poor diet;
- Smoking;
- Alcohol and drug abuse; and
- Congenital infections can lead to a small-for-date baby.

Infections are transferred to the baby from the mother during the pregnancy and can affect the placental function leading to diminished growth. These include infections such as:

- Toxoplasmosis
- Others (chicken pox measles)
- Rubella
- Cytomegalovirus
- Herpes

Taking the first letter of each of these infections spells out TORCH.

Torch screening is the name given to the placental and blood test carried out to detect these infections. Exposure to these infections can also lead to

early miscarriage or foetal abnormalities. Babies born with these infections present a risk to their carers and the use of universal precautions are recommended for all personnel handling newborn infants (Department of Health 1990).

Congenital abnormality for example, Downs syndrome (Trisomy 21) or Edward's syndrome (Trisomy 18) are often associated with a small-for-date babies. Trisomy is the term used to indicate an extra chromosome which leads to an abnormality.

Poor maternal nutrition can occur if the mother is not able to afford a healthy balanced diet. This may also be related to a lack of understanding of normal nutritional needs and how these need to be altered during pregnancy.

The EPICure study (2000) followed the survival, long-term development and health status of very premature and small-for-date babies finding that at 2.5 years, 50 per cent had no disability. In the remainder, 25 per cent had moderate disability and 25 per cent had severe disability, such as cerebral palsy, other neurological problems or developmental delay.

The problems identified were:

- Poor health;
- Slower growth;
- Developmental disabilities;
- Cerebral palsy;
- Visual problems;
- Hearing problems;
- Motor delay and poor motor skills;
- Learning difficulties and academic achievement;
- Poor language skills; and
- Difficulties with visuomotor skills.

Following discharge each baby will be followed up and their developmental progress will be carefully monitored. They will be assessed according to individual health and development needs in order to provide the appropriate care and treatments for the baby as well as support for the family.

Problems of small-for-date babies

Babies who are small for date are at risk of problems occurring at birth which may necessitate admission to the SCBU in order to stabilise, observe and treat them.

The following sections will define and discuss the management of temperature and blood glucose at birth and the subsequent care needed by premature and small for date babies. The cause and management of physiological jaundice will also be discussed. The final section will discuss the use of kangaroo care as an adjunct to care which can be used to help the parents to overcome some of the problems associated with separation and the need to form a bond with their baby.

The management of temperature at birth

The newborn temperature should be maintained between 36.5–37.5°C it is measured using electronic axilla probes (Bailey 2000; Browne et al 2000; Rennie and Roberton, 1999).

Thermoneutrality is the environmental temperature at which minimal rates of oxygen consumption or energy expenditure occur. It is the temperature at which the baby can maintain a core temperature at rest between 36.2°C–37.3°C with a change of only 0.2–0.3°C per hour from the core and skin temperatures. Hypothermia in the newborn is defined as a temperature below 35°C (Rennie and Roberton 1999).

The newborn baby will have the normal physiological mechanisms for keeping warm or cooling down but these may be immature and slower to initiate if the baby is small, premature or ill at birth. Newborns have a limited ability to sweat or shiver (usually developed in the first 3 months), however, they can utilise non-shivering thermogenesis (NST), which is initiated by cutaneous cooling, oxygenation and separation from the placenta. When the cord is cut cold receptors in the skin stimulate the release of noradrenaline and thyroxine which stimulates the metabolism of the brown fat. Increased oxygen is also needed to initiate this system (Fellows 2001).

Brown fat is located

- Around the neck;
- Between the scapulae;
- Across the clavicle line; and
- Down the sternum.

It also surrounds the major thoracic vessels and pads the kidneys. The cells contain a nucleus, glycogen, mitochondria and multiple fat vacuoles in the cytoplasm, which are used for energy production. The presence of thermogin means that when the fat is oxidised it produces heat rather than energy. The metabolism of brown fat liberates 2.5 calories per gram per minute warming the blood flowing through it (Rennie and Roberton 1999).

Non-shivering thermogenesis also needs a good source of glucose and fatty acids for energy all of which are reduced in the small sick newborn baby who also has a high surface area to body mass ratio (Fellows 2001).

Heat is lost during birth, resuscitation and transportation

If the temperature goes below 35°C it affects oxygenation by increasing pulmonary artery resistance and reducing surfactant production. This leads to poor perfusion causing an increase in anaerobic metabolism, worsening acidosis, and increased pulmonary artery pressure, which decreases the amount of flow through the lungs leading to hypoxia. The increased use of glucose because of the increased metabolism can lead to hypoglycaemia which also worsens acidosis and reduces the energy available for growth. Poor cardiac output has an effect on the intestinal blood flow which can cause intestinal ischaemia and necrotising enterocolitis (Fellows 2001).

Care at birth

The temperature of the foetus is at least one degree higher than that of the mother due to heat exchange via the placenta. The drop in ambient temperature at delivery is more marked when the wet infant is delivered into a cool environment.

- A healthy term infant will respond by increasing heat production. Drying and wrapping the infant in warm towels will enable it to maintain its temperature. Kangaroo care can also help the baby to keep warm (Engler et al 2002).
- Premature and small babies will experience difficulties in maintaining their temperature.

The body temp of a 1kg infant can fall 1°C every 5 minutes. Initially the baby will be transferred to a resuscitaire with a radiant warmer to be assessed and resuscitated if necessary. Delivery rooms may be cool and draughty, which increases convective heat loss. Set the radiant warmer to maximum and have warm towels and hat ready as the head is a large surface area for heat loss. (Rennie and Roberton 1999; Yeo, 2000).

Radiant heaters provide heat directly onto the skin. They are used at delivery or during interventions but they increase insensible and convective heat loss and metabolic rate as the infant tries to produce neutral thermal conditions. Once the baby has been transferred to the SCBU it will be nursed in an incubator. Incubators provide an enclosed protected space. Double glazing reduces radiation heat loss surrounding the infant with a curtain of heat even when the doors are open. They have the facility to administer humidity (87 per cent) to help prevent evaporation heat loss through the skin. Evaporation heat losses are higher in premature babies because of immature skin and there is a risk of further cooling and dehydration if nursed under dry radiant heat. Premature babies who are resuscitated and ventilated at birth are put straight into plastic bags without drying. This prevents some of the evaporation heat loss that can occur due to the baby's immature skin especially during transfer from the labour ward to the NICU where they will be taken out of the plastic bag and put straight into a pre-warmed and humidified incubator (Yeo 2000). Oxygen can also be administered into the incubator environment. Incubators reduce oxygen consumption which can be 8.8 per cent higher under a radiant warmer. Once settled in the incubator regular assessment of the temperature will be carried out and recorded. An unstable temperature may indicate that the baby is becoming unwell.

If a baby in an incubator becomes cold turn up temp 0.5 °C and check:

- Colour;
- Heart rate;
- Respiration rate;
- Blood sugar;
- Activity; and
- Feeding/Aspirate.

If still cold after an hour:

- Turn up the incubator temp by another 0.5°C.
- Inform medical staff especially if the baby remains unwell.
- The baby may require an infection screening and antibiotics.

General points:

- Don't keep doors open longer than necessary.
- Check baby's temperature before commencing care/procedures.
- Warm oxygen and air.
- Overhead heaters provide dry heat only.
- Humidity may be required.

- For cot nursed babies who become cold use a hat, extra clothes and covers along with an overhead radiant heater. Closely observe the baby and inform medical staff if the temperature does not stabilise as this can also be an early sign of infection or illness.
- Advice about temperature management is given to all parents of term and premature babies before discharge. This is because overheating has been identified as one of the factors thought to contribute to sudden infant death syndrome (SIDS) (Department of Health 2004; Fleming et al 1996).

It is especially relevant for babies who have been ill and or premature at birth as by the time they are well enough to go home they should be able to maintain their temperature in a normal home environment unlike the intensive care environment which is usually much hotter. The parents are advised on the following points:

- Do not let the baby become over heated while sleeping.
- Back to sleep (supine position).
- Feet-to-foot of the cot.
- Light covers (do not swaddle).
- Maintain a normal room temperature.
- Smoke free zone.
- Prompt medical advice.
- Bed share for comfort not sleep.
- Breast feed. (Department of Health, 1991, 2000, 2004; Fleming, 1996).

Glucose homeostasis in the newborn.

Foetal blood glucose levels are approximately 70–80 per cent of the maternal level, which allows for the process of facilitated diffusion across the placenta. Glucose is stored as glycogen from as early as nine weeks. The rate accelerates during the third trimester (the last few weeks of pregnancy).

Thus the more premature the infant is the smaller the reserves increasing the susceptibility to hypoglycaemia at birth. At birth the baby undergoes a change from an intrauterine anabolic-dominant state to a neonatal catabolic state as separation from the maternal supply occurs.

All newborns have the potential for glucose instability at birth when the neonate has to regulate its own glucose metabolism.

Normal healthy term babies should be able to maintain their blood glucose with no difficulty.

For newborns, who do not show abnormal clinical signs (asymptomatic) the blood glucose concentration should be maintained at or above 2.6 mmol/l. (World Health Organisation 1997).

In the term infant hypoglycaemia is defined as 1.6 mmol/l if less than 48 hours old

(Beresford 2001; Rennie and Roberton 1999; World Health Organisation 1997; Yeo 2000).

Hypoglycaemia refers to a low blood glucose concentration and it exists whenever available glucose fails to meet metabolic requirements (Beresford 2001; World Health Organisation 1997). Neonatal hypoglycaemia is not a medical condition but a feature of illness or a failure to adapt from the foetal state of continuous transplacental glucose consumption to an extrauterine pattern of intermittent nutrient supply. It is likely to occur due to:

- Hypothermia; or
- Delayed initiation of feeding.

Nervous tissue has no reserves of carbohydrate and depends on an adequate level of blood glucose. Low blood glucose levels can lead to convulsions and coma.

The management of hypoglycaemia involves identifying those at risk.

In the premature baby hypoglycaemia is defined as blood glucose of less than 1.1 mmol/l.

Blood glucose levels tend to be lower due to reduced glycogen and fat stores. Differences in fat content are important as fat accounts for only 2 per cent of the body weight at 28 weeks but about 16 percent at term. Although fat is not convertible to glucose, mobilization and oxidation of fat reduces glucose uptake and oxidation. An elevated insulin; glucose ratio and immaturity of ketogenesis persists for some months after birth. This may be due to them needing a greater protein intake for growth. Protein acts as an insulinogenic stimulator.

As premature infants have an immature counter regulatory response to hypoglycaemia it is recommended that they maintain a plasma glucose concentration greater than 2.6 mmol.

Counter regulatory response is the process, which ensures the availability of glucose and other fuels activated by glucagon and adrenaline.

Blood glucose levels in premature babies can be maintained by early feeding or by infusion. Twice daily laboratory estimates should be sufficient to tailor feeding requirements to the individual (Beresford 2001; World Health Organisation 1997).

Premature infants with respiratory distress should not be enterally fed but treated with intravenous glucose until their respirations have settled and then nasogastric feeding can be commenced.

If they continue to experience respiratory problems and are very unstable then total parenteral nutrition (TPN) will be commenced.

A healthy premature infant under 32 weeks will not be able to suck effectively and will require tube feeding. Intravenous 10 per cent dextrose may be used until tube feeding has been established. Total parenteral nutrition (TPN) will be used if feeding cannot be established or if the baby develops abdominal distension and an increase in gastric aspirates indicating that the baby is not tolerating enteral feeding or may be developing necrotising enterocolitis.

Healthy premature infants 32–36 weeks should be able to coordinate sucking and swallowing effectively. They are usually able to attempt breast, bottle or cup feeding. Early feeding with breast milk is preferable for premature and small-for-date babies (Wheeler and Chapman 2000).

The small for date baby has long been identified as at risk of

hypoglycaemia due to high brain–body mass ratio with a corresponding increase in glucose consumption also:

- Reduced fat stores;
- Failure of counter regulation;
- Delayed gluconeogenesis (the production of glucose from non carbohydrate stores); and
- Hyperinsulinism.

Those at greatest risk will be:

- Below the 3rd centile in weight (birth weight two standard deviations from the mean for gestation) (Cornblath and Schwartz 1993).
- Those who are disproportionate (increased head circumference/body weight ratio).

Frequent blood sampling is not necessary to identify those at risk. Laboratory measurements of cord blood glucose and blood glucose at 4–6 hours of age (before second feed) are recommended (Hawdon and Ward Platt 1993). They should start early feeding if otherwise well.

All maternity units will have a protocol that identifies the infants at risk and how the blood glucose of these babies should be monitored and treated.

Persistent hypoglycaemia in any newborn baby can also indicate other problems such as an endocrine disorder or an inborn error of metabolism (Digiacomo and Hay 1992). Therefore further tests for these conditions would be considered for babies with an unstable blood sugar which persists despite the early initiation of infusions or feeding.

Stress Hypoglycaemia may be present in the following conditions:

- Sepsis;
- Perinatal asphyxia;
- Congenital heart disease;
- Heart failure; and
- Severe cyanotic heart disease.

Catecholamine response to stress is a central feature of counter regulation. Peripheral circulatory failure in sepsis and asphyxia may lead to both reduced mobilisation of substrate from the periphery and accumulation of lactate in the presence of anaerobic glycolysis. This leads to exhaustion of liver glycogen and reduced capacity for gluconeogenesis (World Health Organisation 1997).

Hyperinsulinism and increased insulin sensitivity may also be present following the use of maternal glucose infusions in labour. Thes may also occur following the administration of β-Sympathomimetics (Ritodrine, Salbutamol, Terbutaline, Adrenaline and Atosiban) used to prevent labour. These have been associated with the maternal hyperglycaemia which gives rise to fetal hyperinsulism (World Health Organisation 1997).

The signs and symptoms of neonatal hypoglycaemia include:

- Jittery/Tremulous;
- Irritability;
- Unstable Temperature;
- Lethargy/Apathy;
- Hypotonic;
- Poor feeding;
- Weak high-pitched cry;
- Cyanosis/Apnoea; and
- Convulsions/Coma.

Therefore the management of glucose homeostasis at birth is to:

- Identify the babies most at risk.
- Keep the baby warm.
- Assess and treat according to the hospital protocol.

Physiological Jaundice

All babies term or premature, healthy or ill, undergo changes in bilirubin metabolism at birth resulting in physiological jaundice which is seen in 40–50 percent of term and up to 80 per cent of premature neonates. It occurs during the first few days and reaches a peak by three to seven days. The baby will have visible jaundice when the bilirubin level reaches 80μmol (Blackburn 1995).

Other causes of jaundice in the newborn period arise from pathological factors, that alter the usual processes involved in bilirubin metabolism such as blood group incompatibility (rhesus or ABO), sepsis or excessive bruising.

Hyperbilirubinemia refers to bilirubin levels that have exceeded a specific level or rate of rise.

There are two types of bilirubin; Direct and Indirect.

Indirect

Indirect (unconjugated) bilirubin is the end product from the breakdown of the excessive number of red blood cells which have not been conjugated by the liver. It is a fat soluble product and cannot be easily excreted. It builds up in the blood and is eventually deposited in the fatty tissue of the skin, which leads to visible jaundice. If the levels of unconjugated bilirubin in the blood and skin increase beyond normal it can be deposited in the fatty tissue of the basal ganglia in the brain, which can lead to the development of kernicterus. This is a condition where the brain cells become damaged by the bilirubin causing acute cerebral dysfunction which may lead to death. Survivors have cerebral palsy, mental retardation and deafness (Rennie and Roberton 1999).

The body has to metabolise unconjugated (indirect) bilirubin in the liver to change it into conjugated (direct) bilirubin. This is a normal process in all humans due to the continued process of red cell degredation. However it does not usually result in visible jaundice as amounts are usually very small.

Direct

Direct (conjugated) bilirubin is water soluble and can be easily excreted via the biliary system into the intestines and the stools. A small amount can be reabsorbed in the colon and excreted in the urine (Blackburn 1995). Once the baby starts to excrete the conjugated bilirubin into the intestines it will alter the appearance of the stools to a loose dark green consistency.

> Physiological jaundice in the newborn occurs because newborn babies have high haemoglobin levels, (18–19 g/dl) for the foetus to maintain oxyhaemoglobin levels in utero.

This, coupled with the short red cell life, means that there is a high rate of haemolysis at birth. Compared to adults, on the basis of body mass, bilirubin production in the neonate is more than double at 135–170 µmol bilirubin/kg body weight per day. Adult levels are reached by about 14 weeks (Dent 2001). Each gram of haemoglobin produces 34–35 mg of indirect bilirubin (Blackburn 1995). Newborn babies can also be deficient in the Y and Z carrier proteins and albumin for binding which are important in the transportation of bilirubin from the blood to the liver and glucuronyl transferase which is an enzyme in the liver responsible for the conjugation process. Although physiological jaundice is the most common cause, jaundice can present at different times and there are other possible causes.

Infants can be born with jaundice or become jaundiced within 24 hours due to:

- Rhesus disease;
- ABO incompatibility;
- Congenital infection;
- G6PD deficiency.

Infants can become jaundiced after 48 hours due to:

- Physiological jaundice (as discussed);
- Acquired infection; and
- Undetected haemolytic disease.

If jaundice persists beyond 10 days it is described as prolonged and is usually due to factors other than the normal physiological processes such as:

- Breast feeding;
- Chronic infection or late infection;
- Hepatitis;
- Obstruction;
- Inborn errors of metabolism;
- Hypothyroidism.

Investigations for jaundice in the newborn include laboratory estimation of serum bilirubin levels:

- Serum bilirubin levels report as total bilirubin and the direct (conjugated) component; and
- Total bilirubin is an accurate reflection of indirect (unconjugated) bilirubin levels because the direct (conjugated) component is usually very low.

Other investigations include:

- Haemoglobin;
- Haemocrit;
- Reticulocyte count;
- Maternal and infant blood group;
- The Coombs test is a measure of antibody-coated blood cells. Infants with blood group incompatibility (rhesus or ABO) will have received from the mother antibodies that coat and destroy the infant's RBCs.
- The Direct Coombs test is a measure of the amount of maternal antibody coating the infant's RBCs. If the antibody is present then the test will be a positive direct result.
- The Indirect Coombs measures the effects of a sample of the infant's serum (which is thought to contain maternal antibodies) on unrelated adult RBCs. If the infant's serum contains antibodies they will interact and coat the adult RBCs giving a positive indirect test. Infants with Rh incompatibility will have a positive direct result. Infants with ABO incompatibility will have a negative or weakly positive result.
- The Kleihaur test detects the presence of foetal cells in the maternal circulation.
- Cases of prolonged jaundice will also be investigated for liver function and thyroid problems.

The management of physiological jaundice involves the use of preventative strategies such as:

- Early feeding to stimulate intestinal motility ensuring that once the bilirubin has been conjugated and moves into the intestines it is excreted quickly hence the change in the baby's stools.
- Preventing hypothermia because the associated release of free-fatty acids can interfere with albumin binding.
- Avoid trauma during labour and the subsequent bruising which increases the load of damaged red blood cells to be metabolised.
- Ensure that Rh (D) immune-globulin is given to Rh (D) negative women with rhesus (D) positive babies following each delivery.

If the baby is premature, small or ill at birth it may be unable to conjugate bilirubin effectively and the levels of unconjugated bilirubin will continue to increase putting the baby at risk of kernicterus. In these cases treatment will be initiated.

Phototherapy is the most common treatment for hyperbilirubinemia. The light reduces bilirubin by the following processes of photoisomerization, which converts indirect bilirubin to water soluble photoisomers. It does this by rearranging the chemical group of the bilirubin molecule to produce photobilirubin which can be excreted into the bile without conjugation (Blackburn 1995).

The light involved is not ultra violet or infra red but is a blue light measured in the 400–500 manometers range as this is the strength which is the most effective (Edwards 1995; Hey 1995, 1995a).

A unit incorporating a combination of blue and white lights is used to enable effective treatment and good visibility. The units are designed to fit closely over the top of the incubators and are serviced regularly to ensure as high as possible irradiance therefore maintaining the effectiveness of the treatment. Recommended irradiance should be between 5–10 µW/cm (Edwards 1995; Hey 1995, 1995a). The advantages are that it is cheap, effective and non-invasive.

The disadvantages are disturbance to the water and electrolyte balance due to insensible water losses from the diarrhoea caused by the conjugated bilirubin being excreted from the gut and the heat from the lights increasing evaporation heat and fluid losses. The blue colour of the lights can make observation of the baby's colour difficult. The baby's eyes have to be covered with pads as the bright light can damage the developing retina. This can disrupt the parent–infant interactions affecting parents' ability to bond with their baby. Parents can become very anxious during this time and need plenty of reassurance and an explanation of the cause and treatment (Blackburn 1995; Dent 2001).

Factors to consider when caring for a baby requiring phototherapy are indicated in Table 9.1.

Table 9.1 Factors to consider for a baby requiring phototherapy

- The baby will be nursed in an incubator which will need to be turned to a lower temperature as the lights add an additional source of heat.
- The baby will need frequent temperature measurements until the temperature has adjusted to the change in the environment.
- The baby will be naked except for a small nappy.
- Eye pads will be used to protect the eyes from the light.
- Exposure to the light will be continuous and the baby will be turned frequently to maximise exposure.
- If the baby is premature it may require extra fluid to replace insensible water losses.
- Frequent nappy changes are needed because of the diarrhoea.
- Skin creams are not used because of the risk of burning the skin when combined with the heat from the light.
- Close observation of the baby for any signs of distress caused by skin rashes and irritation is also necessary.

To monitor the progress and effectiveness of the phototherapy the levels of bilirubin are plotted onto charts which differ: (a) for the different gestations and sizes of the babies; and (b) whether they are well or sick. Therefore, smaller, sicker babies require phototherapy at lower levels than term, well babies who often do not require any treatment. Incorporated into the charts are levels at which an exchange transfusion may be required if the phototherapy is not enough.

The effects can be lost if the lights are stopped too soon and a rebound can occur requiring further treatment. The treatment will be continuous until the levels of bilirubin start to fall, usually by about 3 or 4 days after commencing treatment.

Other methods used for giving phototherapy include a 'Biliblanket' where the light source is linked to a woven fibre optic pad via a fibroptic cable. This means that the baby can be wrapped in the blanket and nursed by its parents. There is no need to cover the eyes and no temperature problems. This method is usually used for babies who are otherwise well. Also a 'Bliibed' can be used which consists of a unit containing the lights that the baby can lie on wrapped in a baby-gro incorporated into the unit. As with the Biliblanket it eliminates the problems associated with temperature control and there is no need to cover the eyes. This would also be used for babies who are otherwise well. In all cases the parents will need reassurance and an explanation of the treatment used especially if the baby has previously been well and has developed a physiological jaundice which needs treatment.

The use of Kangaroo care (KC)

As identified in both triggers there are many difficulties for the parents of babies who are admitted to the NICU/SCBU soon after birth. It was discovered that forming a bond with their baby can prove difficult within these contexts. An innovative practice which has been recently introduced into neonatal care in developed countries involves the use of Kangaroo care (KC).

Kangaroo care also known as skin-to-skin contact was originally developed to overcome the problems associated with the lack of incubator care in developing countries where low birth weight babies were dying of infection caused by cross-contamination from shared bedding space and equipment in the nursery. These babies were also at risk of being abandoned by their mothers (Bauer et al 1996; Bohnhorst et al 2001; Jones et al 2001).

> Kangaroo care is the practice of holding a baby naked, except for a nappy and hat, against the mother or father's naked chest. It resembles the way that marsupials such as kangaroos care for their young (Bauer et al 1996).

The parent then acts as the main source of heat, nutrition and stimulation (Bohnhorst et al 2001). The concept originally involved having the mothers stay in the hospital and 'incubate' their babies next to their body until the babies were stable enough to go home. This resulted in a reduced rate of infant mortality, decreased infection rates, fewer apnoeic and bradycardiac spells, increased rates of lactation and improvements in bonding and attachment resulting in less abandonment (Jones et al 2001)

In developed countries Kangaroo care is practiced daily for a period of time to help the parents to feel close to their baby. It has been shown to have the same positive outcomes with an improvement in the relationship between the parents and their baby both in the short and long term, decreases in the incidence of apnoea and bradycardia and improved oxygenation (Ludington-Hoe et al 1996). It has been associated with a longer duration of quiet sleep, reduced activity and lower energy expenditure. It helps to stabilize the baby's temperature and helps to improve lactation (Bauer et al 1996). More than 263 published reports exist to date relating to the safety, efficacy and feasibility of KC as a nursing intervention for babies greater than 28 weeks gestation who are relatively stable (Engler et al 2002). There are also studies that suggest that it can be used for babies of lower gestational ages being mechanically ventilated and for those requiring phototherapy (Engler et al 2002). Charpak et al (2001) conclude that growth can be optimized and that the use of KC would humanise the practice of neonatology. The effects for the parents have been positive as expressed by mothers and fathers, with reported feelings of closeness and positive parenting behaviours (Engler et al 2002).

The practice of KC is now becoming more widespread especially within the contexts of the NICU/SCBU where the normal closeness between a newborn and its parents are often denied due to the baby needing to be in an incubator to provide warmth and the need for constant observation and monitoring. Parents seem to enjoy the experience of kangaroo care once they have overcome their initial fears about handling their small baby. In practice nursing staff often need to initiate the idea and explain the concept to the parents moving on to help them to get the baby out of the incubator and to provide a comfortable chair with as much privacy as possible. Once comfortable the parent and baby can be left for 30 minutes to an hour with the nurses within calling distance should the baby or parent experience any difficulties. The positive effects appear to give the parent some feeling of mastery and control, which in turn helps to empower them to feel involved in the day-to-day decisions for their baby and will help them to develop their long term relationship with their baby.

→ Trigger 9.2: Feedback

Go to Chapter 9 Trigger feedback on p. 281 below

? Chapter 9 Trigger feedback: What do you know?

Trigger 1. The context of NICU

When developing an information booklet for parents you need to convey the facts in a clear way, without the use of jargon. Do not make the information too complicated. It may be useful to talk with parents in this situation to find out what sort of information they would find useful.

The booklet needs to consider information on the following:

- What RDS is and what causes it.
- How their baby will be managed.
- Information about surfactant.
- An explanation about the ventilation and other equipment such as incubators and monitors.
- How they can become involved in the care of their baby.
- Breast feeding and expressing breast milk. You may consider developing this aspect within a separate leaflet.
- Visiting policies, including times and who can visit.
- Facilities for parents and family.
- Phone numbers for the Unit and personnel they can access.
- Other members of staff and what their roles are, for example, the physiotherapist.
- Support groups both within the NICU and external agencies such as BLISS who offer support for the families of premature babies.

● Cultural and religious needs also need to be addressed and in some cases it may be necessary to think about providing information in different languages.

Questions 1 and 2: Why are babies born prematurely, how is it defined, where should they be nursed? What are the problems and complications and what care is needed?

For both of these questions see the key text books and fixed resources. Make notes from these sections for useful facts to use in the booklet. Also observe in practice how the care for these babies is planned and managed.

Question 3: What is respiratory distress syndrome; how is it managed?

The information in the fixed resource and practice policies will help you with the information needed for the booklet. In the practice policy you will find the criteria used to determine when a baby needs surfactant, how it is given and the care needed.

Question 4: Why was breast milk needed?

See fixed resource, notes from this page will help to provide information for your booklet. It may also be useful to talk with the infant feeding advisors within the unit where you are working. Visiting the web page for the UNICEF Baby Friendly Initiative will be useful www.babyfriendly.org.uk.

Question 5: How will the parents be supported?

See fixed resource to provide you with some ideas you can make notes from or you could phone around or visit other units to find out what is being done for parents.

Also the following website may be useful www.bliss.org.uk (BLISS is a charity organisation who supports parents of premature babies.)

Trigger 2. Admission to the Special Care Baby Unit

In order to provide an information package for new staff you will need to ensure that the information includes practices which are evidence based. Make notes from the fixed resources and references supplied. It will also be useful to check guidelines and policies being used in current practice.

Questions 1 and 2: Why are babies born small for date, how is it defined? What are their characteristics, causes and problems?

For both of these questions see the references to the key text books and the fixed resources make notes from these sections for useful facts to use in the booklet.

Question 3: Why do small babies have a problem with maintaining their temperature and how is it managed?

See the fixed resource references and practice policy. It may also be useful to find out the different functions that incubators can provide, for example, the use of humidity in conjunction with wrapping a baby in a plastic bag at delivery. Also the different temperature settings used for different size babies in incubators. This needs to be considered in relation to the neutral-thermal environment that has also been discussed.

Question 4: Why do small babies have a problem with maintaining their blood glucose and how is it managed?

See the fixed resource references and practice policy. The current policies for the identification of babies at risk of hypoglycaemia and their management are based on the recommendations made following an extensive review of the literature by the World Health Organisation (1997).

Question 5: Why do newborn babies develop physiological jaundice, how is it managed?

See fixed resource and references. Find out about the charts used in practice to assess when phototherapy should be commenced and how these are used. You will be able to read the policy guiding the use of phototherapy in practice and observe the different methods of using light.

Question 6: What is kangaroo care and how is it managed?

To answer this question you will find some information in the fixed resource. There are also a number of web pages with useful information for parents and nursing staff try www.prematurity.org/baby/kangaroo.html.

Reflect on your learning

- Babies who are premature and small at birth usually require admission to NICU/SCBU for a number of reasons where they will receive highly specialised care from specially trained nursing and medical staff.
- It is important to recognise that at birth maintaining the baby's breathing, temperature and blood glucose levels are fundamental to survival.
- Physiological jaundice is a problem which can affect all newborn babies in varying degrees and can lead to the need for treatment with phototherapy.
- The management of nutrition and especially the provision of breast milk which is important to the baby's long term development.
- Facilitating family centred care and the use of innovative practices such as kangaroo care are ways of involving parents to help them to regain some control over the situation they are in by empowering them to help with the care and decision-making for their baby and to encourage them to develop a bond with their baby in this alien and difficult environment.

References

Acolet, D. (1993) Changes in plasma cortisol and catecholamines concentration in response to massage in premature infants. *Archives of Diseases in Childhood* 68 (1), pp. 29–31.

Affonso, D. D., Hurst, I. (1992) Stressors reported by mothers of hospitalised premature infants. *Neonatal Network* 11 (6), pp. 63–70.

Ainsworth, S. B., McCormack, K. (2004) Exogenous surfactant and neonatal lung disease: An update on the current situation. *Journal of Neonatal Nursing* 10 (1), pp. 6–11.

Als, H., Lawhon, G. T. Brown, E., gibes, R., Duffy, F., McAnulty, G., Blickman, J. (1986) Individualized behavioural and environmental care for the low birth weight preterm infant at high risk of bronchopulmonary dysplasia: Neonatal intensive care unit and developmental outcome. *Paediatrics* 78, pp 1123–32.

Als, H., Longhorn, G., Duffy, F. H., McAnulty, G., Blickman, J. (1994) Individualized developmental care for the very low birth weight preterm infant: Medical and neurofunctional effects. *Journal of the American Medical Association* 272 (11), pp. 853–8.

Als, H., Duffy, F., McAnulty, G. (1996) Effectiveness of individualized neurodevelopmental care in the newborn intensive care unit. *Acta Paediatr Suppl* pp. 416–21.

Als, H. (1998) Developmental care in the newborn intensive care unit. *Current Opinion in Paediatrics* 10, pp. 138–42.

Appleton, S. (1997) Handle with care: An investigation of handling received by preterm infants in intensive care. *Journal of Neonatal Nursing* 3 (3), pp. 23–7.

Bailey, J. (2000) Temperature measurement in the preterm infant: A literature review. *Journal of Neonatal Nursing* 6 (1), pp. 28–32.

Barros, F. Vigtora, C., Semer, T. C., Filho, S. T., Tomasi, E., Weiderpass, E. (1995) Use of pacifiers is associated with decreased breast feeding duration. *The American Academy of Paediatrics* 5 (6), pp. 497–9.

Bauer, J., Sontheimer, D., Fischer, C. H., Linderkamp, O. (1996) Metabolic rate and energy balance in very low birth weight infants during kangaroo holding by their mothers and fathers. *Journal of Paediatrics* 129 (4), pp. 608–11.

Becker, P. T., Grunwald, P. C., Moorman, J. (1995) Effects of developmental care on behavioural organisation in very low birth weight infants. *Nursing Research* 42 (4), pp. 214–20, in Yeo, H. (ed.) (2000) *Nursing the Neonate*, 2nd edn. Oxford: Blackwell Science.

Beresford, D. (1997) Family centred care: Fact or fiction? *Journal of Neonatal Nursing*, 3 (6), pp. 8–11.

Beresford, D. (2001) Fluid and electrolyte balance, in Boxwell, G. (ed.) *Neonatal Intensive Care Nursing*, 2nd edn. London: Routledge, pp. 220–3.

Bildner, J., Krechel, S. W. (1996) Increasing staff nurse awareness of postoperative pain management in the NICU. *Neonatal Network* 15 (1), pp. 11–16.

Blackburn, S. (1995) Hyperbilirubinemia and Neonatal Jaundice. *Neonatal Network,* 14 (7), pp. 15–25.

Blackburn, S. (1998) Environmental impact of the NICU on developmental outcomes. *Journal of Paediatric Nursing* 13, pp. 279–89.

Bohnhorst, B., Heyne, T. (2001) Skin-to-skin (kangaroo) care, respiratory control, and thermoregulation. *Journal of Paediatrics* 138 (2), pp. 193–7.

Boyd, S. (2001) Surgical aspects of neonatal intensive care nursing, in Boxwell, G. (ed.) *Neonatal Intensive Care Nursing*, 2nd edn. London: Routledge, p. 366.

Browne, S., Coleman, H., Geary, E., James, J., Kinsella, S., White, M. (1992) Accurate measurement of body temperature in the neonate: A comparative study. *Journal of Neonatal Nursing* 6 (5), pp. 165–8.

Cameron, J. (2001) Management of respiratory disorders, in Boxwell, G. (ed.) *Neonatal Intensive Care Nursing*, 2nd edn. London: Routledge, pp. 100–3.

Charpak, N., Ruiz-Pelaez, J. G., Figueroade, C. Z. (2001) A randomized controlled trial of kangaroo mother care: Results of follow-up at one year of corrected age. *Paediatrics* 108, pp.1072–9.

Cornblath, M. Schwartz, R. (1993) Hypoglycaemia in the newborn. *Journal of Paediatric Endocrinology* 6, pp. 113–29.

Day, C., Hart, G., Hamsworth, A. (1997) Phototherapy for neonates. *Journal of Neonatal Nursing* 3 (4), (Step by step guide).

D'Appolito, K. (1991) What is an organised infant? *Neonatal Network* 10 (1), pp. 23–9.

Dent, J. (2001) Management of haematological problems, in Boxwell, G. (ed.) *Neonatal Intensive Care Nursing*, 2nd edn. London: Routledge, pp. 165–84.

Department of Health (1990) *Guidance for Clinical Health-care Workers: Protection against Infection with HIV and Hepatitis Viruses: Recommendations of Expert Advisory Group on AIDS*. London: HMSO.

Department of Health (1991) *Sleeping Position and the Incidence of Cot Death*. London: HMSO.

Department of Health (2004) *Reduce the Risks: An Easy Guide*. London: HMSO, FSDI).

Derbyshire, P. (1995) Parents in paediatrics. *Paediatric Nursing,* 7 (1), pp. 8–9.

Digiacomo, J. E., Hay, W. (1992) Abnormal glucose homeostasis, in Boxwell, G. (ed.) *Neonatal Intensive Care Nursing*, 2nd edn. London: Routledge, p. 223.

Downs, J. (1991) The effect of intervention on development of hip posture in very preterm babies. *Archives of Diseases of Childhood* 66, pp. 797–801.

East, P. (2001) Pain and comfort in the neonatal intensive care, in Boxwell, G. (ed.) *Neonatal Intensive Care Nursing*, 2nd edn. London: Routledge, pp. 189–203.

Edwards, S. (1995) Phototherapy and the Neonate: Providing a safe and effective nursing care for jaundiced infants. *Journal of Neonatal Nursing*, 1 (5), pp. 9–12.

Engler, A. J., Ludington-Hoe, S. M., Cusson, R. M., Adama, R., Bahnsen, M., Brumbaugh, E. (2002) Kangaroo care: National survey of practice, knowledge, barriers and perceptions. *American Journal of Maternal Child Nursing* 27 (3), pp. 146–53.

Engerbretson, J., Wardell, D. (1997) Development of a pacifier for low birth weight infant's non nutritive sucking. *Journal of Obstetric, Gynaecological and Neonatal Nursing*, 26 (6), pp. 660–4.

Fay, M. J. (1988) The positive effects of positioning. *Neonatal Network*, 6 (5), pp. 23–8.

Fellows, P. (2001) Management of thermal stability, in Boxwell, G. (ed). *Neonatal Intensive Care Nursing*, 2nd edn. London: Routledge.

Feldman, R., Eiderman A. L. (1998) Intervention programmes for premature infants. How do they affect development? *Clinical Perinatology.* 25 (3), pp. 613–26.

Field, T., Scapidi, F. A. (1990) Massage stimulates growth in preterm babies: A replication. *Infant behaviour and development* 13, pp. 176–80.

Fleming, P. J., Blair, P. S., Bacon, C., Bensley, D., Smith, I., Taylor, E., Tripp, J. (1996) Environment of infants during sleep and risk for SIDS: Results of 1993–5 case-control study for confidential enquiry into still births and deaths in infancy. *British Medical Journal* 313 (7051), pp. 191–5.

Fraser, D. M., Cooper, M. A., (eds) (2003) *Myles Textbook for Midwives*, 14th edn. London: Churchill Livingstone, pp. 1031–5.

Gibson, A. (1997) Surfactant and the neonatal lung. *British Journal of Hospital Medicine,* 58 (8), pp. 381–97.

Hawdon, J. M. and Ward-Platt, M. P. (1993) Metabolic adaptation in small for gestational age infants. *Archives of Diseases in Childhood* 68, pp. 262–8.

Hawdon, J. M., Ward-Platt, M. P., Aynsley-Green, A. (1992) Patterns of metabolic adaptation for preterm infants in the first neonatal week. *Archives Diseases of Childhood* 67, pp. 357–65.

Heimler, R., Langlois, J., Hodel, D. J., Welin, L. D., Sasidharan, P. (1992) Effects on the breathing pattern of preterm infants. *Archives of Diseases of Childhood,* 67, pp. 312–14.

Henson, C. (2001) Family support, in Boxwell, G. (ed.) *Neonatal Intensive Care Nursing*, 2nd edn. London: Routledge pp. 390–411.

Hey, E. (1995) Phototherapy: Fresh light on a murky subject. *Midirs Midwifery Digest* 5 (3).

Hey, E. (1995a) Neonatal jaundice – How much do we really know? *Midirs Midwifery Digest* 5 (1).

Hill, S., Engle, S., Jorgensen, J., Kralik, A., Whitman, K. (2005) Effects of facilitated tucking during routine care of infants born preterm. *Paediatric Physical Therapy* 17 (2), pp. 158–63.

Horgan, M. Choonara, L. et al (1996) 'Measuring pain in neonates: an objective score'. *Paediatric Nursing,* 8(10), pp. 24–27.

Ives, N. K. (1999) Neonatal jaundice, part 1, in Rennie, J. M., and Roberton, N. R. C., (eds) *Textbook of Neonatology,* 3rd edn. London: Churchill Livingstone, p. 719.

Johnston, P. G. B. (1998) *The Newborn Child,* 8th edn. London: Churchill Livingstone, pp. 43–5, 91, 105–22, 138.

Jones, J. E. et al. (2001) Varieties of alternative experience: Complementary care in the neonatal intensive care unit. *Clinical obstetrics and Gynaecology,* 44 (4), pp. 750–68.

Jones, L. (1996) Mother's own expressed breast milk: Guidelines for storage. *Modern Midwife,* pp. 2–29.

Klaus, M. and Kennell, J. (1982) *Parent Infant Bonding,* (St. Louis: Mosby).

Lau, R., Morse, C. (1998) Experiences of parents with premature infants hospitalised in neonatal intensive care units: A literature review. *Journal of Neonatal Nursing* 4 (6), pp. 23–8.

Lawrence, J. Alcock, D. et al (1993) The development of a tool to assess neonatal pain. *Neonatal Network,* 12 (6), pp. 59–66.

Lucas, A. and Morley, R. (1992) Breast milk and subsequent intelligence quotient in children born preterm. *Lancet,* 339, pp. 261–4.

Lucas, A., Morley, R., Cole, T. J. (1994) A randomised multi-centre study of human milk versus formula and later development in preterm infants. *Archives of Diseases in Childhood:* Fetal and Neonatal Edition, 70 (2), pp. 141–6.

Ludington-Hoe, S. M., Swinth, J. Y. (1996) Developmental aspects of kangaroo care. *Journal of Obstetrics, Gynaecology and Neonatal Nursing,* 25, pp. 619–703.

Lynch, A. Y. (1997) Prone to good positioning? The nursing cost of bad positioning of neonates. *Journal of Neonatal Nursing,* 3 (4), pp. 16–20.

McCormick, M. Workman-Daniels, K. Brooks-Gunn, J. (1996) The behavioural and emotional well being of school age children with different birth weights. *Paediatrics,* 97 (1), pp. 18–25.

Morgan, J. B. (1992) Nutrition of the very low birth weight infant. *Care of the Critically Ill,* 8 (3), pp. 122–4.

Nethercott, S. (1993) A concept for all the family. Family centred care: A concept analysis. *Professional Nurse* 8 (12), pp. 794–7.

OSARIS Collaborative Group (1992) Early versus delayed administration of a synthetic surfactant – the judgement of OSARIS. *Lancet,* 340, pp. 1363–9.

Parker, L. (1995) Necrotising enterocolitis. *Neonatal Network* 14 (6), pp. 17–23.

Pederson, D. R. and Bento, S. (1987) Maternal emotional responses to preterm birth. *American Journal of Orthopsychiatry* 57, pp. 15–21.

Peters, K. L. (1996) Selected physiologic and behavioural responses of the critically ill premature neonate to routine nursing intervention. *Neonatal Network* 15 (1) p. 74.

Phillips, S. S. (1994) Introduction, in Phillips, S. S., Benner, P. (eds). *The crisis of caring: Affirming and restoring caring practices in the helping professions* (Washington, DC: Georgetown University Press) pp. 1–16.

Proud, J. (1994) Understanding Obstetric Ultrasound. *Books for Midwives*. Cheshire: Hale.

Pinelli, J., Symington, A. (2000) How rewarding can a pacifier be? A systematic review of non nutritive sucking in preterm infants. *Neonatal Network* 19 (8), pp. 41–8.

Redshaw, M. E. (1997) Mothers of babies requiring special care: Attitudes and experiences. *Journal of Reproductive and Infant Psychology* 15, pp. 109–20.

Reid, T., Freer, Y. (2001) Developmentally focused nursing care, in Boxwell, G. (ed.) *Neonatal Intensive Care Nursing*, 2nd edn. London: Routledge) pp. 14–38.

Rennie, J. M., Roberton, N. R. C., (eds) (1999) *Textbook of Neonatology*,
3rd edn. London: Churchill Livingstone, pp. 289, 389–99.

Roberton, N. R. C. (1993) Should we look after babies less than 800 grams? *Archives of Diseases of Childhood* 68, pp. 326–9.

Smith, L., Coleman, V., Bradshaw, M. (eds) (2002) *Family-centred Care: Concept, Theory and Practice*. Basingstoke: Palgrave.

Soll, R. F. (1999) Prophylactic synthetic surfactant for preventing morbidity and mortality in preterm infants (Cochrane review). *The Cochrane Library*, 3, Oxford: Update Software.

Sparshott, M. (1996) The development of a clinical distress scale for ventilated newborn infants: Identification of pain and distress based on validated behavioural scores. *Journal of Neonatal Nursing*, 2 (2), pp. 5–10.

Stevens, B. J., Frank, L. (1995) Special needs of preterm infants in the management of pain and discomfort. *Journal of Obstetric, Gynaecologic and Neonatal Nursing*, 24 (9), pp. 856–62.

Sweet, B. R., (ed.) (1997) *Mayes' Midwifery: A Text Book for Midwives*, 12th edn. London: Bailliere Tindall, p. 511.

Taylor, B. (1996) Parents as partners in care. *Paediatric Nursing* 8 (4), pp. 4–7.

World Health Organisation (1997) *Hypoglycaemia of the Newborn: Review of the Literature*. Geneva: WHO.

Turrill, S. (1992) Supported positioning in intensive care. *Paediatric Nursing*, 4 (4), pp. 24–7.

Turrill, S. (1999) Interpreting family-centred care within neonatal nursing. *Paediatric Nursing* 11 (4), pp. 22–4.

Vibhuti, S., Ohlsson, A. (2000) Randomised trial of analgesic effects of sucrose, glucose and pacifiers in term neonates. *Journal of Paediatrics*, 136 (5), pp. 701–2.

Vickers, A., Ohlsson, A., Lacy, J. B., Horsley, A. (2000) Massage for promoting growth and development of premature and low birth weight infants (Cochrane review). *The Cochrane Library* 3, pp. 13–19. Oxford: Update software.

Ward-Larson, C., Horne, R., Gosnell, F. (2004) The efficacy of facilitated tucking for relieving procedural pain of endotrachael suctioning in low birth weight infants. *The American Journal of Maternal/Child Nursing* 29 (3), pp. 151–156.

Webster, E. (1999) 'The use of pacifiers for non nutritive sucking by babies in the neonatal unit: A qualitative investigation into neonatal nurses perspectives'. *Journal of Neonatal Nursing* 5 (6), pp. 23–9.

Wheeler, J., Chapman, C. (2000) Feeding outcomes and influences within the Neonatal Unit. *International Journal of Nursing Practice* 6 (4), pp. 196–206.

Wilcox, M. A., Smith, S. J., Johnson, I. R., Maynard, P. V., Chilvers, C. E. (1995) The effect of social deprivation on birth weight excluding physiological and pathological effects. *British Journal of Obstetrics and Gynaecology* 102 (11), pp. 918–24.

Wood, N. S., Marlow, N., Costeloe, K., Gibson, A. T., Wilkinson, A. R. (The EPICURE Study Group) (2000) Neurologic and developmental disability after extremely preterm birth. *New England Journal of Medicine* 343, pp. 378–84.

World Health Organisation (1992) *International Statistical Classification of Diseases and Related Health Problems*, 10th revision. Geneva: WHO.

Yeo, H. (ed.) (2000) *Nursing the Neonate*, 2nd edn. Oxford: Blackwell Science.

Young, J. (1994) Positioning premature babies. *Journal of Neonatal Nursing* 1 (1), pp. 27–31.

10

Children with Life Limiting and Life Threatening Disease

Julia R. Twigg

Learning outcomes

- Examine best practice in how to 'break bad news' to children, young people and parents.
- Discuss childhood cancer, using a case study of acute lymphoblastic leukaemia to devise a care plan.
- Increase awareness of spirituality, and the support of children and young people in distress.
- Develop skills of communication to provide effective support to children and families through life threatening illness.
- Increase knowledge of palliative and end of life care for children.
- Explore the provision of services for children with terminal illness.

Introduction

Mortality rates for children in developed nations have decreased dramatically throughout the twentieth century; figures for the United Kingdom for 2002 record 15 deaths per 100,000 in children aged 1 to 14, the death rate for infants under one year was 5.2 per 1,000. This contrasts with 20 years earlier when the figures for 1980 were 31 children per 100,000 population aged from 1 to 14 and 12 per 1000 infants (Office for National Statistics 2005). Improvements in living standards, advances in medical knowledge, the introduction of vaccination programmes, antibiotics, improved road safety in the 1980s with the introduction of seat belts, have all had a significant impact upon childhood survival. The majority of deaths occur in the first year of life due to congenital anomalies or problems of prematurity. Accidents remain the biggest cause of death in children and young people between the ages of 4 to 24.

Many children who suffer from complex conditions, which previously may have led to early death now survive, for example childhood cancer. By the mid 1990s nearly 75 per cent of children with cancer survived at least 5 years. For the main type of childhood leukaemia (acute lymphoblastic leukeamia) survival was above 80 per cent according to the National Registry of Childhood Tumours, 2005 (Office for National Statistics 2005). Advances in surgery and the possibility of a life saving transplant hold out hope for some young people and their families. New therapies are always being sought to overcome otherwise incurable degenerative conditions. However, this can bring its own challenge and families live with prolonged uncertainty. As supportive therapies become increasingly sophisticated and more treatment options become available, decisions about when palliative care is more appropriate than actively seeking to prolong life can be delayed (Hynson and Sawyer 2001). Despite improvements children, young people and their families may have to face the real possibility of premature death, figures in 2003 suggest that 12 in every 10,000 children in the United Kingdom have a life limiting/threatening illness and approximately half of them will need active palliative care at any one time (Association of Children's Hospices 2005). Acquired Immune Deficiency Syndrome (AIDS) has had a major and increasing impact upon children and young people and is an international concern. Increasing knowledge and skills to provide support and palliative care is important as well as increasing knowledge and providing resources to prevent and treat this disease.

Children and young people need developmentally appropriate care to support them throughout the difficulties created by their illness, as well as the side effects and consequences of treatment. Children's nurses need to be adept at caring for children receiving intense or complex treatment regimes; while caring for the child and family as a whole through critical times, from diagnosis, through treatment, relapse, exacerbations of illness and sometimes to end of life care. Nurses caring for these children work in different environments, in children's homes, acute hospitals, respite and hospice services. The triggers in this chapter aim to help children's nurses explore the dilemmas and challenges of working with children and families with life threatening/limiting conditions.

❗ Trigger 10.1: The Bad News

The intention of this trigger is to help you to consider how best to support a child and family at the time of diagnosis.

The Trigger

Louisa is a five year old child admitted to the children's hospital for investigations into a history of joint pains, lethargy and bruising. The parents are in the office with the doctors and Louisa's named nurse and have been gone for some time.

Louisa has appeared to be pre-occupied playing with her dolls but she looks up as the nurse passes: 'Where's my Mum and Dad gone?'

'They've gone to see the doctor he's talking to them about you and what we need to do to get you better.'

Mum and Dad come out of the office. Mum hurries away. Dad looks towards Louisa and appears concerned, but he smiles when he sees his daughter and says 'they won't be long' and follows his wife.

'Where are mummy and daddy going?'

'They've probably just gone for a cup of tea.'

'Mummy's been crying, did the doctor make her cry?'

Situation

You are a student nurse caring for five year old Louisa, who has been admitted to your ward for investigations into joint pain, lethargy and bruising. Louisa lives with both parents. Her mother is a classroom assistant and her father is a chauffeur. She has an eleven year old sister and a younger brother aged two.

The ward you are working in is a regional centre caring for children with cancer, and from the ward report you know that Louisa is suffering from acute lymphoblastic leukaemia. Her parents are told the diagnosis that afternoon. You are one of the nursing team caring for Louisa throughout the evening shift.

Feedback

As a group of students you are required to devise a nursing care plan for Louisa, who has been newly diagnosed wiith acute lymphoblastic leukaemia. Use the information in Table 10.1 to inform your care plan.

Table 10.1 Nursing Assessment

Name of Patient: Louisa Meredith	**General Information**
Preferred Name: Lulu	**Health** All immunisations up to date No allergies
Age: 5 years **D.O.B**. 26.03.99.	No major health problems until recent admission.
Address: 12, Any Street, Any Town	**Development** All developmental milestones attained Eats with a knife and fork, can dress herself
Religion: Not Baptised	Needs some help with buttons
Consultant: Dr Green	Good language,
Named Nurse: Staff Nurse Jenny Jones	A little shy in new situations.

(Continued)

Table 10.1 (*Continued*)

Presenting Problems

Louisa has wanted to sleep a lot, not wanting to go to school or dance class more irritable than usual.

History of a month of persistent colds and feverish illness. Mother noted that gums have been bleeding and she seems to be bruising easily, complaining of aching in her legs and arms.

General Practitioner referred her to the local hospital, blood tests taken and referral to Regional Children's Hospital.

Louisa understands that she is in hospital to find out why she is always so tired and feeling poorly.

Diagnosis

Acute Lymphoblastic Leukaemia

Communication/information

Parents informed by consultant about diagnosis.

Written information offered, prognosis and treatment explained. Parents have agreed that Louisa will enter trial of treatment.

Family-centred care

Mother and Father feel able to speak to Louisa about diagnosis and treatment but would like a nurse to be present to explain anything they can't answer. Mother feels she needs some time to absorb information before she can share news with other family members and Louisa.

Parents will organise work patterns and discuss with grandmother about sharing care of younger brother and sister so that they can stay with Louisa most of the time (including mother staying overnight).

A booklet was offered to the parents giving information about anticipated sibling responses.

Attends to own toilet needs, needs reminding to brush teeth and help with washing hair.

Usually sleeps through the night from 7 pm until 7 am.

Recently been needing an afternoon nap on return from school

Family and significant others

Lives with Mother and Father. Mother works part time as classroom assistant in a junior school, Father works as a chauffeur for a car hire and vehicle company.

2 siblings – Kate aged 11 attends school, Matthew aged 2 years attends nursery when mother at work.

Maternal Grandmother lives close by and cares for all three children regularly.

Louisa's has a best friend Grace, and several other friends from school that she sees regularly.

The family have a pet dog Bruno.

Favourite Recreations

Louisa likes to read, and to be read to. Her favourite stories are about Angelina Ballerina. She goes to Dance class with her friend Grace and was a fairy in the Dance class Christmas show.

Lulu has her favourite teddy with her. She doesn't like to sleep without him.

Favourite Foods

Quite a fussy eater. Generally likes pizza with pineapple topping, pasta with grated cheese and cottage pie, sandwiches and flavoured yoghurts and ice cream. Prefers cold drinks particularly blackcurrant.

Her appetite is quite poor at present.

Education

Louisa attends the local primary school. She started reception class in September, a bit shy at first, she has settled in well and can read simple books and do simple arithmetic.

The facts

What are the main facts in this trigger? Make a list.

Hypotheses: What may these facts mean?

- Louisa's symptoms are symptoms of leukaemia.
- Leukaemia is a life threatening condition.
- Giving bad news to parents is inevitably distressing to them.
- Children can 'sense' when things are wrong.

Questions developed from the hypotheses

1. What are the signs, symptoms and prognosis of acute lymphoblastic leukaemia?
2. How can we support Louisa's family after the news has been given?
3. How can we best support Louisa during this time?
4. What are the nursing considerations for a child with leukaemia?

Questions 2, 3 and 4 may be answered by providing a rationale for the nursing care plan.

Trigger 10.1: Fixed resource material

Read the following to help you answer the questions. (You may also wish to search and review other up-to-date research and evidence-based literature and seek other relevant resources to provide you with the answers to your questions.)

Alderson, P. (1993) *Children's Consent to Surgery*. Bucks: Open University Press.

Edwards, M., Davis, H. (1997) *Counselling Children with a Chronic Medical Condition*. Leicester: BPS Books.

Faulkner, A., Peace, G., O'Keefe, C. (1995) *When a Child has Cancer*. London: Chapman & Hall.

Gibson, F., Evans, M. (eds) (1999) *Paediatric Oncology: Acute Nursing Care*. London: Whurr.

Haut, C. (2005) Oncological emergencies in the Paediatric Intensive Care Unit, *AACN Clinical Issues: Advanced Practice in Acute and Critical Care* 16 (2), pp. 232–45.

Mack, J. W., Holcombe, G. E. (2004) 'The day one talk', *Journal of Clinical Oncology* 22 (3), Feb. pp. 563–6.

Pearman, K. (2002) Chemotherapy-induced nausea and vomiting: a health promotion resource. *Paediatric Nursing* 14 (6) pp. 30–2.

Ptacek, J. T., Eberhardt, T. L. (1996) Breaking Bad News, a review of the literature. *Journal of the American Medical Association* 276 (6), pp. 496–502.

Sharp, S., Cowie, H. (1998) *Counselling and Supporting Children in Distress*. London: Sage Publications.

Sloper, P. (1996) Needs and Responses of parents following the diagnosis of childhood cancer. *Child: Care, Health and Development* 22 (3), May, pp. 187–202.

Thompson, S. W. (2003) When kids get cancer. *Registered Nurse* 66 (7), pp. 29–34.

Useful websites

http://www.Cancerbacup.org.uk (CancerBACUP)

http://www.cancerwise.org (Cancer wise)

http://www.lrf.org.uk (Leukaemia research organisation)

http://www.nccf.org/childhoodcancer/facts.asp (National Childhood Cancer Foundation and Children's Oncology Group)

Trigger 10.1: Fixed resource sessions

Cancer in childhood (Lecture notes)

Childhood cancer is rare, 1 in 600 children under the age of 15 years develop a cancer and cure rates of over 60 per cent are higher than for most adult cancers (CancerBACUP 2004). The cumulative risk of contracting cancer in the first fifteen years of life is about 1 in 600 (Parkin et al 1998). Research into cancer and its treatments is ongoing and survival rates for acute lymphoblastic leukaemia (the largest incidence of childhood cancer) is above 80 per cent. In 2000, there were around 1,400 new cases of childhood cancer diagnosed in Great Britain. However, cancer accounts for around 20 per cent of all deaths in children aged 1 to 14 years (Office for National Statistics 2005). In the United States in 2005 approximately 9,510 children will be diagnosed with cancer and about 1,585 children will die from the disease (American Cancer Society 2005).

Causes and incidence of cancer in childhood

The cause of cancer in childhood is uncertain. There are some lifestyle and environmental factors that can predict a higher than average risk of cancer in adults, these are *extrinsic factors*. The role of extrinsic factors in childhood cancer is uncertain. The part that environmental factors play in childhood cancers has been widely investigated. Parental, foetal and childhood exposure to different agents including ionizing radiation, power lines, radon exposure, pesticides, maternal cigarette smoking, diet and virus exposure have all been examined but findings are inconclusive (American Cancer Society 2005). Children and young people who have been treated with chemotherapy and radiation for certain forms of cancer have a higher risk of a second cancer.

The vast majority of childhood cancers are *intrinsic*. Of childhood cancers 90 per cent are cancers of the primitive embryonic tissue; arising from the mesoderm and ectoderm germinal layers. Approximately one-third of childhood cancers are Leukaemia (blood forming tissues), with acute lymphoblastic leukaemia being the most common. Central nervous system and brain tumours (neuro ectodermal tissues) are the second most common form of cancer in childhood and the most common solid tumour.

There are links to genetic and chromosomal factors particularly for early childhood cancers. Retinoblastoma, a malignant tumour affecting the retina, for example, is a genetic disorder and is present at birth or diagnosed during the next two years. Children with the chromosomal abnormality trisomy 21 (Down's syndrome) have approximately a 20 per cent higher risk of contracting childhood leukaemia, both acute lymphoblastic (ALL) and acute myeloid leukaemia (AML) (Chesells 2001).

The *incidence* of ALL, neuroblastoma; a cancer of the sympathetic nervous system, and Wilm's tumour, the most common kidney tumour, and rhabdomyosarcoma peak in early childhood. Other types of childhood cancer, including osteosarcoma, Ewing's sarcoma and Hodgkins disease rise in incidence throughout childhood and continue into young adult life.

The nature of cancer

Cancerous cells share certain characteristics, have disordered metabolism and many of the properties of normal cells are no longer present. Differences between cancerous and healthy cells include:

- Normal cells only take in the nutrition they need, while cancerous cells consume an increased amount depriving normal cells around them.
- Normal cells recognise cells of the same type and grow towards each other, and growth will stop when they come into contact with cells not like them, this property is called contact inhibition, in cancerous cells this property is lost. The result of which is the ability to grow outside the cells of origin, infiltrate and spread to surrounding tissues.
- Cancer cells are not able to mature and differentiate to take on the specialist function of the cell in which they arise. In malignant tumours, the cancer cells do not die at the same rate that new ones are produced and, therefore, tumours grow bigger.

Some cancer cells break away and travel via the blood stream to other places (metastases).

In summary the effects of cancer are to do with proliferation of cancerous cells which leads to:

1. Tumour growth and infiltration of other organs.
2. Suppression of normal cell function, replacement of normal cells with cancerous cells
3. Consumption of nutrients depriving healthy cells,

Signs and symptoms

Children may present in a variety of ways according to the site and type of cancer. Cancer in childhood may be difficult to diagnose and abnormalities are not usually visible and can rarely be felt (Thompson 2003). They are fast growing and spread rapidly, disease is often quite widespread on diagnosis, which can often fuel the guilt, or anger of parents who may feel that diagnosis has been delayed due to delay in seeking advice, or delay in recognition by health professionals. Diagnosis is made from history, current symptoms and from the results of investigations, which are carried out to diagnose and stage the disease. The investigations will be carried out as soon as diagnosis is suspected. Investigations may include all or some of the following depending upon the type of cancer suspected: blood tests, bone marrow aspirate, lumbar puncture, x rays, ultrasound scan, bone scan, CT scan, magnetic resonance imaging (MRI), biopsy (CancerBACUP 2004). Minimising the pain or distress caused by these investigations is important through adequate preparation, analgesia and sedation as required.

Children and families will need support throughout this anxious time. Some parents find sources of information available on the Internet or from professional and voluntary organisations, valuable and informative.

Treatment of childhood cancer

The vast majority of children in the United Kingdom are treated in regional centres that specialise in the care and treatment of cancer. Parents are usually asked on diagnosis if they are willing for children to enter a trial of treatment. This is part of the ongoing battle in the fight against cancer, different drug protocols are tried and the data from all children entered in the trial is kept on a central database to help determine the most effective combination of treatments. Cancer Research funds these trials and there are currently 22 centres in the United Kingdom, which together form an organisation called the United Kingdom Children's Cancer Study Group (UKCCSG). Treatment is intensive because of the comparatively rapid spread of the disease.

Treatment includes surgery for removal of solid tumours with chemotherapy and radiotherapy to eliminate remaining cancer cells. As for any child recovering from surgery, attention to wound healing by preventing infection, ensuring adequate nutrition, hydration and pain management is essential. However, for these children recovery may be compromised by their underlying condition, and treatment regimes.

Leukaemia is treated primarily with chemotherapy. The course of treatment has different phases:

- An intensification phase given in three blocks of intensive treatment. This aims to kill off any leukaemic cells which may be left but cannot be detected.
- Induction, involving intensive treatment which aims to destroy as many leukaemic cells as possible. This usually last four to six weeks after which a bone marrow test is taken to check to see if the child is in remission.
- Central nervous system treatment: ALL sometimes develops in the brain and spinal cord. A cytotoxic drug, usually methotrexate, is injected intrathecally into the spinal spinal fluid by lumbar puncture to prevent this.
- Continuing maintenance therapy lasts up to 2 years or longer from diagnosis and involves tablets daily and monthly injections of chemotherapy. Children will normally take part in their usual daily activity throughout the maintenance period.

Chemotherapy works by interfering with the normal cell growth and division. Different drugs affect different parts of the cell cycle. Most childhood tumours, because of the rapidly dividing cells are chemosensitive. Dosages of drugs are relatively higher than those administered to adults and the timing of administration is very important (Burke et al 1999). Different drugs are administered in combination or rotation. Each drug has a different affect upon the cell cycle. Some cancerous cells develop resistance to certain drugs. However, combination therapy reduces the risk of drug resistance. Radiotherapy is a treatment option for some types of childhood cancer although its use is limited as much as possible as it does have significant long-term detrimental effects for growing children.

There are many distressing and potentially life threatening side effects to treatment. Although cancerous cells are more sensitive to chemotherapy due to their rapid division, healthy cells will also be destroyed. The expected side effects are different depending on which drugs are being used, how the drugs are administered, usually orally, intravenously or by intramuscular injection, and for how long the drugs are administered. Three main types of body tissue are commonly affected. Each of these areas depends on the rapid growth of new cells to perform their normal functions in the body. The three areas are:

- The lining of the gastrointestinal tract: leading to burning sensation or pain in the mouth, diarrhoea and constipation; and nausea and vomiting.
- Skin and hair: leading to skin rashes and hair loss.
- The bone marrow: leading to cell count changes, infection and fatigue.

Supportive therapy is very important alongside active treatment. Protective and rescue therapy, intended to support the body's ability to excrete toxins, and minimise damage to healthy cells will be administered along with chemotherapy. It is important that these are administered at the proper intervals.

Infection is one of the biggest risks to the child with cancer, not only does it delay the administration of chemotherapy, it is life threatening, the compromised immune system may be overwhelmed, more children die from infection during cancer treatment than any other cause (Pui 1997, cited in Thompson 2003). The child needs to be protected from infections as far as possible through careful hygiene and maintenance of asepsis and reverse barrier nursing when undergoing bone marrow transplantation or when severely immuno-compromised. Management of nausea, vomiting, gastro-intestinal ulceration, constipation and diarrhoea is important to minimise dehydration and support nutrition as well as minimising these distressing and painful conditions, which may impact upon readiness to comply with treatment. The child will be monitored for any potential complications, for example regular checking of blood counts prior to treatment. Oncological emergencies can occur either as a result of the disease, for example, hyperleukocystosis, and obstructive emergencies due to tumour mass, or as a result of treatment, including severe sepsis and acute tumour lysis syndrome (Haut 2005). As far as possible children are supported in their own homes throughout maintenance therapy and are encouraged to engage in normal activities when they feel well and able to do so.

There are many new therapies being investigated for the treatment of cancer. Current advances in cancer treatment include stem cell and bone marrow transplantation, gene and immunotherapy.

In order to anticipate the care children will need during treatment, it is essential that you access information about the drugs used, mode of action, administration, special precautions, side effects. In order to plan care you need to explore the evidence base for effective nursing interventions to minimise complications, manage pain and other effects of the disease and treatment.

Breaking bad news

A definition of bad news offered by Buckman (1986) is: 'Any news that drastically and negatively alters the patient's view of his/her future'. He suggests that the 'badness' of any news depends upon what the patient already knows or suspects about the future. He later stated that the impact of the bad news depends upon the size of the gap between the patient's expectations and the medical reality of the situation (Buckman and Kason 1992).

'Bad' news in the above context is very much related to the giving of a diagnosis or review of progress, which may happen in hospital, doctor's surgeries or outpatients. Much of the literature that is written about the breaking of bad news is related to the doctor's experience. There is some research into parent's experiences; however, little is focused upon children or nurses' experiences. Nurses often have to deal with the 'run up' to bad news being broken when parents or children may be alarmed or suspicious, often they are present when parents are given bad news. Nurses are frequently the professionals involved in clarifying or simplifying information that has not been fully understood and they may be asked direct questions by children and parents the answers to which may constitute bad news. A common situation that is frequently faced by nurses is giving information which is not perceived as 'major', for example, a delay in discharge or cancellation of surgery. Children's nurses are well aware of the dismay and distress such 'lesser' news can cause to children and parents. The determination of whether or not news is 'bad', apart from in the more obvious and dramatic situations often lies in the mind of the receiver. For example a delay in going to theatre may be welcome for a child but very unwelcome to the parent who will have to go through the process of preparing themselves and their child once again.

It has been stated that there is no way of softening the blow of bad news (Faulkner et al 1995, p. 59) and indeed it might be considered unethical and inappropriate to do so, because to soften the blow may mean telling half truths or offering false hope. However, the experience can be made worse for families through mishandling and insensitive or inappropriate interpersonal skills. Families, and individual accounts all confirm that the events leading up to and the way that bad news was broken to them are always remembered. This is, undoubtedly, a stressful experience for all involved, and the following guidelines, are offered, to provide structure for the giver of bad news, and to meet the needs of recipients of news of serious illness, worsening condition, poor prognosis or in the case of infants a diagnosis which indicates disability. The protocol will offer pointers for any situation a health care worker may meet, not all of the ideal conditions may be present and one may need to adapt, for example, the environment or timing may not be ideal, but the communication skills required of the giver of bad news are the same.

The timing of when to give bad news is important, views are divided as to whether it should be delayed until all the facts are known, and information needed to be given determined; or the giving of piecemeal information, which may create anticipatory but lower levels of tension over a longer period so that when the news is broken, some coping mechanisms are already in place to help the person deal with what is being said. Parents, and indeed children, are often alerted, prior to being told, that the condition is potentially serious from the response of staff, investigations carried out and it may be that the child has already been transferred to a specialist centre or admitted to an intensive care unit. What they often do not know is the extent of the problem or what can be done about it. Many parents may have struggled to get attention for their child, and although undeniably shocked to have news given to them or their fears confirmed, may be relieved that, at last, they have a name for the problem and people were taking steps to 'sort it out'. The majority of parents want to be told as soon as possible, even if the news is 'hopeless'.

The ways in which health professionals present bad or difficult news is an important factor in how it is received, understood and dealt with. Such news must be shared with children and parents in a sensitive non-hurried fashion, away from possible interruptions' (Department of Health 2004).

The setting is important because recipients of bad news need to be told in a place that provides quiet and privacy. Often people react in an emotional way and this can leave them feeling vulnerable. They need to be able to recover from their distress and ask questions free from unwelcome intrusion. The provision of something to drink, tissues, a telephone for them to call whoever they wish and not be overheard by others is helpful. The setting also needs to be a safe place for the news giver, the reactions of people are unpredictable no matter how well situations are handled, help should be close at hand and easy to summon if people are angry and violence is a possibility, or if people are overwhelmed and extra help is necessary.

Who should be present? Both parents should be told together, if at all possible with anyone they wish to be around to support them. The news giver should be a well informed authoritative person, who can answer parent's questions and discuss treatment or other options; this is usually the paediatric consultant. A nurse, preferably the named nurse, should always be present and members of the multidisciplinary team, for example a social worker can be included in the discussion or contacted for further help and support as necessary. A team approach to breaking bad news is important, Davis and Blight (2003) researching problems nurses identify when communicating with the families of patients with cancer found that the most extensively described difficulty was poor team communication. When bad news was communicated poorly, there was a knock on effect on nurse–family communication.

When the news is about an infant it is recommended that the baby is present and referred to by name. If the news involves a young person or child then a decision about whether or not they should be present needs to be made. Mack and Holcome (2004, p. 564) state when giving a diagnosis of cancer:

> The decision of whether to include the pediatric (sic) patient is not always straightforward. However we believe that teenagers should almost always be invited to attend. When adolescents are not part of the discussion, they may assume that the information they later receive is not completely honest and that the actual news about diagnosis and treatment is worse than what they are told.

Mack and Holcome (2004) go on to highlight that including teenagers from the beginning may help to engage them in their own care

Younger children may be excluded from the initial conversation as it may be distressing for children to see their parents upset and seemingly out of control, parents will need some time to recover. Afterwards information and support can be offered to them as to how the news can be given to children. Possibly the most helpful way is for the doctor to tell the child in the presence of the parents. Parents will also need help to inform siblings and other family members not present. Some parents, understandably, want to protect their child from bad news. A quote from Alderson (1993) from a ward sister expressed the view; 'some can't bear to hear things being said to children they can't accept.' She continues to say 'in fact most children can accept more than the parents can, and surprise their parents in how well they can cope' (p. 110). Parents may feel that news which they find overwhelming and distressing will have the same impact upon their child and cause them to lose hope. Children's nurses' work within a family-centred philosophy of care, and the views of parents and the knowledge they have of their child must be respected; however, situations like this are exceptional and outside the range of most people's experience. Parents may seek or rely upon the knowledge of health professionals to guide them as to how to respond. It is helpful to suggest that children will already know that something is wrong and be feeling anxious, that even if parents 'pretend' that everything is all right, that children will observe events around them that will worry them. As long ago as 1978 a study by Blubond-Langner into the private worlds of dying children illustrated quite clearly the process by which children knew they were ill and could die, even if staff or parents did not inform them or tried to protect them from this knowledge. When parents are not able to talk to their children honestly then it is difficult for children to express their fears and concerns and for adults to respond. Edwards and Davis (1997) summarise the reasons why children should be given information these include: enabling more helpful understanding of events and promoting adaptation, helping children to make sense of what is happening, to be actively involved in aspects of treatment such as decision-making and consent, and to dispel misperceptions and inaccuracies. They state that; 'children's imagination and fantasies about what may be happening to them can be far more frightening than reality' (p. 135). Suitable preparation and ways of offering information clearly, simply with honesty and reassurance need to be worked out between health professionals and parents with the use of materials such as diagrams, play situations, stories etc. Knowledge of child development, understanding of health and disease and common concerns around treatment as well as the experiences of the child concerned, for example previous experience of illness of themselves or others, is important when planning what and how to explain the situation to a child. This a situation where parents' expert knowledge about their child and the professional's knowledge of child development and common concerns children have in these situations can work together to provide optimum care.

   How and what to say: Buckman and Kason (1992) offer a 6-step protocol for breaking bad news. The first step covers the above, getting the physical context right and deciding who should be there, and starting off. Starting off is the opening statement where the ground needs to be laid for the news to come. An example may be:

'Thank you for coming, I know you must be anxious about . . . condition and all the tests we have been carrying out, we've been very concerned about . . . and the results we have indicate that we were right to be concerned.'

The next step is to find out how much the patient, or in this case the parent knows, this will give you a starting point so that you are not starting too far ahead of where the parents are at, and does not patronise or create impatience if parents are already well aware and informed. A simple question such as 'How does . . . seem to you?' or 'What do you know already about the tests we have been carrying out? . . . reasons we have asked to talk to you?' The way the parent answers may also indicate how they are feeling, there may be an angry retort, for example 'That's what you are meant to tell us!' Parents may be very fearful, or very calm and have a good grasp of the situation already and have worked out the questions that they want to ask you.

Nurses are unlikely, for the most part, to be the professionals giving the parents the initial diagnosis, however, when asked a question to which the possible answer may be bad news it is as well to remember the above and enquire how much people already know or have been told, and try to gently ascertain why they are asking the question. This is particularly important with children, a question about what is going to happen to them may mean in the immediate future rather than a question about their long-term prognosis.

Find out how much the patient/parent wants to know: Some people want all details, others need time to assimilate information and their initial response may be one of helplessness and reliance on others to know what is best. Some people may feel over-loaded at a time when they are less able to 'take in' what is being said. However, certain information will need to be offered at this time, which leads to the next step of sharing the information.

Giving information: Important information to be conveyed is; the diagnosis, and how certain or uncertain it is; the treatment and goals of treatment, parents will need to know what to expect, and it may be that some treatment decisions may need to be made in a relatively short period of time.

It is recommended that information is shared clearly using easily understandable language, not jargon; giving information in small chunks, the use of diagrams and written material may help. Some parents may want more detailed information; they may have already accessed the Internet and present staff with questions, or can be directed to reliable Internet or other information sources. The presence of a professional interpreter is essential when breaking news of life threatening diagnosis to people who speak limited or no English. The use of a family member, particularly a sibling to interpret is not appropriate when news is difficult. There may be inhibitions and different cultural beliefs about who and how people should be informed, this may be in conflict with staffs' beliefs about good practice, but accommodation for different value systems is important in such sensitive situations.

Check for understanding frequently: that both parent understands the information and clarify that the same meanings are shared. Offer parents or patients the chance to ask any questions or make any requests they wish and again check that you have understood what they have asked and that you have given them an answer. Important information to offer parents and patients is the possible cause of the illness, people often look for causes and want to attribute meaning and find causes for otherwise inexplicable events in their lives. Normal emotional reactions are anger or guilt, telling them at this time that there is no known cause, or that no one is to blame may be important. This is of course made more complex when guilt or anger may be a reasonable response as in the case of an accident, or situation of neglect. It may be inappropriate to explore fully, such feelings however legitimate, at this time, accepting that is how people might feel and identifying what the priorities are right now is a useful strategy.

Responding to feelings in this situation: This is the fifth step described by Buckman and Kason, and as previously discussed people respond in a variety of ways. Many people describe feeling numb and unable to believe what has been said, others feel physically overwhelmed, once reality has set in there may be intense distress or questions about why us? This can lead to expressions of anger, or angry behaviour. Many parents feel helpless and bewildered; others will exhibit severe distress through crying or wailing. Wright (1999) writes about his research into sudden death and identified that carers have particular difficulty when a relative withdraws 'in this state the client becomes inaccessible, mute and appears to be refusing to listen' (p. 72).

Silence can be hard to deal with and can leave the carer feeling they are of no help and vulnerable as they enter their own thoughts. However, in his research Wright found that relatives appreciated the care worker being there and being able to stay with the pain and distress. A quietly accepting response that allows parents time to assimilate information and allows them to express what they need to express is valued by parents.

Sharp and Cowie (1998) summarise the theories of Lazarous and Abramovitz; Cox; and Freeman, which all offer explanation as to why individuals will respond differently to stress, or why at times they may feel able to cope and at others are overwhelmed. The seriousness of a situation will undeniably affect the impact of any event. The individual's experience of stress will be influenced by their primary appraisal of how significant a harmful, threatening and challenging event may be and a secondary appraisal of their ability to cope, a critical imbalance between perception of threat and perceived ability to cope will lead to distress. People's perception of their coping capabilities, will be influenced among other factors, by previous traumatic or difficult events in their lives, how and how well or otherwise they coped then and their assessment of their ability to cope now. An accumulation of stressful events, lack of resources either financial, personal or social, or increased demands such as a high work load, may decrease one's ability to effectively manage a new crisis. Rice et al (1993) propose a model of stress in children and young people that considers the interrelationship of the number and nature of stressful events and the synchronicity with other important developmental events or processes, such as entering puberty or beginning a new school. Social support and or internal resources mediate these.

Ways of helping people include; offering support, involving them in the decision-making process, as soon as they feel able, helping them to begin to take control of events as far as possible in order to maintain and restore self esteem, identifying existing resources; and offering them additional sources of help. These steps offer the start of some restoration of coping capabilities, it can also be the start of working in partnership and a family-centred approach to care.

The way that bad news is broken will not necessarily influence the individual response. Even if delivered with great care and sensitivity parents will still understandably be distressed, carers' responses should be parent or patient led and remain supportive of the individual. Professionals are recommended to describe their emotions not to display them, although signs of being affected by the sadness of the news is appreciated by parents as an indication of really caring about their child. There may be a temptation to try to make people feel better, and parents may try to push the medical team into 'fixing things'. It may well be that some requests can be supported, some fears alleviated and whatever comfort can be offered is offered, however, it is important not to be pushed into agreeing to the impossible, or giving false hope. Most recipients of bad news have identified the need for some hope to be given, painting the bleakest picture possible without offering any hope, thinking that anything positive that may happen will be a bonus, is not helpful to most people in this situation, a fine balance between hope and likely possibility needs to be maintained.

Making plans: This is the final step, parents and patients will need help to plan and organise the future, sensitive listening here is important if we are to identify individual needs as opposed to presuming what they are. It may be as simple as the need to know whom to contact next and arranging this for them by providing a phone number or help making plans to fix what can be fixed, for example both parents may want to stay with their child. Nurses are often the appropriate people to identify and meet these needs. A plan or strategy to deal with the immediate situation needs to be put in place, false hope should not be given and depending upon the reality of the situation preparation for the worst while hoping for the best may be the most appropriate option. In some situations, for example childhood cancer, there is very often real hope for cure and this will need to be emphasized and parents helped to believe and work with this premise. Written information is often highly valued by parents who need time to assimilate what has been said. It has been suggested that audio taping interviews may be a means of improving communication with families (Department of Health 2004) however, Ptacek and Eberhardt (1996) advise some caution, not all families will appreciate or benefit from playing the tape. Information about support groups or other sources of help may be useful at this time and should be incorporated into any written information offered. Further appointments to keep parents up to date, informed and to go through any questions the parents or patients have should form part of the plan.

It is important that all the health care team are aware of what information the parents and or children have been given so that there is consistency of information and approach to the child and family to avoid confusion and conflict.

These situations are undeniably stressful for the health care workers involved. They will need time to recover and possibly time to process such events within the ward team or through clinical supervision.

→ Trigger 10.1: Feedback

Go to Chapter 10 trigger feedback on p. 324

! Trigger 10.2: Why Me?

This trigger requires you to reflect upon expressions of distress, either emotional or spiritual, in children, young people and their families and to consider which responses might be helpful.

The Trigger

A reflective learning journal entry

The incident: 14 year old Martin approached me as I was filling in the nursing records. The conversation was as follows:

Martin: What religion does it say I am on that form?
Me: It says you are a Methodist.
Martin: Well you can cross that out.
Me: Why do you want me to do that?
Martin: I don't think there can be a God, if there is I don't want anything to do with him. How comes he's let me get a disease like this when I've always tried to be a good kid. Some kids at my school are right 'losers', always getting into trouble, bullying people, messing about, but they haven't got this why doesn't he give it to them. Why me?

Background to the incident: Martin is 14 years old and has been treated for a malignant illness, which has meant he needed to undergo investigations, painful surgery and courses of chemotherapy, which he has borne with exemplary courage, co-operation and good humour. However a recent assessment of progress revealed secondary spread of the disease and relapse necessitating further treatment. The other nurses had noted him starting to become withdrawn, less communicative and spending more time alone. He has had angry outbursts towards his parents and told his mother to go home when she wanted to stay with him overnight.

What happened next: I agreed to cross off the religion on his notes, but suggested he might want to talk about it to his parents or one of the sister's on the ward. I spoke to the staff nurse in charge and she said she would go and talk to him later.

What I felt: I felt inadequate and a bit shocked, I didn't know what to say and wondered if what I did was enough and if there was more I could have said to help him. But honestly I don't think I could give him an answer that wouldn't sound trite. I can understand how he feels, and I do wonder why these things happen to children. The staff nurse spoke to Martin, he seemed OK and was playing on the computer, he didn't say much to me and I wasn't sure how to talk with him.

Situation

You are a member of a group of student nurses taking part in a peer supervision exercise, individuals in the group are asked to share with the learning group an incident from practice. This learning journal entry is the incident you have chosen to present to the group to explore further. Within the group you are asked to discuss the incident, identify what the main issues are, explore the literature and make further enquiries to determine appropriate responses should a similar incident happen in the future.

Feedback

Discuss the incident as a group, your feelings and responses to the situation. Using Heron's (2001) six category intervention (a brief description of this is offered in the second fixed resource session) as a framework or model, formulate a helpful response to Martin's obvious distress.

The facts

What are the main facts in this trigger? Make a list:

Hypotheses: What may these facts mean?

- Children and adolescents may think that illness is a punishment and unfair.
- Adolescents get angry.
- Young people may reject religious or spiritual beliefs in times of difficulty or when their lives or bodily integrity is threatened.
- Nurses find it hard to know how to respond in these situations

Questions developed from the hypotheses

The answers to the trigger questions should inform the feedback for this trigger.

1. How do children and young people make sense of a serious and life threatening illness?
2. What is the nurse's role in supporting the child and family's spiritual well being?
3. How can we recognise when children and young people are distressed?
4. Is there any meaningful way of responding in situations when there are no answers?

Trigger 10.2: Fixed resource material

Read the following to help you answer the questions. (You may also wish to search and review other up to date research and evidence-based literature and seek other relevant resources to provide you with the answers to your questions.)

Burnard, P. (1992) *Learning Human Skills, An Experiential Guide for Nurses*, 2nd edn. Oxford: Butterworth Heinemann.

Cook, P. (1999) *Supporting Sick Children and Their Families*. Oxford: Balliere Tindall.

Faulkner, K. (1997) Talking about Death with a Dying Child. *American Journal of Nursing* June, 97 (6), pp. 68–9.

Heron, J. (2001) *Helping the Client, A Creative, Practical Guide*, 5th edn. London: Sage Publications.

Lindsay, B., Elsegood, J. (eds) (1996) *Working with Children in Grief and Loss*. London: Balliere Tindall.

Richardson, J. (1996) Counselling Children, in Burnard, P., Hullatt, I. (eds) *Nurses Counselling:The view from the Practitioners*. Butterworth-Heinemann. Chapter 4, pp. 42–57.

Savins, C. (2002) Therapeutic work with children in pain. *Paediatric Nursing* 14 (5), June, pp. 14–16.

Turner, M. (1998) *Talking with Children and Young People about Death and Dying: A Workbook*. London: Jessica Kingsley.

Useful Websites

http://www.cancerwise.org (Cancer wise)

http://www.tcf.org.uk (The Compassionate Friends)

Trigger 10.2: Fixed resource sessions

Spiritual care and the search for meaning

Consideration of an individual's spirituality as an integral part of holistic care is a concept promoted within nursing. However, apart from noting religious beliefs and identifying religious rituals and specific dietary requirements nursing care plans rarely offer space to explore a person's spirituality in a meaningful way. Spirituality is hard to define, several overviews of literature relating to spirituality in childhood have offered definitions (Pfund 2000; Smith and McSherry 2004), but most agree it is a multi-dimensional concept and each person's spiritual identity is uniquely personal, informed by many influences, family, culture, education and life experiences being equal, if not more important for some individuals, than religious teaching or beliefs. Spiritual belief is in constant flux and it comes into focus during times of crisis. It appears that Martin is trying to make sense of and find some meaning to what is happening to him, when he can find no explanation, or sense of justice in what appears to be an unfair situation.

Children develop concepts of spirituality through secure stable relationships, they often find meaning through simple logic and are often open to spiritual concepts and explanation. However, they are also made vulnerable by their capacity to attribute negative feelings to experiences or hold fearful ideas. Adults as well as adolescents and children find some situations hard to comprehend, but yet still seek meaning to events.

> Our sense of meaning, the framework within which we live our lives, develops over time as a result of a complex interaction between our own psychological development and the experiences we encounter in the world. It is an attempt to give order and predictability to our lives (Kavanagh 1994, p. 10).

However, he goes on to state that a sense of meaning is very subtle, hard to articulate and brought into focus when what we have taken for granted is suddenly no longer.

Young people of Martin's age are starting to find their own identity separate to that of their family. They are on the cusp of moving from a younger child's ready acceptance of adult teaching; towards a questioning of adult ideals and beliefs; 'Children imagine God as a protective, ideal parent figure, magnified by a child's absolute need for care, protection, love and the need to believe that a parent is almighty' writes Pfund (2000 p. 144), whereas adolescents question adult values and beliefs. Children's spirituality is linked to cognitive, moral and social development. Adolescents are according to Erikson's (1963) stages of development working through the developmental crisis of forming a sense of identity separate to their parents; they come to see themselves as distinct individuals, unique and separate from any other individual. Group identity is an important precursor to finding a personal identity, and the adolescent distances himself from his family and finds support and identity within his peer group (Geldard and Geldard 1999). This move away from family and questioning of family values may also be reflected in examining and rejecting or accepting religious beliefs. Old certainties of family, of adults appearing to be in control, 'almighty' are shaken. Adolescence can be characterised by ambivalence, adolescents want to grow up, but may feel fearful at times and want to regain the security of the family, and that, which is familiar and safe. There is often conflict in the home as adolescents frequently create tensions. Richardson (1996) states that adolescents provide particular challenges for nurses and other health care workers, with regard to purposeful and satisfying mutual understanding and communication. Adolescents usually possess the ability to understand and reason like an adult but will have less life experience to guide decision-making. They may also be more volatile and erratic emotionally. This time of life is tumultuous for the child following a 'normal' transition to adulthood, for the child with chronic or serious health problems the necessary dependence upon parents can create tension for young people, parents and carers. Where the young person accepts without struggle the interventions of adults this is often to the cost of individual and peer identity.

Many people remain in an early stage of moral development where the good are rewarded and the bad are punished, the severity of the punishment often determines for many children the seriousness of the deed. This idea may be translated by young people into religious beliefs around the necessity to be good and not to misbehave in order to be loved by God. This belief framework makes no sense in a situation in which a child is suffering. Faulkner et al (1995), researching into children's experience of cancer, recorded that a child stated that 'God couldn't love them' (p. 41). Where there is no logic, the sense a child and indeed many adults may make of it is that they must have done something wrong, or they are bad. Many adolescents and adults are outraged at the apparent injustice when they can perceive of no known bad behaviour on their part, which merits such a punishment. Feelings of betrayal are also possible, as Martin appears to feel, when having kept his side of the bargain, always trying to be a 'good kid', appeared not to be enough. Spiritual well being is sometimes only evident in its absence, spiritual distress is characterised by alterations of mood shown in crying, anxiety, hostility, withdrawal, apathy and feeling of pointlessness. Young people may be afraid of rejection, of being ridiculed or censored when they express powerful feelings and so may feel isolated, or withdraw more after an 'outburst'. If a young person, or indeed a parent exhibits or expresses such feelings the nurse can accept and acknowledge how they must feel and offer opportunities for the young person to say more when they are ready.

Erikson (1987) identifies the final life conflict as integrity v despair, although this is placed in older age, which is when people usually face loss and death, it may be brought into premature focus when a young person is facing their own mortality. The successful resolution of this conflict, integrity, arises from the sense of a complete life lived with meaning, with some of the grief engendered by the despair of losing the future, reaching some resolution; this may be possible for the adolescent, or indeed a child, facing death but is the more poignant filled as it is with expectations and possibilities which will not be realised, the question of who am I and what will I become not answered. A young person's spirituality can be respected and nurtured by not withdrawing love and affection despite rejection, respecting their autonomy, allowing them to freely express freely how they are feeling but maintaining the safe boundaries of acceptable behaviour, providing a listening space for the exploration of ideas. Often the nurses closer in age to the young person will be the ones they feel most comfortable speaking to, this is demonstrated by Martin in that he expressed his thoughts to someone close in age, who had spent some time building a relationship with him.

He may be less comfortable speaking to a chaplain or counsellor, although a chaplain, religious or community leader used to working with patients and relatives in hospital will be supportive and open to speaking to the young person without necessarily criticising his anger with God, and used to withstanding the anger and rebuffs they might encounter. Someone immediately outside the family and day-to-day caring encounters may also be useful in that there will be less sense of 'emotional payback' if the young persons wants to express ideas and emotions which they feel may hurt, upset or embarrass someone closer to them.

In our pluralistic society nurses work with children and families from different cultures and faiths to their own, knowledge about and respect for different belief systems is important even if parts of it conflict with the nurse's own. It is important that nurses don't label or assume religious or cultural beliefs before working with a child or family. The nurse may also be working through the spiritual crises that arise from the challenges of caring for children with life threatening diseases and may seek support, the same considerate listening should be offered to them.

Suggested Activities

- Explore different belief systems
- Explore your own spiritual beliefs.
- Discuss and share your spiritual beliefs with another student within your group. How are they similar? Do your family and upbringing; religious beliefs or events in your life influence your spiritual beliefs?

The use of counselling skills for nurses

Counsellors work within a code of ethics and within agreed boundaries and structures; formal counselling requires a contract which involves agreeing frequency of meetings, number of meetings, a time frame usually 50 minutes, discussion about boundaries with relation to confidentiality and an explanation about the purpose of counselling (British Association for Counselling and Psychotherapy 2002). It would be both inappropriate, because of role boundaries, and unlikely that a children's nurse working in an acute care setting would work in this way. However, nurses are involved in caring for people and are often the people in whom patients and parents confide. They are also the workers who will identify distress or uncertainty through the assessment process or noting changes in behaviour and response to different situations. Nurses are taught the importance of and encouraged to develop self-awareness, communication, interpersonal and observational skills, and patients value the qualities of unconditional positive regard, warmth, genuineness and empathy from nurses, which were identified by Carl Rogers (1967) as the necessary personal qualities of an effective counsellor.

Counselling skills are useful for nurses in that they promote therapeutic interaction, good listening and questioning skills, which will encourage clients to talk about how they are feeling, help clients identify their problems and help clients work out a solution or mutually agree what actions to take. This is in contrast to offering advice or information based upon what the nurse perceives as the problem or appropriate action, or rescuing people by solving problems based upon your own assessment of a situation within your own terms of reference.

An important skill of counselling is first of all attending to the child or parent. In a very busy ward situation with several children to care for and a list of things to complete it is very easy to miss or overlook signals for attention or that people need to say or confide something important. Too often small issues can become large, or vital information can be lost or overlooked until a crisis occurs. Children and parents will pick up signals from the nurse that they are too busy or occupied, they may wish not to intrude or bother anyone and worries, upsets and misunderstandings can increase. Frequently it may be that parents or children find a 'gap' when nurses appear to have time for them to ask important questions. This is not always at opportune times, and can be unexpected. I recall taking a child for a bone scan after she had treatment for osteosarcoma, I explained what would happen and what the scan was for, the girl knew she had cancer, but I felt on the spot when she asked, 'What happens if the cancer has spread?' I collected myself and answered in terms of additional treatment, but felt momentarily at a loss, as I knew that further spread meant a poorer prognosis.

Paying attention is important in all interactions with children and family members, you convey to children and parents that you are there for them and that they are important. You convey this by appropriate body language; speaking directly to people maintaining eye contact, adopting an open posture and positioning yourself at the persons level, for example sitting or standing whenever possible so that eyes are level. Some children and indeed some parents may not be comfortable with too much eye contact and may find it difficult to start a conversation directly about what is troubling them. Playing alongside a child may help, and inconsequential conversation may turn into something more meaningful, children often use metaphor and play to communicate quite important feelings, children's nurses need to be sensitive to this and respond appropriately. Parents may use the opportunity to talk while engaged in social chit chat or day-to-day contact with nurses. A regular opportunity for daily contact and communication may be more beneficial than a series of planned meetings to discuss problems.

Listening skills

The value of listening skills cannot to be over estimated: 'Listening is the beginning, middle and end of helping. It hears what is spoken and what is implied. To hear another person is perhaps the biggest gift we can ever give' (Tschudin 1995, p. 39).

Different levels of listening can be identified:

- *Cosmetic listening*: when we put on the appearance of listening but we are not really, our thoughts are somewhere else. This can happen frequently when we are distracted or short of time, or are only focused on what it is we want to achieve from an interaction.

- *Listening in conversations*: here we listen and engage in a conversation, but often we equally busy talking and thinking about our own concerns.
- *Active listening*: here we are paying attention, we are focused and mentally recording facts about what the person is saying, body language, congruence etc. and we check with the other person that we are 'getting it right'. The person talking feels heard.
- *Deep listening*: this is where we are totally focused on the person, when we listen at this level we gain a sense of who the person is and experience empathic understanding. This can be a very powerful and experience for both parties and can in itself be therapeutic.

Therapeutic encounters involve active and some deep listening. Most people would feel uncomfortable being 'counselled' all the time, and indeed if used inappropriately this can be intrusive and unwelcome. If used inappropriately then people will indicate they do not wish to speak further and outside of a formal counselling situation it is important this is respected, unless it is felt that the situation warrants further exploration. Children will often only tolerate short periods of 'counselling' and it may be that they will return to the 'problem' later, once they realise you are comfortable with them and gauged your reaction. To gain children's trust and confidence it is important that you do not display emotion too overtly (Geldard and Geldard 2002), if they perceive that you are shocked, distressed or uncomfortable they may feel that what they are saying is wrong, or feel responsible for your upset, or that the situation is one which is too difficult for anyone to hold. People, adults and children but particularly adolescents, often think that how they are feeling is unique to them and to share this with someone may open them up to ridicule; to have their feelings heard and accepted in a calm manner, which nevertheless acknowledges the importance of their feelings and experiences, is immensely reassuring even if no action is taken or necessary.

It may be that the child or parent is unclear about what is causing them to feel as they do, and nurses may need to help them clarify the issues. If some action is necessary, or possible, to help resolve problems, then the patient, parent or nurse will need to be clear about what the real problem is, and if possible the parent or child will need to be helped as appropriate to work out their preferred solution. Skills of reflecting, clarifying, paraphrasing and summarising are essential to do this.

An example of talking with a parent is offered below:

Reflecting (sometimes called echoing): is the process of reflecting back the last few words, or a paraphrase of the last few words, that the client has used, in order to encourage them to say more, echoing the client's thoughts and that echo serves as a prompt.

Mum: 'It was after she started school things started to go wrong'
Nurse: 'Things started to go wrong?'
Mum: 'Yes she seemed to enjoy going to school at first, then she started waking up with all these aches and pains, saying she didn't want to go to school, but I just thought she was playing me up'.

Statements can be made which is empathy building. These are statements that demonstrate that you have understood the feeling the client may be experiencing, careful listening is necessary here and the use of intuition, checking what is implied rather than what is said, for example:

Nurse: 'It sounds as if you feel guilty . . .'
Mum: 'Yes I do, I made her go to school when she must have been feeling really poorly, I was too busy thinking about getting off to work myself, getting Matthew to Nursery, I really thought it was just school, she's quite shy, and I was worried she wouldn't settle into school, and thought if I gave in she'd never settle down. Now I feel I've got to make it up to her and I want to stay with her but her baby brother is being difficult at home, my mum does a lot, I can't keep expecting her to. . . . Her Sister isn't saying much to me when she visits, I would love to go home for a short while but I really can't let her down, but I am so exhausted I don't know if I'm any help here, I keep snapping at everyone including the staff and I really don't want to and that makes me feel worse.'

Clarifying and paraphrasing: what appears to be a complex and multifaceted problem can help to make the situation clearer and restates the problem using different words:

Nurse: 'So you feel tired, that you need to go home to sort things out there, but you feel guilty about leaving, it sounds as if you are being pulled in too many directions and this is tiring you out.'

Mum: (sighing) 'Yes that's just it'.

Nurse: (Visibly relaxing) 'Things have been busy but I've got ten minutes right now, perhaps I can help you sort something out?'

Simple problem solving can work here; different solutions or courses of action can be examined. It is better if the client can decide what actions to explore, the possible advantages of each solution can be listed and discussed alongside the potential disadvantages, and an unexpected or combined course of action might be the result. Although people can do this for themselves it is often useful to work things out loud or writing them down with another person. Going through things in your head time and again can be confusing and add to tiredness.

An example in this situation could be:

Action One: Staying in the hospital and hoping things will be ok at home:

Advantages	Stay with daughter, she won't get upset
	Husband will learn to cope with family problems
	I will know what is happening here
Disadvantages	I will remain worried about other children
	I will get more tired due to broken nights
	Situation at home might get worse

Action Two: Bringing the whole family to stay in a hospital house:

Advantages	We'll all be together
	Help and distraction for daughter
Disadvantages	Loss of income from Husband's work
	Sister will miss school

Action Three: Asking husband or grandma to stay:

Advantages	Different company for daughter
	I could spend time with the other children
	Dad would get to spend time with her
	Opportunity for Dad and Grandma to help me over a long period of time
	I might be able to sleep better and get some strength back
Disadvantages	I'll feel guilty about leaving her, and might not sleep anyway
	She might want me and no one else
	Loss of income from Husband's work

Summarising: This can be used at the end of a conversation so that both people can agreed what has been said and actions agreed. .

For example:

Nurse: 'Let me see if I can sum up what we've talked about. You're very tired and upset, and you are concerned about things at home, you would like some time at home to sort things out but you know your daughter will fret if she's left alone, and you can't bear for her to be more upset. But you really need to see what's happening at home with the other kids, so you are going to talk to dad or grandma and see if they can stay over for a couple of nights while you are at home, you will come in during the day time.'

Mum: 'Yes, I'm going to telephone my husband and my mum and discuss arranging for them to come and stay in hospital for a couple of nights while I sort things out and take stock of the situation. I'll phone every day and at the weekend I'll bring her brother and sister in for the whole day and take over again. Perhaps her dad could stay at least one night another weekend. If I can get some sleep I'm sure I'll be less irritable and be able to cope better.'

Nurse: 'It's not surprising you feel tired, I can see you are trying to do the best for everybody. I'll introduce you to one of the mums who's part of the support group. I can introduce your partner to one of the dads. I know they have regular meetings, and go out sometimes to relax and have a chat. The social worker can give you some information about helping with travelling costs, and perhaps help her dad to find out about taking time out of work for a short spell. We could, if you would like, contact the health visitor and the school nurse to see if they can offer some advice and support for your other two children. Would you like me to see if there's a family room for the weekend?'

From the above example you can see that as well as skills of listening and questioning there are a number of *categories* of response which are helpful. This suggests that Heron's (2001) conceptual model is useful format for understanding a range of useful and therapeutic responses. Heron described six categories, below is a synopsis of the categories:

1. *Prescriptive*: To offer advice or make suggestions; an example would be:
   'Perhaps you would like to talk it over with your partner.'
2. *Informative*: To give information, instruct, impart knowledge; an example would be: 'Many parents feel that way, there is a support group run in the hospital, here is the number, if you call in the afternoon there is usually someone there.'
3. *Confronting*: To challenge restrictive or compulsive verbal or non-verbal behaviour An example would be: 'I know it's a difficult time for you, but you refuse all offers of help, its hard for me to know how to help you.' Nurses may find it difficult to

confront and allow potentially harmful behaviour to continue because they don't want to upset or make a situation worse, confrontation can however be very helpful provided it is done in a non threatening, non judgemental way, using 'I 'statements, with the intention to be helpful rather than accusatory, and ensuring you are in an appropriate place and have time to respond to the impact of the intervention.

4. *Cathartic*: To enable the release of emotion, this may be released through angry language, tears or sometimes laughter. Some examples are: 'what do you really want to say to . . . ?' 'That sounds really sad . . . '

5. *Catalytic*: To be reflective, to 'draw out' through the use of questioning, reflecting and paraphrasing. The use of open questions is most useful here, an example is: 'How do you feel?' rather than 'Are you unhappy?'

6. *Supportive*: To offer support; to validate, to confirm. This intervention should be present in all nursing situations, it is integral to any therapeutic conversation, it makes confrontation possible and maintains mutual positive regard; an example is: 'I can see you want the best for your child, you've done a great job so far. She is such a bright and lovely child.'

Morrison and Burnard (1989) who researched nurses' confidence in the above interventions found that nurses are most at ease with prescriptive and informative interventions which are identified as being authoritative interventions, and supportive interventions which are more facilitative. Catalytic, cathartic, (facilitative) and confrontation (authoritative) interventions were the ones with which nurses felt least comfortable.

When working with children you often may need to work through the media of toys or play, you need to offer more information and explanation to reflect the child's limited experience. It is important to think like a child in order to access how they may see the world. Young children often have feelings or fears, which aren't obvious to an adult, reality and fantasy, can't always be distinguished for the child, they can only understand things from their own frame of reference. Knowledge of child development, or at least sensitivity to the way children think and feel, coupled with respect for what they are trying to express is important. Knowledge of stages of development may help you to tune into the logic behind the thinking and behaviour of children of different ages, and to provide appropriate comfort and reassurance in difficult situations. It is, however, important to respect their experience. Children do not all have the same experiences, a child who has experienced treatments and the side effects, whose life is in the balance will have more lived experience, will be more expert in some instances than the nurse or parent. Many children with life threatening illness, going through sometimes painful surgery or treatment, have special needs, and may be profoundly handicapped with cognitive as well as physical difficulties. (Brearley 1997). They may have communication difficulties, and sensory deficits, which will add to their distress and bewilderment. It is important, that health care professional in partnership with parents, help inform, support and comfort these children.

Suggested Activities

Practise listening to each other, experience how it feels to really be listened to. How do you know when people are really listening? Listen to friends and family, note how they respond to you. Practise different responses, using different interventions as appropriate. People are often self-conscious when they begin to use these skills but as people talk to you and you appreciate what they have to say, it will become more natural. Communication skills are like any other, they need to be practiced and developed over time until they become a spontaneous unreserved response to the people in your care, or to those you care about.

! Trigger 10.2: Feedback

Go to Chapter 10 Trigger feedback on p. 324

→ Trigger 10.3: Palliative and Terminal care for Children

The Trigger

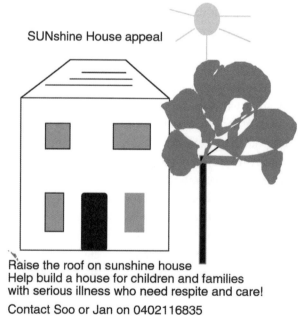

Figure 10.1 Sunshine House appeal

Situation

The poster is displayed in the School of Nursing and throughout the local hospital. You are an interested group of children's nurses, wanting to contribute to the fundraising events.

Feedback

Identify the information you will need to 'sell' a proposal for a new children's hospice in the area. Formulate ideas around gaining support and fundraising for the hospice proposal.

The facts

What are the main facts in this trigger? Make a list.

Hypotheses: What may these facts mean?

- Hospice provision for children is not considered important enough for statutory provision.
- A hospice for children would be valued by the local population.

Questions developed from the hypotheses

1. What is the function of a children's hospice?
2. What population does it serve?
3. How are the services of a hospice different to other services offered by the hospital?

Trigger 10.3: Fixed resource material

Read the following to help you answer the questions. (You may also wish to search and review other up-to-date research and evidence-based literature and seek other relevant resources to provide you with the answers to your questions.)

Dominica F., Hunt, A. (1993) 'Children's Hospices' in Glasper, E. A., Tucker, A. (eds) (1993) *Advances in Child Health Nursing*. Oxford: Scutari, Chapter 3, pp. 27–39.

Davis, R. (2003) Children's nursing. Establishing need for palliative care services for children/young people. *British Journal of Nursing* 12 (4), pp. 224–30.

Hill, L, (ed.) (1993) *Caring for Dying Children and Their Families*. London: Chapman Hall.

Hurwitz, C., Duncan, J., Wolfe, J. (2004) Caring for the child with cancer at the close of life. *Journal of American Medical Association*, 292 (17), Nov 3, pp. 2141–9.

Hynson, J. L., Sawyer, S. M. (2001) Paediatric palliative care: Distinctive needs and emerging issues, *Journal of Paediatrics and Child Health* 37 (4), pp. 323–5.

Useful websites

http://www.jrf.org.uk (Joseph Rowntree Foundation)
http://www.childhospice.org.uk (Association of Children's Hospices)
http://www.ippcweb.org/ (The Initiative for Pediatric Palliative Care)

Trigger 10.3: Fixed resource sessions

Palliative care for children

> Palliative care is an approach that improves the quality of life of patients and their families facing problems associated with life-threatening illness, through the prevention and relief of suffering by early identification and impeccable assessment and treatment of pain and other problems, psychosocial and spiritual (World Health Organisation 2005, http://www.who.int/cancer/palliative/definition/en/).

Death in childhood, in the developed world, is relatively rare. While much of the expertise and knowledge surrounding palliative care is focused on caring for terminally ill adults, many of the principles are relevant to the care of children. However, there are some significant differences. Expertise in paediatric palliative care is building, however more research and sharing of knowledge is needed (Hynson and Sawyer 2001). Internationally, Acquired Immune Deficiency Syndrome (AIDS) is a major and current concern and increasingly children and young people are facing premature death and requiring palliative care services.

With many gains in the knowledge of childhood diseases and promises of cures generated by research, the move from curative to palliative care is less clear for children and adolescents. Decisions to discontinue active treatment may be difficult and complicated, and for some ill children hope for cure and active treatment may be still in existence until the last few hours of life. 'Prognostic uncertainty and continued hope for survival make the shift to palliation difficult' (De Graves and Aranda 2005, p. 132). In the United States Haut (2005, p. 232) states: 'despite the national trend towards hospice and palliative care, children with chronic and life threatening illness, continue to die in the hospital setting, often in the intensive care unit'.

For children with cancer or other acute life threatening illness, pain and symptom relief and supporting children and families through social, psychological and spiritual problems will be part of the active phase of treatment. However, when the illness is acknowledged as terminal, it may undergo a qualitative change in emphasis. For many families end of life care may be best delivered by the staff within the hospital, or from the community or outreach team with whom they have often built a strong and trusting relationship over time.

The largest group of children cared for in hospices are born with or develop long-term disorders for which the prognosis of progressive deterioration and a premature death is considered inevitable. Many have profound handicaps and complex needs. These families require support not only in the terminal phases of their children's illness but throughout their children's lifetime and sometimes beyond. Coping with their children's increasing disability, nursing requirements and the demands and stresses this creates in their everyday life and relationships can be exhausting. Such families' value respite services, and families may be in contact with and receipt of hospice services for many years. This prolonged respite service is a function of children's hospice services, which may differ to that of adult care. A report into children's hospice services in the United Kingdom for the Joseph Rowntree fund found that approximately 20 per cent of children in hospices had conditions, which were likely to lead to death in childhood. (Robinson and Jackson 1999). The majority will survive into adult life and transition to adult services is an important current consideration.

Thus the definition of palliative care for children is further elaborated on by the World Health Organisation:

Palliative care for children represents a special, albeit closely related field to adult palliative care, a definition of palliative care for children and their families is as follows; the principles apply to other paediatric chronic disorders:

- Palliative care for children is the active total care of the child's body, mind and sprit, and involves giving support to the family.
- It begins when illness is diagnosed, and continues regardless of whether or not a child receives treatment directed at the disease.
- Health providers must evaluate and alleviate a child's physical, psychological and social problems.

- Effective palliative care requires a broad multidisciplinary approach that includes the family and makes use of available community resources; it can be successfully implemented even if resources are limited.
- It can be provided in tertiary care facilities, in community health centres and even in children's homes. (World Health Organisation 2005 http://www.who.int/cancer/palliative/definition/en/).

The diagnoses of children admitted to Hospices in the United Kingdom include: children with progressive and non-progressive disorders of the central nervous system; inborn errors of metabolism; neoplastic disorders (cancers); neuromuscular disorders; and other congenital anomalies. Many families will not have a hospice within easy travelling distance and would choose anyway to care for their children at home. Hospice provision offers outreach services, which support in families in their own homes. Families using the services of the hospice for respite may still prefer their child to die at home, there are some paediatric community services which provide palliative care to children and families (Andrews and Hood 2003).

In order to support a good quality of life remaining for the child, good symptom control is vital. A key area is pain management: pain is one of the most feared and distressing symptoms, pain is also a common symptom which needs to be prioritised and treated meticulously' (Collins 2005, p. 77). A combination of pharmacological and non-pharmacological methods is used. The use of opioids is recommended, supplemented by non-opiod analgesia such as anti-inflammatory medication. Anticonvulsants and antidepressants may be prescribed as an adjunct to analgesia. Mode of administration is important; oral routes and the use of syringe drivers are preferred to intramuscular injections. According to Collins (2005 p. 77): 'the vast majority of children of children have satisfactory analgesia using conventional doses of opioids; and only a minority require massive opioid doses or invasive approaches.' The aim is to maintain adequate pain control balanced with minimal side effects and a reduced burden of treatment interventions. For children with cancer the use of radiotherapy or chemotherapy to reduce tumour mass may alleviate pain.

Other physical symptoms at the end of life include dyspnoea, fatigue, poor appetite, nausea and vomiting, constipation and diarrhoea, some or all of which may be amenable to intervention and relief.

The child may also suffer from psychological symptoms, which the family will find equally distressing to manage. Anxiety, restlessness, insomnia and depression can all be helped by appropriate medication along with a supportive presence, reassurance and alleviation of fears. The family, particularly parents, are the best people to offer this loving support. However, they themselves will require support and expert advice from the palliative care team. Children may also find reassurance from familiar figures and trusted professionals they have seen regularly.

There is an increasing awareness of the needs of brothers and sisters (De Maso et al 1997; Evan's and Kelly 1995; Faulkner et al 1995; Simms et al 2002). Siblings will also be affected by the events around them, they are aware of what is happening and they may will be filled with anxiety and sadness. They have complex needs, which may include a wish to contribute in some way to the care of their sibling, reassurance and explanation about what is happening. They need someone to listen to their concerns and deal with ambivalent feelings; jealousy, resentment, fear, love, which they may feel towards the dying child, who is the main preoccupation of their parents' life during this time, in an accepting and non-judgemental way. Children and young people also need time out to play, or be with friends, keep up with schoolwork and lead a normal life. This may be difficult for parents who are emotionally drained and physically too tired to support or understand. The palliative care team can offer support to siblings and advise parents, extended family, friends, schools and communities about the likely impact of a sibling's terminal illness. Palliative care teams often continue to keep in contact with families after the child has died, families may need some help to plan and organise the funeral. It can be very difficult for families who have worked so closely with professionals during this time to suddenly be left without their support and companionship.

The above is a brief and non-exhaustive resumé of some of the features of good palliative care. To compete this section; palliative care requires good teamwork, however, the balance between support and intrusion into families lives should be considered. Treatment interventions need to be aimed at reducing troublesome symptoms to provide a good quality of remaining life, interventions need to be effective but the treatment regimes and modalities should not become intolerable to the child and family. Professional expertise and support should be readily available on a regular and also emergency basis; symptoms may occur or worsen unpredictably, families need to know they can get support when they need it. Each individual child and family is respected and care is tailored to meet their needs as far as possible. Good communication is essential in assessment of needs, for good symptom control, to alleviate anxieties, to provide a supportive environment for the whole family and to co-ordinate care within and between agencies. Palliative care can be offered even in difficult settings, The World Health Organisation (2005) has produced guidelines for first-level facility health workers in low-resource settings with particular emphasis upon the care of people suffering from AIDS.

The needs of the palliative care team or those providing palliative care in acute or community teams should not be overlooked, care and support for each other should be a feature of any team working in such a demanding area of work.

→ Trigger 10.3: Feedback

Go to Chapter 10 Trigger feedback on p. 324

? Chapter 10 Trigger feedback: What do you know?

Trigger 10.1: Bad News

Question 1: What are the signs, symptoms and prognosis of acute lymphoblastic leukaemia?

There are many sources of information to answer the above question including text books and information for professional's, parents and children available on websites. Acute Lymphoblastic leukaemia is responsible for up to one-third of childhood cancers. Treatment is successful in up to 70 per cent of cases; in some instances a cure of 95 per cent can be expected. Even when the child is considered higher risk there is still good response to more aggressive treatment regimes (CancerBACUP 2004).

In normal health the body produces lymphocytes to protect the body from infections; in leukaemia cells do not mature properly and become too numerous in the blood and bone marrow. The normal functions of the bone marrow i.e. to produce red cells, white cells and platelets are reduced. The leukaemia cells may infiltrate the central nervous system (CNS).

Signs and symptoms are related to:

- Infiltration and replacement of normal cells.
- A lack of red blood cells leads to anaemia; the child is generally tired and lethargic and may be breathless on exercise.
- A reduction in platelets will lead to increased clotting time and the child may have bleeding from gums into the gastro-intestinal tract and bruising into the skin, petechiae.
- Low normal white cell production may lead to frequent and persistent infections; the child often has a fever without clear signs of infection.
- The child may also complain of aching bones and joints as leukaemic cells begin to invade the bone periosteum.
- With CNS infiltration the child may complain of headaches and sometimes signs of raised intracranial pressure may be present.
- The spleen and liver and lymph nodes are enlarged due to extra medullary infiltration.
- The child may have weight loss due to hypermetabolism and competition for Nutrients.

Lymphocytic leukaemia can be further classified by the type of cell involved, most commonly, in approximately 80 per cent of ALL cases the cancerous cells are precursor B-cell origin. This is associated with a good prognosis, some leukaemias originate in the differentiated beta or t cells with a much less good prognosis. There are other forms of leukaemia some chronic, which rarely affect children. Other acute forms involving non lymphocytes constitute 25 per cent of childhood leukaemia, of these acute myeloid leukaemia forms 20 per cent. The prognosis is generally less good for acute myeloid leukaemia. All children are treated as a matter of urgency with intensive chemotherapy and the majority gain a remission where almost all of the leukaemic cells have been killed, and it is hoped that with further treatment to completely eradicate the disease and achieve a cure. Children are graded as high or low risk on the results of laboratory investigations, and the speed of their initial response to treatment (Leukaemia Care 2005).

Usually treatment for ALL is two years for girls and three years for boys, providing there are no complications (CancerBACUP.org.uk; children's cancer).

Suggested Activity:

- Revise the immune system.
- Revise the formation and function of blood,

This information will considerably enhance your understanding of the disease process and affects of leukaemia.

Questions 2, 3 and 4

The answers to these questions will provide a rationale for the nursing care plan that is developed (see Table 10.2).

Table 10.2 Nursing Care Plan: Louisa Meredith

Activities of living	Actual/potential problem	Action	Rationale
Communication	Emotional distress: • Parental distress on diagnosis • Potential distress of Louisa and siblings	• Support parents and offer them contact numbers of counsellor, parent support group and social worker • Offer age-appropriate information and toys for Louisa and her siblings, involving the play specialist. • Using a family-centred care approach negotiate with the family their involvement in care.	To enhance coping capability of Louisa and her parents and siblings.

(Continued)

Table 10.2 (*Continued*)

Activities of living	Actual/potential problem	Action	Rationale
Maintaining a safe environment	1. Risk of infection	● Minimise contact from external sources of infection. Careful hand hygiene and aseptic procedures (especially when accessing venous access lines).	Louisa has a compromised immune system that increases her susceptibility to infection. Prophylactic treatment may limit the severity of any infectious diseases contracted.
	2. Bleeding	● Check urine and stools for blood ● Note bruises, nose bleeds, or bleeding from the gums ● Avoid vigorous nose blowing or teeth brushing ● Handle gently and promote rest ● May require blood or platelet transfusion	To detect any further bleeding
	3. Pain management ● Complaining of limb pains ● Investigations may cause distress and decreased tolerance for treatment regimes	● Introduce pain assessment chart to Louisa and parents. ● Regularly assess pain status. ● Administer analgesia as prescribed. ● Apply topical anaesthetic as prescribed prior to blood tests etc. ● Provide reassurance, support and age-appropriate explanation prior, during and after investigations	Pain symptoms to be alleviated as much as possible to reduce distress and the potential problems of hospitalisation and treatment, decrease fear and increase confidence of child and family. Pain may be a symptom of infection or caused by treatment. (*Continued*)

Table 10.2 (*Continued*)

Activities of living	Actual/potential problem	Action	Rationale
Temperature control	• Persistent pyrexia	• Record temperature four hourly. • Infection screen: throat swabs, urine, stools. • Chest X-Ray.	Due to reduced immunity there is a need to detect infection and provide early treatment.
Breathing	• Breathlessness • Increased pulse rate	• Record pulse and respirations four hourly.	To observe any further deterioration/ difficulty in breathing. Increased pulse rate due to anaemia.
Eating and drinking	• Poor appetite at present as a result of treatment. • Nausea, vomiting and changing taste due to treatment. • May have insufficient calorie and fluid intake to maintain normal growth, to support the immune system and repair.	• Encourage and offer small meals and treats to Louisa when she wants to eat and drink. • Fortified drinks when her appetite is poor. • Contact dietician for further advice. • Explain reasons for changes in appetite and taste to parents.	Maintain adequate calorie intake to promote normal growth and to support recovery from illness and treatment.
Elimination	1. Additional intravenous fluids to support excretion of waste products of metabolism that is due to cell breakdown induced by chemotherapy.	• Record urine output while induction treatment is in progress. • Daily urinalysis. • Check for blood in urine • Record and report any cystitis or difficulty in immediately passing urine.	To ensure that the intake and output of fluids is in balance. Early detection of complications of chemotherapy.

(*Continued*)

Table 10.2 (*Continued*)

Activities of living	Actual/potential problem	Action	Rationale
	2. Bowel irregularity; diarrhoea or constipation	● Record frequency of bowel actions. ● Stool softeners administered as appropriate.	Constipation is a side effect of opiate administration and some chemotherapy agents. Straining may cause rectal bleeding, fissures and infection. Diarrhoea also a side effect of treatment regime, and possibility of opportunistic infection.
Rest and sleep	● Tiredness due to anaemia and treatment regime. ● Aches and pains in the legs.	● Support sufficient rest. ● Establish a regular routine of naps and activity to encourage a normal sleep routine.	To provide appropriate balance between activity and rest to support recovery and prevent boredom.
Work (education) and play	Louisa may 'miss out' on education and fall behind in her expected educational attainment	● Attend Hospital School. ● Hospital School Teacher to contact Louisa's school for work for to do.	To minimise educational disadvantage due to long absence from school.
Hygiene care	● Dry sore skin. ● Risk of stomatitis. ● Rashes caused by reaction to chemotherapy. ● Increased risk of infection.	● Wash or bathe gently using hydrating products and creams afterwards. ● Check that skin creases etc. are dry. ● Note any rashes or sensitive areas. ● Use sun block if going outside. ● Assess oral cavity daily for soreness and support good oral hygiene. ● Use of soft toothbrush and mouthwashes.	Chemotheraphy causes sore mouths and dry skin in the majority of children. Therefore, avoiding, preventing problems and providing early treatment for problems that arise is important.

(*Continued*)

Table 10.2 (*Continued*)

Activities of living	Actual/potential problem	Action	Rationale
Sexuality (body image)	• Hair loss may cause distress. • Loss of appetite leading to weight loss. • Insertion of long line for administration of fluids etc. • Change of body image due to disease.	• Reassure Louisa and parents that body changes are temporary and that she will recover after the treatment is completed. • A shorter hairstyle is planned for Louisa so that her hair loss doesn't appear too dramatic. Prepare by helping her choose a wig, hat or scarf.	To support morale, prepare for bodily changes and to minimise distress. To avoid negative reactions provide information for parents, siblings and peers.
Dying	• Parents are aware that leukaemia is a form of cancer and potentially life threatening. • Parents are understandably anxious and concerned. • Mother is quite tearful at times and finds it hard to concentrate. • Father is keen to collect as much he information as can about treatment options. Louisa is aware and asking why her parents are 'upset'.	• Named nurse to arrange regular meetings with parents to provide opportunities to talk and to organise meetings with medical staff and others as necessary. • Parents will be updated regularly re progress of disease, and optimistic prognosis emphasised while acknowledging losses and difficulties diagnosis and treatment pose for parents and Louisa. • Advice offered to parents about how to answer/ give information and answer any questions Louisa may have. • Play worker and Named nurse will support parents when giving information to Louisa. • One or both parents will be present when Louise is undergoing treatment.	Prognosis in this instance is good, however parents will be fearful and aware that leukaemia is a potentially life threatening disease. Parents also have to deal with what will feel like the loss of 'normal life' and normal life expectations for their daughter. Louisa may become aware of her parents concern; being open to answering her questions and addressing her concerns may help to alleviate her worries. Minimising separation from parents will provide comfort and alleviate Louisa's fears of being left alone.

Trigger 10.2: Why me?

Questions: The trigger questions should inform this work

As a member of group of students you were asked to rehearse and offer suggestions for how you might respond using the six categories of therapeutic interventions identified by Heron (2001). Some examples of responses to Martin's request are offered below. You may have alternative and possibly more helpful suggestions within each category, it would be a worthwhile activity to practice responding to questions using different interventions in a group or with a partner, identifying which intervention is most helpful. Below are some suggested interventions within the categories you may have other, more useful ideas.

- *Prescriptive*: I think we need time to discuss this further, perhaps you would like your parents there, or would you like Sister, or the counsellor to come and talk with you?
- *Informative*: Many young people feel that God is unfair when something like this happens, the chaplain is always willing to come and talk to you, or I can contact the counsellor. I can ask Staff nurse to see you this afternoon if you want to talk it over more with her.
- *Confronting*: I've noticed you've appeared to be angry with a lot of people recently not only God, would it help to talk?
- *Cathartic*: You sound really upset and angry, you are going through a lot at the moment, it must be frightening.
- *Catalytic*: Tell me more about how you feel . . .
- *Supportive*: I think you are really brave, you have dealt with everything so well, I know all the staff your parents and friends feel the same. I'm not surprised you are feeling so bad at the moment, would you like to talk more?

You may wish to complete the learning journal entry, or write one of your own, reflecting on the situation in light of what you have learned, to identify the way forward, and how you will develop your skills to deal with similar situations which will occur throughout your nursing career.

Trigger 10.3

Question 1: What is a hospice?

A Children's Hospice service supports children and young people who are expected to die before, or shortly after, reaching adulthood. Through the provision of help at home or in a purpose built building, highly trained staff help the children and their whole family with the medical and emotional challenges that having a life-limiting or life threatening illness or condition brings, and help them to make the most of life (The Association of Children's Hospices 2005).

Sister Frances Domenica describing the innovation of hospice care for children (Glasper and Tucker 1993) writes about the first hospice for children in the United Kingdom, and probably the world which was opened in Oxford in 1982, in which she took the major role. The inspiration for the hospice arose from her involvement with Helen a very sick little girl who had undergone surgery for removal of a brain tumour; Sister Frances was, at the time, the Superior General of the Anglican order of All Saints. She offered support and a willingness to be alongside the family. Recognising that there was a physical as well as an emotional burden of care and hoping to give the family a rest she offered to care for Helen at weekends. The care provided was a close to possible to that Helen received at home, with attention paid to the details of Helen's likes and dislikes; the song she liked to have sung to her, the food she preferred and her companion cat. Respect and care for Helen as an individual and the importance of her routine being recognised meant that her family could relax and trust Helen to the care of Sister Frances. The value of this service led to the idea of offering the same support to other families and eventually fund raising to build Helen House. This led to fund raising and the building of more children's hospices. In the United Kingdom in 2003 there were 35 established children's hospice services with seven more at the project stage. These services are funded by charitable donations with approximately 5 per cent of funding from statutory sources, with a higher percentage of statutory funding in Scotland and Wales. (The Association for Children with Life-threatening or Terminal Conditions and their families (ACT) and the Royal College of Paediatrics and Child Health (RCPCH) 2003)

Question 2: What population does a children's hospice serve?

A map of Children's hospices throughout the UK can be obtained from the Association for Children's Hospices (2005) website. There is a greater concentration of children's hospices in the Midlands and South Eastern area with fewer in the north east and only one in Northern Ireland. This may reflect a greater concentration of population, or the existence of other community and hospital services which meet the needs of the local population. However, a study of the use of hospice services by families for respite care by the Joseph Rowntree Fund in 1999 discovered that one of the few complaints families had was that the hospice was not sufficiently local and involved long journeys with children and any equipment required. Another complaint was poor availability of breaks, as more established hospices become over-subscribed, often due to increased uptake of services, which are filling an unmet need, or bed occupation by established children. There has been some criticism that often hospice's are being used to fill the gap in respite services for children with long-term illness, but who do not fulfil the category because of some physical illness which excludes them from social care services. The majority of children using hospice services will survive into adult life, and the move to adult services is an important transition. The number of hospice services has increased since the research in 1998, with the criteria for entry being looser in newer hospices than established ones.

The groups of children offered or requiring hospice services has been identified (ACT and RCPCH 2003), as falling into four categories as follows:

1. Life threatening conditions for which curative treatment is feasible but may fail, palliative care may be necessary when treatment fails, e.g., malignancy, irreversible organ failure.
2. Conditions where there may be long periods of intensive treatment which may prolong and enhance life and allow participation in normal activities, but premature death still occurs. e.g., cystic fibrosis.
3. Progressive conditions where cure is not an option, but where palliative care may extend over many years, e.g., Batten's disease, mucopolysaccharidises, muscular dystrophy.
4 Non-progressive but irreversible conditions, where the child is susceptible to health complications which increases the likelihood of premature death, e.g., severe cerebral palsy, multiple disabilities following brain or spinal cord injuries.

Hospices are often affiliated with religious orders, and spiritual care is recognised as important to children and families, however, services are non-denominational and open to all irrespective of religious belief. A study of United Kingdom services (Robinson and Jackson 1998) found that only 12 per cent of the children using the service were from ethnic minority groups, the majority of these accessed one hospice.

Suggested Activity

- Explore your local children's hospice care provision,
- What is the criteria for this service?
- Who can and who does access the service?
- Who can refer?
- Does the hospice serve the needs of the whole population?
- Are there other palliative services?
- Are there any significant gaps in palliative care provision?

Question 3: How are the services of a hospice different to other services?

Hospices are usually associated with a building, but many hospices provide outreach and community services as well as residential care. There are other care teams, hospitals and community teams that provide palliative and end of life care. Why do we need a service separate or in addition to the acute care services offered to children? Some of the answers offered by a review of the literature include:

- To increase the knowledge base around appropriate care for children, medication, treatment regimes, etc.

- To provide care for families that is more relaxed and free from the pressures of acute care wards.
- To provide a service that is available on a 24 hour basis through telephone contact, and that can provide a rapid service either in the home or with admission.
- To provide parents with an environment away from home, where they can relax often with their other children and where some of the caring responsibilities can be taken on for a while by staff who know and respect their child's individual needs.
- Hospices may provide a safe place where parents can leave their sick child to gain some respite and for a while gain some semblance of normal family life for themselves and their other children.
- Hospices work in a multidisciplinary way with experienced staff on site and easily available, staff use their expertise and knowledge to provide holistic care for the child, his family including siblings and extended family.
- Holistic care is emphasized with emotional and spiritual needs taking equal priority with physical care needs.
- There is a planned response to grief and loss, which provides a positive model for families, children and staff. Capewell (1996, p. 83) writing about the planned response model states 'the need to prepare for dealing with loss and grief throughout the organisation and in relation to services offered to staff, children, their families and the wider community is understood.'
- Support continues after the child has died. Many hospices provide care and advice for siblings and other family members. This model of care has been adapted by some children's acute hospital services particularly paediatric intensive care units, and children's cancer wards where children may spend their last days.

Not all families choose hospice care for their children. Many families prefer to care for their child at home and for some families a sense of normality is important, not all families will be comfortable with the presence of other children and families with serious conditions. A hospice service ought to be one of the options available to families if they so choose.

Suggested Activity

- Explore the literature and contact your local hospice to find out how parental satisfaction with the service is identified.
- Discover what other palliative care services, and bereavement support exists with the children's hospital, secondary and primary care services.
- Contact the local hospice support group to discover how you can help raise funds or awareness of the needs of children with life threatening or life limiting illness.

Reflect on your learning

- Increasing numbers of children survive with life threatening illness, this although providing hope can lead to long-term uncertainty for children and families, and the move from active to palliative care is less clear.
- Internationally, increasing numbers of children and young people are affected by AIDS and face the prospect of early death. Knowledge and skills dissemination is essential not only to find a cure but also to relieve suffering at the end of life.
- The development needs of children need to be considered as they continue to live with life threatening illness.
- A family-centred approach, with consideration of the needs of siblings is important.
- Knowledge of appropriate palliative care regimes for children is still developing.
- Caring for children with life threatening illness is both challenging and rewarding.
- A high level of nursing knowledge and skill is required to care for a child and support families' physical, emotional and social needs.
- Excellent inter-disciplinary teamwork is essential to ensure the highest quality of care for all children and families.
- Voluntary organisations play a key role in provision of palliative care.
- Staff working with children and families in these situations need support for and between themselves.

References

Alderson, P. (1993) *Children's Consent to Surgery.* Bucks: Open University Press.

American Cancer Society (2005) *Cancer Facts and Figures 2005* http//www.cancer.org/downloads (accessed 22nd April 2005).

Andrews, F., Hood, P. (2003) Shared care: Hospital, hospice, home. *Paediatric Nursing* 15 (6), pp. 20–2.

Association for Children with Life-threatening or Terminal Conditions and their Families and The Royal College of Paediatrics and Child Health (ACT and RCPCH) (2003) *A Guide to the Development of Children's Palliative Care Services*, 2nd edn. Bristol: ACT.

Association of Children's Hospices (2005) www.childhospice.org.uk (accessed October 2005).

Blubond-Langner, M. (1978) *The Private Worlds of Dying Children.* Oxford: Princeton.

Brady, M. (1993) Symptom control in dying children, in Hill, L. (ed.) *Caring for Dying Children and Their Families.* London: Chapman Hall. Chapter 9, pp. 123–61.

Brearley, G. (1997) *Counselling Children with Special Needs*. Oxford: Blackwell Science).

British Association for Counselling and Psychotherapy (2002) *Ethical Framework for Good Practice in Counselling and Psychotherapy*. Rugby: BACP Publications.

Buckman, R. (1986) '*How to Break Bad News*', (Mississauga: University of Toronto, Medical Audio Visual Communications (video series)).

Buckman, R., Kason, Y. (1992) *How to Break Bad News – A Practical Protocol for Healthcare Professionals*. Toronto: University of Toronto Press.

Burke, G. A., Estlin, E. J., Lowis, S. P. (1999) The role of pharmacokinetic and pharmocodynamic studies in the planning of protocols for the treatment of childhood cancer. *Cancer Treatment Review* 25 (1), p. 13.

Burnard, P. (1992) *Learning Human Skills, An Experiential Guide for Nurses*. Oxford: Butterworth Heinemann.

CancerBACUP (2004) Children's Cancers, http://www.cancerbacup.org.uk/Cancertype/Childrenscancers (accessed 13 July 2004).

CancerWise (2002) Communcating with a child who has cancer. *The University of Texas MD Anderson Cancer Center*, http://www.cancerwise.org (accessed 3 February 2004).

Capewell, E. (1996) Planning an organisational response, in Lindsay, B, Elsegood, J. (eds) *Working with Children in Grief and Loss*. London: Balliere Tindall, Chapter 5, pp. 73–96.

Chesells, J. (2001) *Down's Syndrome: Blood Disorders/leukaemia Key Points*. (based on conference paper) available on web page of the Down's Syndrome Medical Interest Group www.dsmig.org.uk (accessed 29 August 2005).

Collins, J. J. (2005) Pain control options in palliative care. *American Journal of Cancer* 4 (2), pp. 77–85.

Davis, S., Blight, J. (2003) 'Communicating with families of patients in an acute hospital with advanced cancer: Problems and strategies identified by nurses. *Cancer Nursing* 26 (5), October, pp. 337–45.

De Graves, S., Aranda, S. (2005) When a child cannot be cured – reflections of health professionals. *European Journal of Cancer Care* 14 (2), pp. 132–40.

De Maso, D. R., Meyer, E. C., Beasley, P. J. (1997) What do I say to my surviving children?' *Child and Adolescent Psychiatry* 136 (9), pp. 1299–302.

Department of Health (2004) *National Service Framework, Children, Young People and Maternity Services*. London: Department of Health.

Edwards, M., Davis, H. (1997) *Counselling Children with Chronic Medical Conditions*. Leicester: BPS Books.

Erikson, E. H. (1963) *Childhood and Society*. New York: Norton.

Erikson, E. H. (1987) *Childhood and Society*, 35th anniversary edn. New York: Norton.

Evans, M., Kelly, P. (1995) Bringing support home for families of children with Cancer. *British Journal of Nursing*, 4 (7), pp. 395–8.

Faulkner, A., Peace, G., O'Keefe, C. (1995) *When a Child has Cancer*. London: Chapman and Hall.

Fallan, G., Hanks, G. (eds) (2005) *ABC of Palliative Care*. London: BMJ Publishing.

Geldard, K., Geldard, D. (2002) *Counselling Children: A Practical Guide*, 2nd edn. London: Sage.

Geldard, K., Geldard, D. (1999) *Counselling Adolescents*. London: Sage.

Gibson, F., Evans, M. (eds) (1999) *Paediatric Oncology: Acute Nursing Care*. London: Whurr.

Glasper, E. A., Tucker, A. (eds) (1993) *Advances in Child Health Nursing*. London: Scutari Press.

Haut, C. (2005) Oncological emergencies in the paediatric intensive care unit. *AACN Clinical Issues: Advanced Practice in Acute and Critical Care* 16 (2), pp. 232–45

Heron, J. (2001) *Helping the Client, A Creative Practical Guide*, 5th edn. London: Sage publications.

Hopkins, M., Pownall, J. (1999) The role of radiotheraphy in palliation, in Gibson, F., Evans, M. (eds) *Paediatric Oncology, Acute Nursing Care*. London: Whurr, Chapter 24, pp. 463–70.

Hynson, J. L., Sawyer, S. M. (2001) 'Pediatric palliative care: Distinctive needs and emerging issues', *Journal of Paediatric and Child Health*, 37 (4), pp. 323–5.

Kavanagh, R. (1994) Spiritual care, in Hill, L. (ed.) (1994) *Caring for Dying Children and Their Families*. London: Chapman Hall, Chapter 8, pp. 106–22.

Leukaemia Care (2005) http://www.leukaemiacare.org.uk (accessed 17th October 2005).

Mack, J. W., Holcombe, G. E. (2004) The day one talk. *Journal of Clinical Oncology* 22 (3), February, pp. 563–6.

Morrison, P., Burnard, P. (1989) Students' and trained nurses' perceptions of their own interpersonal skills: A report and comparison. *Journal of Advanced Nursing* 14, pp. 421–6.

Office for National Statistics (2005) National Registry for Childhood Tumours, http://www.statistics.gov.uk (accessed 14 August 2005).

Parkin, D. M., Kramarova, E., Draper, G. J., Masuyer, E., Michaelis, J., Neglia, J. (eds) (1998) *International Incidence of Childhood Cancer*, Vol. II. Lyons: IARC Scientific Publications No. 144, International Agency for Research on Cancer.

Pfund, R. (2000) Nurturing a child's spirituality. *Journal of Child Health Care* 4 (4), Winter, pp. 143–8.

Ptacek, J. T., Eberhardt, T. L. (1996) Breaking bad news, A review of the literature. *Journal of the American Medical Association* 276, pp. 496–505.

Pui, C.-H. (1997) Acute lymphoblastic leukaemia. *Pediatric Clinic North America* 44 (4) p. 831.

Rice, K. G., Herman, M. A., Peterson, A. C. (1993) Coping with challenge in adolescence; A Conceptual Model and Psycho-educational Intervention. *Journal of Adolescence* 16, pp. 235–51.

Richardson, J. (1996) 'Counselling children, in Burnard, P., Hullatt, I. (eds) *Nurses Counselling: The View from the Practitioners*, Oxford: Butterworth-Heinemann, Chapter 4, pp. 42–57.

Robinson, G., Jackson, P. (1999) *The Role of Children's Hospices in Providing Respite Care,* Joseph Rowntree Foundation. http://www.jrf.org.uk/knowledge/findings/socialcare (accessed 2 March 2005.

Rogers, C. R. (1967) *On Becoming a Person.* London: Constable.

Sharp, S., Cowie, H (1998) *Counselling and Supporting Children in Distress.* London: Sage Publications.

Simms, S., Hewitt, N., Vevers, J. (2002) Sibling support in childhood cancer. *Paediatric Nursing* 14 (7), September, pp. 20–2.

Smith, J., McSherry, W. (2004) Spirituality and child development: A concept analysis. *Journal of Advanced Nursing* 45 (3), pp. 307–15.

Thompson, S. W. (2003) When kids get cancer. *Registered Nurse* 66 (7), pp. 29–34.

Tschudin, V. (1995) *Counselling Skills for Nurses,* 4th edn. London: Balliere Tindall.

World Health Organisation (1998) *Cancer Pain, Relief and Palliative Care in Children.* Geneva: World Health Organisation.

World Health Organisation (2005) 'Palliative Care:symptom management and end-of-life care', *Integrated Management of Adolescent and Adult Illness*, http:// www.who.int/cancer/palliative/definition (accessed 25/09/2005).

Wright, B. (1999) *Sudden Death, A Research Base For Practice*, 2nd edn Edinburgh: Churchill Livingstone.

11

Long-term Care

Valerie Coleman

Learning outcomes

- Analyse the potential physical, psychological and social effects of living with a chronic illness for children, young people, parents, siblings and significant others.
- Outline the implications of the effects of chronic illness for healthcare and management by children's nurses and the multi-disciplinary team.
- Utilise a family-centred care approach to work in partnership with children or young people and their families with long-term care needs to promote optimum health.
- Discuss the need for resources and respite support for children or young people and their families with long-term care needs.
- Plan a transition protocol for vulnerable children and young people making transitions in life and healthcare.

Introduction

This chapter focuses on children/young people and their families with long-term care needs. Some of these children endure illnesses or injuries that affect them for a prolonged period of time. However, they do recover and regain their health in due course. While other children with long-term care needs have a chronic illness from which there is usually no recovery. Chronic illness is defined as being:

> Conditions that affect children for extended periods of time, often for life. These diseases can be managed to the extent that a degree of pain control or reduction in attacks, bleeding episodes or seizures can generally be achieved. However they cannot be cured (Eiser 1990, p. 3).

In the context of this chapter the main focus is on children and young people that do have a chronic illness. Nurses require the appropriate knowledge, skills and attitudes to care for these children, working in partnership with their families, and the multi-disciplinary team. Children with chronic illness are not a homogeneous group (Cooper 1999) and attempts have been made to categorise these illnesses. Bradford (1997) describes three such categories:

1. Chromosome aberrations, abnormal hereditary traits or inter-uterine factors.
2. Impact on the children, for example on their mobility, the visibility of the illness, and their cognitive and sensory functioning.
3. The severity of the illnesses with regard to such issues as the financial burden on the family and their contribution to the disruption of family life.

Cooper (1999) also states that there is diversity among children with a chronic illness in terms of, the nature of the disorder, the progression and severity of the disease and the ability of the child and family to adapt. The triggers topics in this chapter have been chosen to mirror some of this diversity, but inevitability they are small in number. However, similar to other examples that could have been included: 'They all share the need to have the technical and medical aspects of [the children and young people's] care balanced with their need and that of their families for some sort of "normal life"' (Cooper 1999, p. 1).

Therefore this chapter explores the child or young person's and family's ability to cope with the common effects of a chronic illness and at the same time to develop strategies to manage specific conditions. The three triggers facilitate learning about living with a chronic illness; resources and respite care for children/young people and their families with complex health needs/severe disabilities; and vulnerable children/young people making transitions in life and the healthcare services. It is intended that the learning of knowledge and skills in relation to these triggers may be transferred to children/young people with different chronic illnesses.

❗ Trigger 11.1: Living with a Chronic Illness

This trigger is intended to facilitate learning with regard to living with one particular chronic illness. It encourages you to develop strategies to use in partnership working with the families of children and young people with cystic fibrosis (and other chronic illnesses) to promote their optimum health.

The Trigger

Ben and his family

Ben age ten years: 'My name is Ben and I have Cystic Fibrosis. I've been in hospital 4 times in the last 6 months. It means I miss a lot of school, but that's OK because I don't like it very much anyway. Rob's a bully and I don't have many friends and the teachers always give me boring work to catch up on.

I don't mind it at home really but mum's nagging me this year about doing more and taking more responsibility round the house, like tidying my room remembering to take my drugs and spending ages doing boring physio, which takes ages and Lucy and Jo moan if I do it downstairs when we watch the telly. Nobody seems to listen to what I want!'

Ben's Mum: 'Our family have a lot to cope with what with Ben having cystic fibrosis, my husband working away from home frequently and me with three kids trying to hold a part time job. I get no time for myself.

Lucy's good now she's older but Ben's not making an effort to do more for himself like she did at his age. I know his needs are different, but he is not trying. Ben's care takes up a lot of time. He has done since he was a baby and had to have surgery for his meconium ileus. Now they want him in hospital again because his chest is bad and he's not pulling his weight like he should. It would just be the week that his dad's got the car as well.

It takes ages to get to the hospital and there's the girls to think about. Thank goodness that Lucy is old enough to baby sit now and my neighbour will sometimes get Jo from nursery for me. My mum-in-law comes over to 'help' a couple of times a week. I'm really grateful, because she gets on with Ben and does his physio well, but she's so critical. I have to bite my tongue so as not to upset her when she tries to tell me what to do. I think she blames me for Ben's illness although we've explained it enough times.'

Ben's Dad: 'I try to help with everything as much as I can, but it's difficult when I'm away from home. I try to give my wife a break from doing Ben's physio but I'm really tired when I get in. It's good to see Mum and that she can come and help, but I hate it when both her and my wife constantly want to bend my ear about what's best for Ben. Their views are so different. It's quite awkward sometimes.

I also worry about the girls sometimes, we have such divided loyalties especially when Ben's ill.'

Lucy age 14 years: 'It's difficult at home sometimes with Ben having cystic fibrosis. I really feel sorry for him because it's a horrible disease and I know some children die from it. I don't mind helping with his physio at weekends. It gives mum a break, but my mates get bored of waiting for me sometimes and he's so lazy he never does anything to help himself.

It's so difficult when he's in hospital because I have to look after Jo a lot. I can get my schoolwork done when she is in bed and I do like playing with her, it's just that she always wants my attention and sometimes really annoys me. She thinks of nobody but herself and you can't explain things to her.'

Jo aged 4 years: 'We're always at the hospital with Ben. I like the toys to play with there, there are lots. Mummy and Daddy are always talking about Ben. I cry when they don't play with me. I like giving the money to the man on the bus, he gives us tickets. I hold them.'

Grandmother: 'I do my best to help my daughter-in-law with Ben. She doesn't listen to me though! Now she's trying to get him to take responsibility for his medication and to do some of his own physio, but it's not right, he's only a child. I'm going to talk to his Dad about this. We've not had anything like this in our family before. It must be to do with her side of the family, but she says it's both.'

Ben's Nurse: 'I've known Ben and his family since Jo was born. He's been in hospital on numerous occasions but more often this year with recurrent chest infections like now. He also needs his poor weight gain investigating. So this time he'll have a thorough multi-professional assessment to determine how we can best help him and his family.

Ben quite likes being in hospital especially if some of the other children he knows are here.'

Situation

You are a third year student nurse. A junior nurse on your ward on her first clinical placement keeps asking you to explain about Ben and his family. Your mentor suggests that you do a teaching session with this student nurse about cystic fibrosis and caring for Ben and his family. This should enable you to achieve a Standard of Proficiency (Nursing and Midwifery Council 2004) with regard to teaching in the clinical area for your practice assessment.

Feedback

You are required to prepare a lesson plan for this teaching session, which you will discuss with your mentor. You will also write some detailed notes based on the questions that arise from this trigger. The content of your lesson should draw on these notes.

The facts

```
What are the main facts in this trigger? Make a list:




```

Hypotheses: What may these facts mean?

- Cystic fibrosis is an inherited condition.
- Children with cystic fibrosis can be born with meconuim ileus and may require neonatal surgery.
- Cystic fibrosis causes repeated chest infections and lack of weight gain.
- Children and young people with cystic fibrosis take medication and have regular physiotherapy.
- Children and young people with cystic fibrosis have crises and remissions.
- Children and young people with cystic fibrosis experience frequent hospitalisation and miss out on their education.
- A multi-professional team manage the care of children and young people with cystic fibrosis.
- Living with a child or young person with a chronic illness affects family life, including that of their siblings.
- Children with cystic fibrosis are expected to gradually take more responsibility for managing their own care as they get older.
- Listening to children and young people with cystic fibrosis will promote their health.
- Children and young people with cystic fibrosis may be bullied.

Questions developed from the hypotheses

1. How is cystic fibrosis inherited?
2. How is cystic fibrosis diagnosed and managed?
3. How does listening to children/young people (and their families) that are living with a chronic illness promote their health?

Trigger 11.1: Fixed resource material

Read the following to help you answer the questions. (You may also wish to search and review other up-to-date research and evidence-based literature and seek other relevant resources to provide you with the answers to your questions.)

Coyne, I. (1997) Chronic illness: The importance of support for families caring for a child with cystic fibrosis. *Journal of Clinical Nursing* 6 (2), March, pp. 121–9.

Fisher, H. (2001) 'The needs of parents with chronically sick children: A literature review. *Journal of Advanced Nursing* 36 (4), November, pp. 600–7.

Hodgkinson, R., Lester, H. (2002) Stresses and coping strategies of mothers living with a child with cystic fibrosis: Implications for nursing professionals. *Journal of Advanced Nursing* 39 (4), August, pp. 377–83.

Pillitteri, A. (1999) Child Health Nursing: Care of the Child and Family. Philadelphia: Lippincott, Chapter 19, 'Nursing care of a child with a respiratory disorder'.

Rudolph, M., Levene, M. (1999) *Paediatrics and Child Health*. Oxford: Blackwell Science, Chapter 5, 'Common symptoms and complaints of childhood.'

Sartain, S., Clarke, C., Heyman, R. (2000) Hearing the voices of children with chronic illness. *Journal of Advanced Nursing* 32 (4), October, pp. 913–21.

Smith, L., Coleman, V., Bradshaw, M. (eds) (2002) *Family Centred Care: Concept, Theory and Practice*. Basingstoke: Palgrave. Chapter 5, 'Empowerment: Rhetoric, reality and skills' and Chapter 6 'Negotiation of care'.

Useful websites

http://www.cftrust.org.uk (Cystic Fibrosis Trust)

Trigger 11.1: Fixed resource sessions

Patho-physiology of cystic fibrosis

> ### Suggested Activity
>
> Prior to reading this fixed resource session it is suggested that you 'revise' the anatomy and physiology of the following systems:
>
> - Respiratory system; and
> - Gastro-intestinal system.

The trigger provided us with some information about the patho-physiology of cystic fibrosis. Ben's mother tells us that he had surgery for meconium ileus when he was a baby. His nurse states that Ben has recurrent chest infections and that his weight gain is poor. The intention is now to explain why Ben and other children/young people have these and other problems by explaining the patho-physiology of cystic fibrosis.

There is dysfunction of the pancreas and the lungs that results in mucous having difficulty flowing through gland ducts (Pillitteri 1999). There are also electrolyte changes in the secretions of the sweat glands.

Pancreas involvement

Pancreatic cells normally produce lipase, trypsin and amylase enzyme secretions that flow into the duodenum to digest fat, protein and carbohydrate respectively. These enzyme secretions in cystic fibrosis become so tenacious that they block the ducts. The consequence of this is that there is backpressure on the acinar cells of the pancreas and eventually they become atrophied and can no longer produce these enzymes (Pillitteri 1999). The ducts become obstructed and fibrosis develops. The disease does not influence the islets of Langerhans and insulin production initially because they have endocrine activity (ductless glands) (Pillitteri 1999), although later complications may occur because of increasing pancreatic disease causing deficient insulin production

Due to the absence of pancreatic enzymes in the duodenum, fat, proteins and some sugars are not digested by children with cystic fibrosis. The children may have steatorrhea, which is when the faeces are large, bulky and greasy. The faeces also have a foul odour due to an increase in intestinal flora caused by undigested food combining with the fat in the faeces. Children may also have a protuberant abdomen, due to the bulk of faeces in the intestine. Children will only benefit from about 50 per cent of the food that they ingest and therefore they show signs of malnutrition that is emaciated extremities and loose flabby folds of skin on their buttocks. Fat soluble vitamins, particularly A, D and E cannot be absorbed because fat is not absorbed, so children develop low levels of these vitamins. Therefore, these children may fail to thrive. Weight gain may be poor, which is the situation with ten year old Ben.

The meconium in a newborn infant is normally thick and tenacious. However in 10 per cent of children with cystic fibrosis the meconium is excessively thick because of the lack of pancreatic enzymes. It can cause an obstruction of the bowel (Rudolf and Levene 1999) that may require surgery to relieve it. The newborn infant with meconium ileus develops abdominal distension and does not pass faeces. This happened to Ben. A prolapsed rectum from straining to pass hard stools is another common finding in infants that have cystic fibrosis.

Lung involvement

Thick mucus secretions will obstruct the small airways in the lungs of the child with cystic fibrosis and this predisposes towards infection (Rudolf and Levene 1999). This is the reason for Ben's recurrent chest infections. The organisms most frequently cultured from the sputum of children with cystic fibrosis are:

- Staphyloccocus aureus
- Pseudomonas aeruginosa
- Haemophilus influenzae

Secondary emphysema (overinflated alveoli) and also pneumonia may occur in children with cystic fibrosis. This is because the air cannot be pushed past the thick mucus on expiration, when the bronchi are narrower than they are on inspiration (Pillitteri 1999), Children's chests may become distended and barrel shaped in the antero-posterior diameter.

Children with cystic fibrosis may also develop clubbed fingers due to inadequate peripheral tissue perfusion (Pillitteri 1999).

Sweat gland involvement

The electrolyte composition of sweat changes. The level of chloride to sodium is increased two to five times above normal (Pillitteri 1999). The children may actually taste of salt if they are kissed.

Prognosis

The average life expectancy for those with cystic fibrosis is now 30–40 years. With good treatment most children are able to lead relatively normal lives in childhood, although some infants who have severe lung disease may die early. In later childhood growth may slow down and puberty is delayed.

Chronic deteriorating lung disease becomes disabling in adulthood. The lung transplantation success rates for patients with cystic fibrosis are encouraging with a 70 per cent survival rate one or two years after transplantation and the longest surviving patients had their surgery 12 years ago (Cystic Fibrosis Trust 2004). Heart-lung transplantations have been carried out for some children with cystic fibrosis and techniques have improved considerably, with the success rate for all patients being reported as approximately 85 per cent at one year after surgery (British Heart Foundation 2005).

Cystic fibrosis may affect other body systems:

- Diabetes may develop in adolescence due to increasing pancreatic disease causing deficient insulin production.
- Biliary atresia due to the blockage of small ducts in the liver.
- Male infertility due to blockage of tubes that carry sperm.
- Irregular menstrual cycles in underweight females.
- Osteoporosis due to nutritional problems and also the adverse effects of steroids taken to control inflammation in the airways.

Madge (2002) stresses that it is essential that the paediatric cystic fibrosis nurse [and other nurses] are aware of these complications. This is because many of the complications can be identified in childhood and early treatment has the potential to reduce further difficulties in later life.

The Negotiated-Empowerment Framework

The Negotiated-Empowerment Framework (Coleman et al 2003) provides a toolkit of skills (Figure 11.1) that will be helpful in the management of care for children like Ben and their families. Successful negotiation and empowering strategies can be incorporated into everyday practice using a systematic approach to care and support children/young people and families living with a chronic illness.

Overlaying a negotiation approach on to an empowerment framework links the two concepts together hence the Negotiated-Empowerment Framework (Figure11.1) that has the following stages to promote new skill acquisition and partnership working.

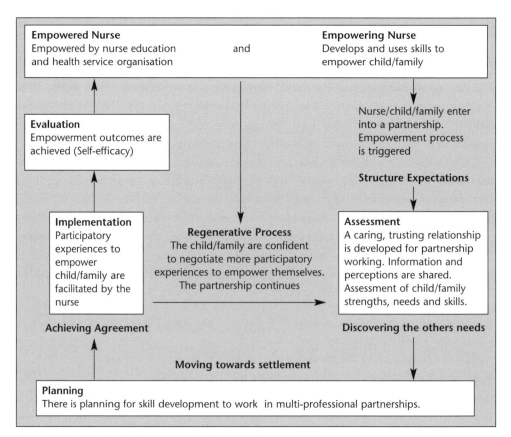

Figure 11.1 Negotiation-Empowerment Framework

Entry stage: Structuring expectations

At this stage on initial diagnosis, or later in the course of living with a chronic illness, a family may recognise that their situation has changed, which engenders feelings of disempowerment and an awareness of the need for new skill acquisition. On the other hand another family may not demonstrate any awareness that their situation has changed and that they need to develop new skills. The nurse will then use his/her communication skills to ask open-ended questions to create a family awareness of the need to develop new skills to cope and care for their child in the long term, working in partnership with the multi-disciplinary team (Coleman 2002).

Structuring of expectations is a requisite of this stage to identify boundaries and minimise the gaps between the hopes of both parties (Smith 2002). This will provide the family with some idea about the potential for involvement; the nurse might for example use some guidelines or a philosophy. This reduces the potential for misunderstanding as everyone is clear about what is on offer and the process of negotiation rather than assumptions being made.

Assessment

During the assessment stage there is a 'discovering of the other's needs' in negotiation terms (Smith 2002). The focus here is what do they (the child/young person and family) want from the negotiation rather than what I (the nurse or other healthcare professional) want. In empowerment terms, the nurse will be assessing the family's strengths as opposed to weaknesses in order to help them develop existing competencies and skills for partnership working to meet their needs (Coleman 2002). It is essential that a caring, valuing, respectful and trusting relationship be built up at this stage between the nurse and family (or other professionals and the family) for this communication to happen. There is a two-way sharing of information to help this relationship building, which according to McWilliam et al (1997) results in nurses and families mutually knowing about each other to enhance partnership working. The nurse will listen, ask open-ended questions and paraphrase to check understanding. This facilitates the family critically reflecting on their new situation leading to an assessment of their needs, competencies and skills.

Planning

This, to use negotiation speak, is the moving towards settlement stage. Both parties need to be empowered to make decisions. They need to understand what is on offer and to avoid pitfalls, through open and honest communication, identifying any points that are not acceptable. It is important to record the points agreed, as this will facilitate care between the nurse, child/young person and family as the nursing shift changes (Smith 2002). The achievement of short-term goals is more likely to promote the self-confidence, self-efficacy beliefs and self-esteem necessary for empowerment than long-term goals (Coleman 2002). The nurse and family plan short-term goals to develop existing and new skills for caring for the child/young person and working in partner-ship with multi-disciplinary team members.

Implementation

Achieving agreement leads in nursing practice to the production of the care plan (Smith 2002). Consideration needs to be made of how negotiated care is documented, by whom, when, verbally or in writing. This may depend on local policy and the individual wishes of the child/young person or parents. It is important that the agreements are summarised so that both parties understand and that there are no loose ends. Responsibility and accountability for delegated care needs to be considered and there-fore facilitating the teaching of skills required by those undertaking some aspects of negotiated care needs is an important aspect of this process. The nurse then acts as a teacher, mentor, supporter and role model to facilitate participatory experiences (psycho-social and physical) during the implementation stage (Coleman 2002). This is to help the child/young person and family to develop their communication skills so that they are empowered to participate in care, and the multiple partnerships that have become part of their lives due to the chronic illness. These skills include those for having their voices heard, assertiveness, decision-making and advocacy, in addition to physical 'nursing' care skills.

Evaluation

It is not possible to know how things will work out, so it is important, in negotiation terms, that a review of the agreement takes place. If it does not work change it. This gives both parties confidence in the process and may support different levels of involvement if families know that it is not a continued expectation or that they may try other aspects of care later as they wish (Smith 2002). The evaluation stage is about measuring the empowerment outcomes that have been achieved or not with regard to the goals that have been set at the planning stage (Coleman 2002). An outcome of empowerment is reached if the child/young person and family are able to confidently use their newly developed skills for care and to participate in some partnership working. Empowerment is a regenerative process and with confidence and belief in self being able to do, the child/young person and family are more likely to re-enter the process to negotiate and develop further skills to empower themselves for care and partnership working (Coleman 2002).

Listening to children and young people (and their families) that are living with a chronic illness

Ben and his family all have perspectives on living with a chronic illness. It is important that nurses and other members of the multi-disciplinary team listen to these perspec-tives because we need to be aware that:

Living with long term conditions for the individuals concerned and their families can often mean physical, psychological difficulties, socio-economic problems, reduced quality of life and sometimes social exclusion. (Department of Health 2001, p. 5)

Contemporary policy and literature supports the need to listen not only to the adult members of the family, but also to children and young people. The *National Service Framework for Children, Young People and Maternity Services* states that: 'Particular efforts are made to ensure that children and young people who are often excluded are actively encouraged and supported to give their views' (Department of Health 2004, p. 15).

The Department of Health (2004) emphasises that high quality services for children and young people are to be co-ordinated around their individual and family needs and take account of their views. Child-centred care, which is central to the *National Service Framework* (Department of Health 2004) seems to encompass many of the principles of family-centred care. Whatever the terminology used it is important to listen to children/young people to enable them to participate in their own care and management at an appropriate developmental level. Listening by nurses and other members of the multi-disciplinary team has the potential to promote optimum health for children/young people and their families living with a chronic illness. The health care team may use the Negotiated-Empowerment Framework (Coleman et al 2003) at each stage of the nursing process to facilitate listening as care is negotiated and planned with children, young people and families, to empower them to live with a chronic illness.

When using the Practice Continuum Tool (Smith et al 2002) that is explained in Chapter 3, individual family members are likely to be in different positions on the continuum at the same time ranging from non-involvement to parent-led care. It may be assumed that care for families living with a chronic illness will always be parent-led (with increasing responsibility being taken on by the child/young person) and most of the time it is likely to be the case. However, it is important to listen to the child/young person and family to make accurate assessments of their current position on the continuum because their situation may alter. This is due to the child/young person either being in crisis or in remission. It may also be because new nursing and/or medical care is being implemented and the family need to develop new physical, and psycho-social skills to empower them to care, and to remain in control of their lives.

For a child/young person it would seem reasonable to associate their position on the continuum with both their experiences of the illness and their developmental age and maturity. Hence nurses and other health care professionals should listen to children/young people and use strategies to enable them to participate in their own care and to move along the continuum towards 'child-led care'. This is especially important as children move into their adolescent years, as 10 year old Ben will soon be doing. However child-centred care seems to be about adults doing things in the child's best interest and protecting them as opposed to listening to them and assisting them to develop competency and autonomy. Ben's mother seems to be aware that he should be taking on more responsibility for his own care, but it is not obvious that Ben is being listened to and helped to develop more independence.

The United Nations Convention on the Rights of the Child (United Nations 1989) and The Children Act (Department of Health 1989) both stressed the importance of listening to children and taking their views seriously (Lowden 2002). However, despite this, the interpretation of children's rights has continued to be influenced by adult perceptions of childhood with regard to what is in the child's best interests and their level of competency to participate. Therefore, the importance of listening to children and their views has not always been a reality in practice. Adults should listen to the views of children like 10 year old Ben old with cystic fibrosis. You will recall that he expressed that 'no-one ever listens to me.'

One of the barriers to listening to children/young people is the meaning given to the concept of childhood rights by adults. The National Children's Bureau (1992) outlines three main approaches to children's rights:

1. *The protectionist approach*: which reflects the view that children should be protected from themselves for their own good (Fulton 1996) and, therefore, it assumes that children, particularly young ones are too incompetent to consent to treatment (Lowden 2002). It effectively marginalizes and objectifies children according to Fulton (1996) and acknowledges their parents as the consumers of health care. This is not likely to promote the child's health especially as they approach adolescence and require developmental opportunities to make the transition into adulthood.

2. *The liberationist approach*: takes a completely opposite view point, believing children to be an oppressed minority group that are deprived of their civil rights. Fulton (1996) states that children will believe these views about themselves and the lack of recognition they receive, including being listened to, becomes a self-fulfilling prophecy with them feeling repressed and subservient in the health service to adult family members. Liberationists consider that children should be empowered by not treating them as children (Lowden 2002). Empowering children like Ben should in theory promote their health, because the concept of empowerment is a central tenet of health promotion (World Health Organisation 1998). However, there has been criticism of this approach as it fails to recognise that developing children do require some degree of protection, although some younger children with a chronic illness will show mature understanding compared with their peers because of personal experiences (Lowden 2002).

3. *The pragmatist approach*: is a balance between the other two approaches recognising that although the child needs protection there should be allowance for the

child's emerging knowledge (Fulton, 1996). This is a more positive approach that values children for who they are and this is a characteristic of an empowering approach so consequently its use in practice should promote child health.

The literature also suggests that there is a lack of clarity in practice about what it means to consult and listen to children. Alderson and Montgomery (1996) identify that children may be consulted at four levels:

1. Being informed;
2. Expressing a view;
3. Influencing the decision-making; and
4. Being the main decider.

Flatman (2002) suggests that healthcare professionals sometimes assume that participation by a child only takes place at the fourth level of being the main decider and they conclude that it is too risky for this to happen. Therefore, the child is kept as a passive recipient of care. However, the other three levels are also methods of participation that should precede the fourth level (Flatman 2002). In other words the developing child should be helped by the nurse and others to acquire the necessary skills to enable them to gradually move up the levels to eventually be the main decider, perhaps in the same way as they can be helped to move along the Practice Continuum Tool (Smith et al 2002).

Sartain et al (2000) assert that children with a chronic illness who have continued contact with health services throughout childhood must be listened to. This view was supported by their research study about hearing the voices of children with chronic illness. The results of this study using semi-structured interviews and drawing techniques provided evidence that children can competently communicate their experiences of ill health and health care. It was found that the children with cystic fibrosis that were included in the study enjoyed the company of others in hospital who also needed intravenous antibiotics like themselves. These children also liked being in hospital because home was boring and it was lonely receiving care from their parents.

Research and data collection with children is, therefore, effective and it gives them a voice (Miller 2000; Sartain et al 2000). This is important because young people are experts regarding their own health and we need to listen to them (Smithies 1998). Health care professionals also need to respond to the children's views to enable them to become empowered to take some control of their chronic illness to achieve optimum health.

Flatman (2002) provides some guidelines for consulting with children/young people in relation to the planning of local services. It is suggested that these guidelines are also applicable to consulting with and listening to an individual child like 10 year old Ben:

- Use age-appropriate communication and methods. This may include play.
- Check comprehension using verbal and non-verbal cues.

- Motivate the child to speak by conveying that you value their viewpoint and want to hear from them.
- Represent the child's views accurately in planning their care.
- Maintain confidentiality.
- Appreciate parental concerns and keep them informed about the consultation with their child.

Children and young people are central to family-centred care and as such contemporary literature is advocating that they should be active participants in this care at the appropriate developmental level. The motivation and communication skills of the health care professionals involved and their beliefs about children's rights are essential for moving from a protectionist approach to children's rights (Fulton 1996) to a pragmatic approach that will ensure that children are listened to. It is evident that all members of Ben's family have a viewpoint that needs listening to and responding to, including Ben. Listening to the child/young person in the context of the family is likely to promote their health because of it's potential to contribute to empowering the family unit as a whole. Empowerment enables individuals to take control over factors that affect their lives (Gibson 1991). This is health promoting and can be deemed as crucial to a child/young person and family living with a chronic illness.

➡ Trigger 11.1: Feedback

Go to Chapter 11 Trigger feedback on p. 376

❗ Trigger 11.2: Resources and Support for children/young people and their families with complex health needs/severe disabilities

This trigger is intended to create an awareness of the current resources and support available for children/young people and their families with complex health needs/severe disabilities (especially respite services).

The Trigger

Extracts from a local newspaper report

Child 1 is an 11 year old girl who has severe disabilities. She is immobile and has frequent fits that may last as long as 20 minutes. Her mother has to give her anticonvulsant drugs to stop her fitting. This 11 year old is living at home with her parents and siblings. The family are waiting for news from the council to see whether the child has been given a place in a residential special school, which would provide some respite for them.

Mother of Child 1: 'I wouldn't wish a child with disability on my worse enemy. Nothing can prepare you for how much you have to fight. It's a long and lonely journey.'

Child 2: is an 8 year old girl who is disabled and has fits at least once a day. This child is mobile though and is able to feed herself although she makes a 'mess'. The child has just been provided with one overnight stay per month with foster parents to give her mother some respite, but this means that some of the other care that she should be getting will be reduced. However, the mother is not getting all the care that has been agreed to.

Mother of Child 2: 'They've cut down what I'm not getting. I don't see how they can reduce 10 hours [care] a month when I'm not getting that much.'

Concluding comments in the report: Disabled children in Britain appear to be invisible in government statistics, so its not surprising that there is not adequate respite care provision for these disabled children and their families.

Situation

There has been a great deal of adverse publicity in the local media recently with regard to parent's complaints (like those in the trigger) about the lack of resources and support for their children/young people with complex health needs/severe disabilities especially for respite care. The health authority has responded by setting up a working group to prove or disprove these complaints.

You are the nurse representative in the group. The remit of the working group is to evaluate the current provision for these children/young people and families. You need to:

- Find out what resources are available *in your locality* to support these children/young people and families, especially for respite care.
- Critically analyse the strengths and weaknesses of the current provision by health, social and education services and also voluntary organisations considering relevant bio – psycho-social, spiritual and ethical perspectives.

Feedback

You have to prepare a briefing paper for the next working group meeting with the key points identified as bullet points for discussion.

(The findings of the working group will be used in the report that the health authority will write to address the family's complaints.)

The facts

> **What are the main facts in this trigger? Make a list:**

Hypotheses: What may these facts mean?

- Media reports are not always accurate.
- The government and local authorities support for families with children with disabilities is poor.
- Families who are very unhappy and frustrated with their situation have to fight for services.
- It takes a long time for decisions to be made by social services.
- Parents are not informed about progress with decision-making.
- Families are left alone to care for children with disabilities.
- Parents are expected to give medical care.
- Emotional strain put on families adds to suffering.
- Governments do not prioritise the needs of the families with a disabled child or young person.
- Reduction in funding leads to reduction in services.

Question developed from the hypotheses

1. What respite provision is there for families of children and young people with profound disability in your locality from the following:

- Health services;
- Social services;
- Education services; and
- Voluntary organisations?

(The extent of your investigation to find out about respite provision in your locality will depend upon your previous knowledge and experiences.)

Trigger 11.2: Trigger resource material

Read the following to help you answer the questions. (You may also wish to search and review other up-to-date research and evidence-based literature and seek other relevant resources to provide you with the answers to your questions.)

Ford, K., Turner, D. (2001) Stories seldom told: Paediatric nurses' experiences of caring for hospitalised children with special needs and their families. *Journal of Advanced Nursing* 33 (3), February, pp. 288–95.

Hall, S. (1996) An exploration of parental perception of the nature and level of support needed to care for their child with special needs. *Journal of Advanced Nursing* 24 (3), September, pp. 512–21.

Olsen, R., Maslin-Prothero, P. (2001) Dilemmas in the provision of own-home respite support for parents of young children with complex health needs: Evidence from an evaluation. *Journal of Advanced Nursing* 34 (5), June, pp. 603–10.

Watson, D., Townsley, T., Abbott, D. (2002) Exploring multi-agency working in services to disabled children with complex healthcare needs and their families. *Journal of Clinical Nursing* 11 (3), May, pp. 367–75.

Useful websites

http://www.cafamily.org.uk (Contact a Family: for families with disabled children)

http://www.dfes.gov.uk/qualityprotects (Department of Education and Skills, Quality Protects)

http://www.dh.gov.uk (National Service Framework Children and Young People)

http://www.drc.org.uk (The Disability Rights Commission)

http://www.jrf.org.uk (Joseph Rowntree Foundation)

http://www.ncb.org.uk (National Children's Bureau)

http://www.scotland.gov.uk (Making it work for Scotland's Children)

Trigger 11.2: Fixed resource sessions

Cerebral palsy: Resources and support for long-term care

The children identified in this trigger have cerebral palsy, a disorder of movement and posture, caused by an early and non-progressive cerebral lesion (Rudolph and Levene 1999). It occurs in approximately 1 in 400 births and has multiple and complex causes (Contact a Family 2005). Rudolph and Levene (1999) state that the underlying brain lesion is the result of it being subject to different insults on various occasions as it develops in the prenatal, perinatal and post-natal (before 2 years old) periods. The causes can include infection, difficult or premature birth, cerebral bleeds, infection or accident in early life or abnormal brain development.

Cerebral palsy may be suspected in neonates who have difficulty sucking, are irritable, experiencing convulsions or have abnormal neurological examinations. However, because most of these neonates develop normally, diagnosis is usually not made until later in the first year of life based on the history and clinical presentation of abnormal movement and posture. Further investigations are not always necessary, however computed tomography (CT) or magnetic resonance imaging (MRI) scans may be useful to demonstrate cerebral malformations, delineating the extent of structural lesions and ruling out tumours (Rudolph and Levene 1999).

Cerebral palsy affects children in various different ways, which influences the amount of support and resources that are required for individual children and their families. The disorder is hardly noticeable in some, while others are more severely affected, like the two children in the trigger. The condition may be conveniently categorised into three main types with many children actually having a combination of all of them. Rudolph and Levene (1999) describe the categories:

Spastic cerebral palsy

This is the result of damage to the cerebral motor cortex or its connections. It is the commonest type of cerebral palsy and causes muscles to be stiff and tight. It is classified according to the extremities affected:

- Spastic hemiplegia paresis only affects one side of the body. Most commonly the arm is more involved than the leg. Decreased spontaneous movements are seen on the affected side during infancy and subsequently walking is usually delayed until 18–24 months. When the child does commence walking there is a characteristic gait with him/her often walking on tiptoes because of increased tone. The affected arm is held in a dystonic posture during running.
- Spastic diplegia predominantly involves both legs and the arms are less affected. The condition is likely to become apparent when the infant starts to crawl. Also there is excessive adduction of the hips with the parents perhaps experiencing difficulties

when putting on a nappy. Walking is delayed and it is characterised by the feet being held in the equinovarus position (plantar-flexion of the ankle and the forefoot is adducted and inverted) and the child walking on tiptoes.

- Spastic quadriplegia is the most severe type of cerebral palsy. This is because of marked motor impairment of all extremities. There is a high association with severe learning disabilities and fits. Other common problems are swallowing difficulties and gastro-oesophageal reflux that often lead to aspiration pneumonia, also microcephaly, flexion contractures of the knees and elbows and associated disabilities especially speech and visual problems.

Athetoid or dyskinectic cerebral palsy

The child displays involuntary movements and there is a change of tone in muscles from floppy to tense.

Ataxix cerebral palsy

The child is likely to be unsteady and have uncoordinated shaky movements and irregular speech

Resources and support

A multi-disciplinary assessment and management approach is integral to the long-term care of children/young people with cerebral palsy and their families. Rudolph and Levene (1999) state that this approach is best provided by a child development team to facilitate good liaison between parents and professionals, and to develop a structured co-ordinated programme to meet all the child's needs.

The team will regularly review the child/young person and family to ensure that their needs are being met and that appropriate resources and support is provided. Team members may include paediatricians, children's nurses, community children's nurses, school nurses, health visitor, physiotherapist, occupational therapist, social worker, educational psychologist, play leader, dietician and teacher thus testifying to the extent of human resources required for long-term care of children with cerebral palsy.

The following resources and support are needed to promote optimum health of the child/young person and family with cerebral palsy:

1. To minimize the effects of spasticity and contractures:

   - A physiotherapist advises on handling and mobilisation to limit the effects of abnormal muscle tone and performs a series of exercises intended to prevent the development of contractures. The physiotherapist may also initiate the provision of boots, splints and walking frames for the child. The family will be taught by the physiotherapist how to do the exercises and to handle the child during activities such as feeding, dressing, carrying and bathing.

- An occupational therapist complements the input of the physiotherapist and advises on special equipment such as wheelchairs and seating. Also the occupational therapist will advocate play activities and materials that will encourage the child's hand function.
- Orthopaedic surgery may be required to correct deformities such as dislocation of hips, and deformity of the ankle that develop as a result of long standing muscle weakness or spasticity. The child is likely to be immobilised in plaster following surgery and to require appropriate nursing care post-operatively.

2. To provide the child/young person with appropriate support for their special educational needs:

- Mainstream school provision is required for children with milder forms of cerebral palsy who will cope providing that minor learning difficulties and issues with physical access are addressed.
- Special schooling either in a school for children with physical or severe learning difficulties is required by other children with more severe cerebral palsy.

3. To manage associated problems: It is common for children with cerebral palsy, especially those with spastic quadriplegia, to have some associated problems that require additional resources and support, namely:

- Learning difficulties;
- Epilepsy;
- Visual impairment e.g., Squint;
- Hearing loss;
- Speech disorders;
- Behavioural disorders;
- Feeding difficulties;
- Under nutrition and poor growth; and
- Respiratory problems.

The two children with cerebral palsy identified in this trigger both had 'fits'. Epilepsy is often associated with cerebral palsy and may require anticonvulsant drugs to control the fits.

4. To promote adequate financial support for the family: There is often increased expenditure for the families of children with cerebral palsy due to travelling costs, special equipment, the need for extra clothes due to incontinence, feeding difficulties and mothers often have to give up work (Ross and Parkes 2004). The families are likely to be entitled to disability benefits. Community Children's Nurses now need to be familiar with disability benefits so that they can advice families how to initiate an application, which is a role that has traditionally been seen as the remit of social workers (Ross and Parkes 2004).

5. To promote practical support for the family: It is essential that children/young people with cerebral palsy and their families have access to practical support particularly respite care. Ross and Parkes (2004) state that knowledge regarding statutory, voluntary and charitable organisations, support groups and sources of grants is essential. However it seems that it is often difficult for parents to access respite services.

6. To promote emotional support for the family: Ross and Parkes (2004) argue that it is not acceptable to expect parents to demonstrate technical competency in care without providing them with the appropriate psychological support to do this in the home environment. Emotional support for the family may be provided by community children's nurses and school nurses, who should also assess the psychological 'readiness' and coping abilities of families with regard to them undertaking complex skilled nursing tasks at home (Ross and Parkes 2004).

Respite care

Respite care is the shared care of a person with difficulties and/or disabilities either at home or in a residential setting in order to give the family a break from ongoing care (Treneman et al 1997). All parents need respite or a break from their children and families and friends are usually prepared to help out. However, this help is not always so easy to obtain for the parents of children with severe disabilities/complex health needs. Parents of these children may also be reluctant to ask for respite care from professionals because they feel it will be viewed as an admission that they cannot cope (Miller 2002).

Respite care is essential in care packages. Olsen and Maslin-Prothero (2001) assert that respite care is an integral part of maintaining the well-being of the whole family including parents, siblings and the child with severe disabilities/complex health needs. It is important that respite care meets the needs of the child/young person as well as giving the parents/carers a break. To gain from a period of respite care for their child, the parents need to feel confident in the respite provision to enable them to gain from the break; to give them time to recover both physical and emotional strength; and also to spend time with each other and siblings. On the other hand accordingly to the Children Act 1989 the child with severe disabilities/complex health needs should have respite care that provides additional opportunities for the child with 'special needs' to meet his/her developmental and social needs (Department of Health 1989). Respite care, therefore, should be a positive experience for both child and family (Miller 2002).

Miller (2002) identifies three types of available respite care, stating that different types of respite care are likely to meet the needs of different families:

1. Institutional respite care in hospital, a residential care unit or a hospice (see Chapter 10).

2. Shared care/link family, which involves formal arrangements being made for the child to stay with another family for respite care. The aim being to develop long-term relationships between families.
3. Home-based respites with care being provided by a limited number of carers in the family home.

The value of the different provision has to be considered in the context of individual families to some extent because what suits one family may not suit another Therefore, it is suggested that you reflect on your personal experiences of respite care especially in the community (hospital provision will be explored in the next fixed resource session) to identify the advantages and disadvantages of the different types of respite care.

It is evident that despite the potential diversity of respite care that there are insufficient resources to meet the needs of families in many areas (Muir and Dryden 2000). There is recognition of this shortfall, for example Quality Protects, a government plan in 1999, identified a need to transform children's services in England including improving respite provision (Department of Health 1999). An initiative by a nursing team in Leeds has been the development of a dependency scoring tool to help match the respite 'needs of children and their families with appropriate provision in the context of finite resources' (Escolme and James 2004, p. 30).

Respite care provision is now increasingly dependent on health service support as part of an integrated children's service (Muir and Dryden 2000), while in the past it may have been considered to be solely the domain of social services. The National Health Service Executive (1998) recommended that nurses should co-ordinate respite care for children with complex health needs. Therefore, children's nurses need to be well informed about respite provision so hence the work you need to do for this trigger in respect of finding out about respite support in your locality for families of children/young people with profound disability from health, social, education services and voluntary groups.

Respite Care in the hospital setting

The intention of this fixed resource session is to first suggest that you reflect on your own experiences of the provision of respite care in the hospital environment, identifying the advantages and disadvantages. This reflection will then be followed by the sharing of good practice from your own experience and the literature in respect of respite care provision in hospital. Respite care in hospital is not an uncommon provision still, despite the emphasis on care of children in the community, and it is important that children's nurses provide quality respite care to meet the needs of both the child and family.

It is likely that you will have identified advantages and disadvantages that are similar to the following.

Advantages

Morris (1998) found that some families value hospital respite provision because they felt that the carers in this setting are most likely to have the skills to meet their children's needs. It is possible that the child/young person and family develop a trusting relationship with the hospital staff due to frequent admissions, which is another reason why they may favour hospital respite care. Hospital respite care may also act as a bit of a safety net for families in the absence of alternative sources of respite care being available, particularly in emergency situations. Olsen and Maslin-Prothero (2001) found in their study that several parents talked about the need for a more responsive and immediate type of respite service, because a system of pre-booked respite did not meet their needs in a crisis. This results in families using the hospital for respite care.

Disadvantages

These seem to outweigh the advantages with hospital respite care being considered inappropriate (Olsen and Maslin-Prothero 2001). Hall (1996) argues that the use of acute beds for respite care is an inappropriate use of hospital facilities. You may agree with this from your own experiences with regard to issues like the difficulties in prioritising and meeting the needs of children admitted for respite care in addition to other children with acute physical care needs. Inevitably the needs of children with acute physical care needs are likely to take precedence over those in for respite care. Yet respite care should benefit the child/young person with severe disabilities/complex health needs providing opportunities to meet their developmental and social needs (Department of Health 1989)

Respite care is also about providing the parents, siblings and other significant family members with a break, but hospital respite care may militate against this happening. Parents may feel guilty about leaving their child alone on a busy acute children's ward and continue to visit. It is also possible that parents may feel pressurised to stay and care for their child by nursing staff.

An advantage was the family knowing the staff well, but on the other hand there will be changes in staff and transient staff such as student nurses on placements for them to re-adjust to.

Good practice – Strategies for effective respite care in hospital

- Recognise that admission to hospital may be a real crisis point for the family (Warner 2000).
- Work in partnership with the family and share information.
- Acknowledge the parents as the 'expert' on their child and listen to them.
- Appreciate that parents may seem to be overprotective and that this is a not an unusual outcome of having a disabled child.
- Nurses should focus on what the child/young person can do rather than what they

cannot do to ensure that their developmental needs are met during respite care (Warner 2000).

- Maintain normal home routine providing care as the parents would do at home so that it is still parent-led care (Smith et al 2002).
- Use databases to avoid having to ask for the same information every time the child/young person is admitted to hospital.
- Named nurse/key worker to co-ordinate and provide continuity of care.
- Appropriate liaison and input by the multi-disciplinary team: physiotherapist, occupational therapist, play therapist, speech and language therapist to be continued.
- Provision of appropriate specialist equipment.
- Identify how the child/young person communicates.

This list is not exhaustive and it is likely that you will be able to add to it from your personal experiences.

It is important that nurses recognise that respite care is vital in the provision of temporary relief for all family members from the continuous demands of caring for a child/young person with special needs, even if it is happening in the unsuitable environment of a hospital (Warner 2000).

➡ Trigger 11.2: Feedback

Go to Chapter 11 Trigger feedback on p. 376

❗ Trigger 11.3: Vulnerable young people making transitions in life and health care

This trigger is intended to enable you to prepare young people to make transitions in life and from child to adult health services. It highlights that young people with many different long-term care needs (physical, mental and social) make these transitions. Young people, like Becky below, are often vulnerable.

The Trigger

Becky age 15 years has Type 1 (Insulin Dependent) diabetes mellitus. She is in her GCSE year at school. Below are extracts from her diary.

Monday 12th

'What a day, everything's awful again. Why doesn't it ever go right? I'm really *fed up* now with having diabetes. It is getting in the way of me having a good time with my friends, because I always have to think about what I'm eating and not forget my insulin. Mum and Dad are always on at me about it. It makes me feel different from my friends. I've been in hospital more recently due to my diabetes being unstable because I have not been 'complying with my treatment' as Sue the Paediatric diabetes nurse specialist says. I've missed quite a few days at school because of being in hospital. Becoming a bit anxious about this because of my GCSE's later this year, I do want to go to university eventually that will be great, although I'm a bit worried about managing my diabetes away from home! The lessons in hospital are not the same.

Saturday 17th

I'm back in hospital on the children's ward and Jill is on duty. She's been talking to me about, her daughter doing her GCSE's, she's at university now. Sue the diabetes nurse calls to see me and we talk again about me having to make the change to adult health services when I'm 17 and going to some different clinics to prepare for this change–transition clinics she calls them. I don't always like being on the children's ward especially with a lot of crying babies, but I'm not so sure about moving to adults yet and neither is my mum. I've known Sue and Jill ever since I was little and first knew I had diabetes–I'll miss them.

Situation

Becky's nurse (Jill) and the paediatric diabetes nurse specialist (Sue) are co-opted onto a working group in the children's hospital National Health Service Trust that is developing a transition protocol. This Trust encompasses acute in-patient services for children with physical health problems, Community Child Health and Child and Adolescent Mental Health Services (CAMHS). The protocol, therefore, should be based on broad principles that may be applied to all young people regardless of their particular condition. Hence the working group has representation from all the services provided by this Trust.

Feedback

To develop a transition protocol for the Children's Hospital National Health Service trust. This protocol will be informed by your work on the questions that you formulate for this trigger.

The facts

> What are the main facts in this trigger? Make a list:

Hypotheses: What may these facts mean?

- Making transitions in life is difficult especially from adolescence to adulthood.
- Transitions from child health services to adult health services are stressful for young people and their families.
- Effective transition programmes are essential for young people in the health service.
- Young people with diabetes and other chronic illnesses may not comply with treatment and experience more regular hospital admissions.
- Developing peer friendships is important to young people.

Questions developed from the hypotheses

These will depend on your previous knowledge, but may include the following:

1. What factors make transitions in life and to adulthood difficult?
2. Why is it difficult for young people to make the transition between child and adult healthcare services?
3. What are the key elements of a transition programme in the health service?
4. What support is available for children/young people that are not complying with treatment?

(The answers to these questions will inform the Transition Protocol that you are to develop for feedback.)

Trigger 11.3: Fixed resource material

Read the following to help you answer the questions. (You may also wish to search and review other up-to-date research and evidence-based literature and seek other relevant resources to provide you with the answers to your questions.)

Cowlard, J. (2003) Cystic fibrosis: transition from paediatric to adult care. *Journal of Advanced Nursing* 18 (14), 8 October, pp. 39–41.

Esmonde, G. (2000) Cystic fibrosis: Adolescent care. *Nursing Standard* 14 (52), 13 September, pp. 47–52, pp. 54–5, 57.

Fleming, E., Carter, B. Gillibrand, W. (2002) The transition of adolescents with diabetes from children's health care services into the adult health care service: a review of the literature. *Journal of Clinical Nursing* 11950, September, pp. 560–7.

Miller, S. (1996) Transition of care in adolescence. *Paediatric Nursing* 8, November, pp. 14–16.

Viner, R., Keane, M. (1998) *Youth Matters: Evidence-Based Best Practice for Care of Young People in Hospital*. London: Caring for Children in the Health Services/Action for Sick Children.)

Ward, L., Mallet, R., Heslop, P., Simons, K. (2003) Planning for health at Transition. *Learning Disability Practice* 6, 3 April, pp. 24–7.

Useful websites:

http://www.barnados.org.uk (Barnados)

http://www.doh.gov.uk/vpst/papers.htm (Department of Health (2001) *Valuing People: A New Strategy for Learning Disability for the 21st Century*) http://www.dh.gov.uk

Department of Health (2003) *National Service Framework Mental Health*

Department of Health (2003) *National Service Framework Diabetes*

Department of Health (2003) *Getting the Right Start: National Service Framework for Children Standard for Hospital Services*, (Growing On and Moving Onto Adult Services, 33–4, Mental Health, pp. 26–7)

Department of Health (2003) *Emerging Findings*, London: Department of Health (transition and Growing Up 20–21)

http://www.jrf.org.uk (Joseph Rowntree Foundation)

http://www.ncb.org.uk (National Children's Bureau)

Trigger 11.3: Fixed resource sessions

Diabetes mellitus: Children and young people

> ### Suggested Activity
>
> Prior to reading this fixed resource session it is suggested that you 'revise' the anatomy and physiology of the following systems:
>
> - Gastro-intestinal
> - Endocrine

The young person identified in the trigger scenario has Type 1 Diabetes mellitus (insulin dependent), which until recently has been the only type to affect children and young people. However some children and young people as a consequence of childhood obesity are now developing Type 2 Diabetes (non insulin dependent) that has previously only affected adults. The ability to produce insulin is not totally abolished with Type 2 Diabetes, but there is an increased insulin resistance, which can be improved by medication that increases the sensitivity to insulin in the cells or by increasing the release of insulin from the pancreas.

This session will first briefly review Type 1 Diabetes mellitus in relation to pathophysiology and management principles, prior to exploring specific issues for young people making the transition to adult health services.

Type 1 Diabetes mellitus

Type 1 Diabetes mellitus results from insulin deficiency. It occurs as a failure of destroyed beta cells in the islets of Langerhans of the pancreas to produce insulin or to produce it in such minute quantities that it has no effect on blood glucose levels. Destroyed beta cells in the Islets of Langerhans produce no or insufficient insulin to enable carbohydrate metabolism. Rudolph and Levene (1999) explain that the process by which the beta cells are destroyed is yet to be established but it is likely to be viruses that will affect genetically susceptible individuals or an autoimmune response.

Normal physiology

The blood glucose range in the healthy child stays between 4–6 mmol/l. Following a meal the nutrients are digested and broken down by the gastro-intestinal tract enzymes into simple monosaccarides sugars, for example, glucose. The simple sugars are absorbed into the blood stream. With the help of insulin, glucose is transformed into glycogen and stored in the liver. This reserve can be later mobilised in between meals, at night time or when starving.

This is done with the help of glucagon, which converts the glycogen back to glucose. Before glucose can be used as a substrate for energy it needs to get into the cell and requires insulin for this to happen. The role of insulin is, therefore, to allow glucose to enter the cell and also to help the liver store glucose as glycogen. Normally insulin is secreted in response to a rise in blood glucose. Insulin is important to the metabolism of fats and protein. Changing glucose levels that are based on exercise levels and carbohydrate intake controls the release of insulin in the well child/young person. Insulin release is also under hormonal and neural influences.

The presence of gastro-intestinal hormones such as gastrin is important because these also stimulate the pancreas to produce the necessary insulin. There is a fall in blood glucose when the child/young person is in a fasting state and this decreases insulin secretion resulting in the metabolism of fat with resultant ketone production.

Pathophysiology

Insulin deficiency in children/young people with Diabetes mellitus leads to them being unable to use glucose, causing hyperglycaemia (high blood glucose levels) and the breakdown of fat. Glucagon has a reciprocal action with insulin. The insulin is the most important one, as it is insulin that channels the glucose into stores in the cells ready to be used as energy. Without insulin, the body is starved of glucose in the cells because glucose is excreted in the urine. Without insulin glucose levels remain high in the blood stream and the blood glucose level rises, especially after meal times, and some of it will then be excreted in the urine.

The body attempts to get energy from the breakdown of fats and proteins, which elevates the blood glucose even more and ketone bodies are produced from the breakdown of fat. A large amount of ketone bodies from fat metabolism are very toxic to the body and can lead to keto acidosis, which in turn can lead to hyperglycaemic coma.

Initial presentation of Type 1 Diabetes mellitus

The onset of this condition is usually abrupt in childhood diabetes. Symptoms are present for only a few weeks prior to the diagnosis being made. The most common presenting symptoms are likely to be polyuria (which may present as secondary enuresis), polydispia and weight loss. It is rarer, but some children may present in diabetic ketoacidotic coma. Rudolph and Levene (1999) identify that other accompanying symptoms may include lethargy, anorexia and constipation and if recognition of the condition is delayed vomiting, abdominal pain, dehydration, ketotic smelling breath and other features of diabetic ketoacidosis may be evident.

The diagnosis is confirmed by random blood sampling and testing the urine for the presence of glucose and ketones.

Management of care

The goals of management in diabetes, as for any chronic condition of childhood, are to encourage the child to live as normal a life as possible, while accepting the limitations that good management of the condition allows (Rudolph and Levene 1999, p. 126).

Insulin administration: The goal is to approximate insulin levels to match physiological insulin secretion, which is achieved by mixing short and intermediate acting insulin (Rudolph and Levene 1999). The insulin is usually given twice daily during childhood, although it may have to be increased in adolescence. Insulin is given as a subcutaneous injection by syringe or alternatively pre-loaded insulin 'pens'. Children should be encouraged to rotate the injection site between upper arms, thighs, abdomen and buttocks. This is to avoid lipoatrophy and lyphohypotrophy, which can affect absorption rates as well as being unsightly (Rudolph and Levene 1999). The dose administered is usually given prior to breakfast and evening meals so that the rise in insulin can match the rise in glucose taken into the body.

Monitoring of blood glucose: Blood glucose measurements need to be monitored regularly by using a spring loaded puncture device for finger pricking to minimise pain and an automatic readout machine such as a glucometer. This provides a more accurate reading than matching the shade of blood on a glucose testing strip (Pillitteri 1999) This monitoring is needed so that the insulin dose prescribed can be adjusted and symptoms of hypoglycaemia or hyperglycaemia confirmed. Blood glucose is usually monitored 3–4 times per day, 2 days per week and whenever the child has symptoms of hypoglycaemia or hyperglycaemia (Rudolph and Levene 1999). Informed adjustments to insulin doses may be made based on these regular recordings of blood glucose.

Urine testing: is not as accurate as blood glucose monitoring (Pillitteri 1999) The family are taught to test for ketones in the urine if blood glucose measurements are high for a time, especially if the child is ill.

Diet: Children with diabetes need to consume a normal healthy diet, which is high in fibre in amounts sufficient to promote normal growth (Rudolph and Levene 1999). Meals should be eaten at regular times throughout the day in consistent amounts; Pillitteri (1999) suggests three spaced meals a day with regular snacks in between. This is to prevent blood glucose levels dropping in between meals (Rudolph and Levene 1999).

Education and support for the child and family: Education and support for the family, including the child at the appropriate developmental level, is crucial on initial diagnosis, especially as early discharge happens so that stabilisation on insulin matches with the child's normal routine at home. Diabetes mellitus is a life long condition and the family and child need to develop knowledge and understanding about this medical condition. There are also several practical skills for them to learn in relation to insulin injections, blood glucose monitoring, urine testing and dietary requirements.

The school attended by the child with diabetes will also need to understand the implications of the condition to prepare them for the return of the newly diagnosed child. The diabetes nurse specialist will undertake this preparation.

Learning about potentially life threatening hypoglycaemia and ketoacidosis episodes is essential for the family (and also the school). The family are likely to need extra emotional support to cope from the health care team during these crises.

Management of acute problems: *Diabetic ketoacidosis*. This is precipitated when insulin levels fall below the child's requirements. Infection may be a cause of diabetic ketoacidosis because it increases the body's requirements for insulin. Non-compliance with treatment is likely to be the other cause for this emergency. The lack of insulin leads to the mobilisation of fat and the production of ketones, which in large amounts are very toxic to the body leading to ketoacidosis. This in turn can result in a hyperglycaemic coma. It is a medical emergency that must be treated immediately with rehydration, insulin administration, electrolyte replacement and the treatment of any infection.

Hypoglycaemia: occurs over a few minutes as opposed to ketoacidosis that occurs over hours to days. It can result from the administration of too much insulin, excessive exercise that uses up glucose or failure to eat sufficient carbohydrate that may occur in illness (Pillitteri 1999). This means that there is too much insulin relative to carbohydrate intake and energy expenditure. Typical signs and symptoms of hypoglycaemia include pallor, hunger, sweating, trembling and tachycardia (Rudolph and Levene 1999). Drowsiness, mental confusion, seizures and coma could result if treatment is not promptly given. The conscious child needs to be given dextrose tablets or a carbohydrate containing snack or drink immediately. A glucose gel may be squeezed on to the buccal mucosa if the child is unable to drink. Glucagon may be injected intramuscularly to release glucose stores from the liver if the child is unconscious or alternatively medical staff may administer intravenous glucose. Longer term it is important that the family and child develop an understanding of the precipitating causes of a hypoglycaemic attack so that adjustments in carbohydrate snacks and/or insulin doses may be considered (Rudolph and Levene 1999).

The National Institute of Clinical Excellence has produced guidelines for the diagnosis and management of Type 1 Diabetes in children, young people and adults (National Institute of Clinical Excellence 2004) and while none of the recommendations are new they do reinforce previous documents (Houghton 2004). National

Institute of Clinical Excellence (2004) identifies implementation priorities for managing diabetes from diagnosis, which will inform practice.

Complications of Diabetes mellitus

Rudolph and Levene (1999) state that there are 4 major long term complications:

1. Retinopathy;
2. Neuropathy;
3. Nephropathy; and
4. Heart disease.

These complications are likely to occur some years after the onset of Diabetes mellitus, in adulthood. However, the complications are directly related to the degree of long-term glycaemic control. Therefore, every effort must be made to ensure that children/young people and their families understand their condition and management and are able to comply with treatment. Fleming et al (2002) identify from their literature review that the added pressures of diabetes frequently causes young people with diabetes to rebel, non-complying with treatment and/or use food as an easy option for manipulation leading to poor glycaemic control that is likely to result in long-term complications.

Compliance

Young people with diabetes have to deal with the challenge of making the transition from child to adult health services in addition to coping with the developmental stage of adolescence. Young people with diabetes are expected to take on the extra responsibility for managing their own care, which may prove to be difficult for some because of the nature of this stage of development, which may lead to non-compliance with treatment. Kyngas (1999, p. 74) defines compliance as 'an active, intentional and responsible process of care in which the individual works to maintain his or her health in close collaboration with the health care personnel'.

Others use the alternative terminology of adherence believing the term compliance to be laden with connotations of paternalism, coercion and acquiescence (Kyngas and Rissanen 2001). Whatever terminology is used there seems to be agreement that there are internal and external factors that influence compliance. Stewart and Dearmun (2001) found in a literature review that the internal factors were associated with adolescent bio-psycho-social development and intra-personal dynamics. The external factors were linked to interpersonal dynamics between the adolescent, family, peers, health care professionals and the whole of society. Becky's diary extracts suggest that both internal and external factors may be influencing her non-compliance with diabetic treatment. She is at the adolescent stage of development and it is evident in the extracts that managing her diabetes has been getting in the way of her spending time with her peers. The extract also suggests that her parents were pressurising her to comply with her treatment, which may well have the opposite effect on her at this stage of development.

Becky's apparent non-compliance concurs with that of other adolescents with a chronic illness. The highest incidence of non-adherence (or non-compliance) to health advice occurs in adolescence (Stewart and Dearmun 2001), with chronically ill adolescents being a particular challenge for health care staff (Kyngas and Rissanen 2001).

In a study to describe the factors that predict compliance among adolescents with a chronic illness, Kyngas and Rissananen (2001) found that support was the crucial predictor of good compliance. The recommendations of this study are to:

- Give positive feedback to adolescents as they endeavour to manage their chronic illness and normal developmental crises.
- Involve the family in care whenever possible (providing it is acceptable to the adolescent).
- Encourage the family to provide emotional and physical support to adolescents with a chronic illness.
- Use good communication skills, listening to the adolescent's needs and individualising treatment.
- Encourage adolescents to participate actively in planning and decision-making processes relating to transition planning.

It is important, therefore, that adolescents with a chronic illness are given frequent support and encouragement during the transition period to promote compliance with treatment.

Transition for young people with Diabetes mellitus

Transitions occur at certain times in childhood for all children. These may be transitions concerned with starting school and then changing schools as certain ages are reached. Transitions are potentially stressful times for children and young people ensuing in a cycle of phases namely shock, provisional adjustment, inner contradictions leading to an inner crisis before re-construction and recovery occurs to enable a successful transition. Children and their families with a chronic illness such as Diabetes mellitus and long-term care needs have also to make several other transitions (Figure 11.2) culminating in the transition from child to adult health services.

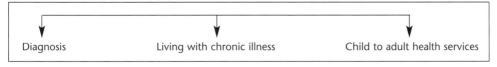

Figure 11.2   Transitions for children with a chronic illness

According to Viner and Keane (1998, p. 41) the American Society for Adolescent Medicine's definition of transition is the most useful: 'The purposeful planned movement of adolescents and young adults with chronic physical and medical conditions from child-centred care to adult-orientated health care systems'.

The *Emerging Findings of the National Service Framework for Children, Young People and Maternity Care* (Department of Health 2003) state that there was evidence that shows that the transfer of young people from child to adult services requires special attention. In the full *National Service Framework* (Department of Health 2004, p. 119) it states that 'All transition processes are planned in partnership and focused around the preparation of the young person.'

This includes processes involving: social care; education; and employment and not just health care. Royal College of Nursing (2004) identifies that transition is a lengthy process, which should continue on into adult care and provides some comprehensive guidelines about the process.

Young people with uncommon conditions are only now surviving into adulthood due to medical advances and there is sometimes a lack of an adult service, which may result in a delayed transfer from the child service. Other young people with long-term conditions that are very common in adulthood such as Diabetes move from the child health service where they have been 'special' (Department of Health 2003) to an environment with many older patients. Here clinicians have less time for social support and the family may be excluded.

The concept of making a transition is relatively new. Previously the terminology solely referred to transferring to adult health services. The changed terminology denotes that this transfer in health care services for the young person is not immediate as it was with just transferring because transition suggests a period of time. This period of time is to allow for planning to promote a smooth transition. Department of Health (2003) found some evidence that well planned transition programmes lead to better disease control and improved patient satisfaction as opposed to the young person dropping out of the medical services.

The transition period

The transition period may cause instability in already vulnerable young people. Therefore, the healthcare team has to ensure that the transition process is a positive experience, building, developing and empowering young people to become well-balanced independent individuals (Fleming et al 2002).

The *Diabetes National Service Framework* (Department of Health 2003, 2.26) highlights the issue of transitions stating that 'Managing the process of transition and having an adult service, which is able to meet the specific needs of teenagers and young adults is therefore key for young people with diabetes and their long term health.'

The transition involves a move between two very different health care systems according to Fleming et al (2002). Family-centred care is integral to children's nursing 'providing professional support for the child and family through a process of involvement, participation and partnership, underpinned by empowerment and negotiation' (Smith et al 2002, p. 22). Children/young people in this system are usually seen at consultations with an adult family member and hence they are not necessarily encouraged to be independent and self-managing in relation to diabetes. At these consultations paediatricians emphasise family and social life, school and work progress, while adult physicians have been found to emphasise the risk of long-term complications, importance of exercise and the maintenance of strict glycaemic control (Eiser 1993). Conversely, within the more formal adult health care system, consultations without a parent will be expected, with the assumption that the young person is cognitively able to manage their own care (Fleming et al 2002). There is the potential for a very abrupt change in the move between these health care systems if the transition is not planned.

There are other barriers to a successful transition that affect parents, young people and the health care professionals. Nurses need to be aware of these to promote optimum transitions.

Parents
- Perceived parental exclusion due to promotion of adolescent independence by adult health care providers.
- Anxiety about long-term disease complications and being 'a step closer to complications and death' (Viner 1999).
- Difficulty 'letting go' of the young person as parents have to gradually relinquish decision-making for their children.

Health care professionals
- Paediatricians may be resistant to transition and 'letting go' because many childhood conditions are unknown to adult physicians. While adult physicians are knowledgeable about diabetes itself, they may be less aware of the emotional turmoil.
- Adult physicians may find adolescents medically challenging, emotionally demanding and financially draining and, therefore, not wish to take responsibility for them (Rosen 1994).

Adolescents
- Anxiety about long-term disease complications and being 'a step closer to complications and death' (Viner 1999).
- Disruption of continuity of care and loosing support from familiar health care professionals.
- Reluctance to take responsibility to manage own health care.
- Anxious about more formal health care environments and likely elderly patients encountered.

(Models have been developed for transition programmes to overcome these barriers and to ensure a smooth transition.)

Suggested Activity

1. There are three major transition models: primary care based; generic adolescent health service; and disease-focused transition. Read Esmonde (2000) to find out about these models.
2. Miller (1996) also outlines three possible models for enabling young people to move from child to adult clinics. You should find out about these models to help with developing your transition protocol.

Models of community children's nursing

Community children's nursing is essential to child health services in the 21st century in the U.K. This is to support the increasing number of children/young people with long term care needs, and also to meet government agendas and targets in relation to caring for children in the community in their own homes as opposed to in hospital.

Samwell (2000) outlines a simple model of the children that constitute the caseload of community children's nurses:

- Children with serious chronic conditions.
- Children with common chronic conditions, for example diabetes (the subject of this trigger) and asthma.
- Children discharged home after acute intervention in hospital.
- Children managed in the community with an acute illness.

There are many diverse models of community children's nursing services (Samwell 2000) that are likely to be managed either by acute healthcare services or a primary care services in the community. Alternatively the service may be part of an integrated children's service incorporating both primary care and acute healthcare services, which is advocated by contemporary policy as the way forward (Department of Health 2004). Children's community nurses may have either generic or specialist roles or conversely they combine these roles (Winter and Teale 1997).

Eaton (2001, p. 32) identifies the aim of most community children's nursing teams as being: 'To reduce the length of stay in hospital or avoid admission altogether and to provide a service which is of high quality and which is cost effective.'

It was highlighted though in the House of Commons Health Select Committee (Healh Committee 1997) report that there was no research-based model to underpin the practice of community children's nursing, suggesting that evidence of a cost effective and quality service was lacking at this time. Proctor et al (1999) subsequently investigated preparation for the developing role of the community children's nurse and different service models. Eaton (2000) suggests that there has been a rise in implementing different models recently and evaluating them to ensure that practice is actually based on best evidence. There are six models of care identified by Eaton (2001), varying according to location and the team's level and area of specialisation:

- Hospital outreach – generalist;
- Hospital outreach – specialist;
- Community – based team;
- Hospital at home: Children receive treatments at home (traction or renal dialysis for example) that would normally be carried out in hospital;
- District nursing service; and
- Ambulatory or assessment unit: usually within a hospital setting, designed for children to be treated or observed for a period of time, but not admitted.

Eaton (2001) stresses that each model has its strengths and weaknesses that need to be considered in relation to local constraints and conditions, and the availability of appropriately qualified staff in the planning of services.

The hospital outreach – specialist model describes the service that was available to Becky the adolescent with diabetes in this trigger. In the diary extract Sue the Paediatric Diabetes Nurse Specialist (PDNS) is identified as being involved in Becky's care. The majority of nurse specialist's roles developed in areas that have a clear association with medical specialities such as diabetes (Marshall et al 2002). Initially the role was medically orientated to improve standards and quality of patient care. Marshall et al (2002, p. 427) however found in a critical review of the literature that the PDNS role has now developed into a more holistic nursing model 'with the paediatric diabetes nurse specialist role being central to the child's diabetes self-management and disease control'. Lowes' (1997) evaluation of the effectiveness of a specialist service for children with diabetes supports this finding and describes the PDNS role as encompassing:

- Managing care at home;
- Reducing the length of stay in hospital for children with established diagnosis;
- Preventing admission to hospital on initial diagnosis;
- Belonging to the specialist diabetic team based in the hospital;
- Outpatient clinic role;
- Education sessions with child, family and colleagues; and
- Setting up support groups.

Marshall et al (2002) emphasise the need for the PDNS to use family-centred approaches and that the most successful education programmes are those given over a long period of time, involving frequent contact and reinforcement. Becky states in her diary extract that she has known Sue (and Jill the hospital nurse) since she was 'little', and it seems apparent that a trusting relationship has been built up over this period of time.

Samwell (2000) identifies that the PDNS is likely to work collaboratively with others and devolve essential skills to health visitors, school nurses and practice nurses who have an existing remit with the children. Therefore, in some respects the PDNS is a facilitator with the expertise and clinical overview ensuring that high standards of care are delivered across all healthcare settings (Samwell 2000). However, it is likely that contact with children/young people with diabetes and their families is maintained by the PDNS, especially at critical times such as in adolescence when the transition to adult health services is to be planned. Transition to adult healthcare services is encompassed in the *National Service Framework for Diabetes* (Department of Health 2003).

Marshall et al (2002) suggest that the PDNS needs to apply psychosocial constructs to understand the personal and social meaning of diabetes and the individual family's attitude towards treatment and health. This understanding informs the delivery of family-centred care using adaptation and negotiation models (Marshall et al, 2002) following initial diagnosis of diabetes and at critical times in the healthcare journey of children/young people. Becky's diary extract suggests that adolescence is a critical time for her with making transitions in life and the health services. Contact with the PDNS will be necessary at this time to enable her to adapt and self-manage her diabetes. Carter (2000), in a study that explored the role/skills used by children's community nurses caring for children with a chronic illness, found that participants viewed the preparation of young people for transition as an important element of their care.

 Trigger 11.3: Feedback

Go to Chapter 11 Trigger feedback on p. 376 below

Chapter 11 Trigger Feedback: What do you know?

Trigger 11.1: Lesson Plan: Nursing care and management of a child and family with cystic fibrosis

Aim

To explain how cystic fibrosis is inherited and the rationale for the nursing care and management of a child with cystic fibrosis

Learning outcomes

At the end of this session the junior student will be able to:

- Explain how cystic fibrosis is inherited.
- Assess, plan, implement and evaluate nursing care for a child with cystic fibrosis.
- Recognise the importance of listening to children and families with cystic fibrosis.

Table 11.1 Lesson plan: Nursing and care management of a child management of a child and family with cystic fibrosis

Time	Content	Teacher Activity	Student Activity	Resources
14.00–14.05	*Introduction* - Reviewing students' previous learning - Explaining content of lesson	Asking questions	Listening. Answering questions	
14.05–14.10	*Development* 1. Inheritance of CF	Explanation Using diagrams	Listening Using examples	Diagrams/ Examples
14.10–14.25	2. Nursing care/ Management and listening to Ben and his family	Use Ben's Care plan and give rationale for care/ management Ask questions	Listening Ask questions Give Answers	Ben's Care Plan
14.25–14. 30	*Conclusion* - Summing up - Asking Questions - Future learning about CF	Summarise key issues Questions to check understanding Establish practical skills that need to be learned to care for Ben	Listen Answer questions Identify personal learning needs for practice	

You discuss the lesson plan in Table 11.1 with your mentor with regards to the learning outcomes, structure and timing. Teaching and learning theory should underpin your plan. You may find it useful to read:

Nicklin, P., Kenworthy, N. (1995) *Teaching and Assessing in Nursing Practice*, 2nd edn. London: Scutari Press, Chapters 3 and 4, pp. 22–67.

You check the content of your lesson plan with your mentor.

Question 1: How is cystic fibrosis inherited?

Cystic fibrosis is inherited as an autosomal recessive condition, one in 25 of the population being carriers. In northern Europe the commonest mutant gene is delta F508. This gene codes for a protein that controls sodium and chloride transport across the apical membrane of secretory epithelial cells. It is this mutation that causes the high salt content of sweat and thick secretions produced by the epithelial cells of some organs.

There is a family history of cystic fibrosis (Rudolf and Levene 1999). A defective gene must be inherited from both parents for the disease to occur. In a family in which both parents are carriers there is a 1 in 4 chance of their children having cystic fibrosis (see Figure 11.3).

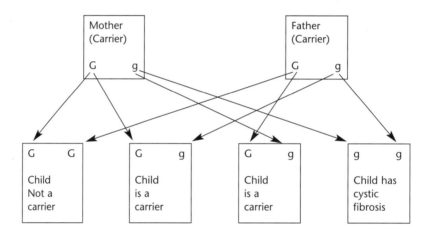

Notes: G = carrier gene. g = cystic fibrosis gene

Figure 11.3   Cystic fibrosis inheritance

The cause of the disorder is an abnormality of the long arm of chromosome 7. It is inherited as an autosomal recessive trait. It occurs in 1 in 2,500 live births, most commonly in White people, and more rarely in Black and Asian people

Question 2: How are children with cystic fibrosis diagnosed and managed by nurses and the multi-disciplinary team?

You may have referred to the National Consensus Standards for the Nursing Management of Cystic Fibrosis (Madge et al 2001) in preparing your care plan. These helpful guidelines make recommendations for best evidence-based practice and offer standards of care within the broad areas of advocacy, clinical management, education, support, advice and research (Madge 2002).

Diagnosis: Neonatal screening for cystic fibrosis, as part of the heel prick test at birth, is being made available for all new mothers and pregnant women. The development of universal screening for cystic fibrosis means that all parents will be offered the choice of whether to have their baby screened.

When babies are not screened at birth cystic fibrosis is diagnosed by the presenting patho-physiology (see the fixed resource session).

The following investigations are undertaken to confirm the diagnosis:

- Sweat test;
- Duodenal analysis;
- Stool analysis for fat content and trypsin content;
- Pulmonary testing – Chest X-ray; and
- Sputum culture.

Management and nursing care: *Goal 1*: To ensure the child absorbs an adequate nutritional amount daily.
Care:

1. A high protein, high calorie diet, supplemented with fat soluble vitamins is required. Extra dietary supplements may be required at time of illness.
2. Extra salt is needed during hot weather to prevent heat stroke and if the child is febrile. Take measures to avoid the child developing a high temperature.
3. Breastfed babies require supplementary formulas because there is not sufficient protein in breast milk for them. This is because breast fed babies cannot use all the protein that is ingested.
4. Pancreatic enzyme supplements (eg pancreatin, cotazym, pancrease) have to be taken with all meals and snacks, although these may not control the malabsorption entirely. These synthetic enzymes are supplied in large capsules that are to be taken before or with meals. They can be swallowed whole, or opened and the powder is sprinkled onto a small amount of food for young children to swallow.
5. The family need to be informed of the possible side effects of pancreatic supplements for example nausea, abdominal cramps, diarrhoea, hypersensitivity.
6. Mouth care.

Evaluation: Child's health and weight follow centile growth curves and the quantity, size and foul odour of the child's faeces decreases.

Goal 2: To prevent the child's airway becoming blocked by infected mucous. secretions
Care:

1. Regular chest physiotherapy and postural drainage to drain secretions from the lungs. Moistened oxygen and aerosol therapy.
2. Antibiotics are administered intravenously or orally at high dosage for long periods to prevent infection and to treat infections when they occur. Bronchodilators and mucolytics are also often prescribed.
3. Change of position.
4. Frequent monitoring of respiratory rate, temperature and pulse rate.
5. Provide respiratory hygiene; frequent mouth care, tooth brushing and mouthwash to make the mouth feel fresh (the sputum coughed up has a foul taste and odour).
6. Organisation of care to ensure adequate rest and to prevent exhaustion.

Evaluation: Child's airway remains patent and temperature is maintained within normal range.

Goal 3: To prevent risk of altered skin integrity due to the nature of stools passed.
Care:
1. Change wet/dirty nappies immediately to avoid skin irritation or breakdown in the nappy area. Prior to children becoming regulated on pancreatic enzymes the stool with its high fat content is very irritating.
2. Check for a prolapsed rectum following bowel movements. (The mucosa must be replaced promptly before the blood supply is compromised.) The incidence of prolapsed rectum decreases when child is receiving pancreatic enzymes.

Evaluation: The skin remains intact in a healthy condition.

Goal 4: To promote child/family-centred care enabling them to work in partnership with the multidisciplinary team.
Care:
1. Listen to the child/young person and family.
2. Negotiate and plan care with the child/young person and family.
3. Develop child and family competencies in care and decision-making skills to empower the family.
4. Facilitate partnership working with the child/young person, family and multi-disciplinary team.

Evaluation: The family participate in the child/young person's care and effective partnership working occurs.

Goal 5: To educate the child/young person and family in order to promote optimum health.
Care:
1. Explain the condition of cystic fibrosis to the child/young person and family.

2. Teach the child/young person and family how to perform nursing care.

3. Create an awareness of the side effects of treatments.

Evaluation: The child/young person and family understand the condition and develop physical and decision-making skills to care. Optimum health is promoted as they are empowered to take control of their lives.

Question 3: How does listening to children and young people (and their families) that are living with a chronic illness promote their health?

The fixed resource session for this trigger about listening to children and young people provides some of the answers to this question, emphasising the need to listen in order to empower the child/young person and family to take control of their lives and to live healthily with cystic fibrosis.

Your answer may also have identified some of the reasons why it is helpful to listen to children/young people with cystic fibrosis and other chronic conditions. Ben in this trigger for example stated that Rob was a bully and that he did not have many friends at school. The reason for this is likely to be connected to Ben having cystic fibrosis. He is away from school quite often due to hospital admissions and he is likely to feel different from his peers when he is at school. This is because of physiotherapy and medication treatment that will need to continue during school hours. Children/young people with cystic fibrosis may also suffer from body image problems due to poor growth and delayed puberty that again make them feel different from their peers and reluctant to participate in sports activities. These factors can limit the opportunities for friendship and make children and young people with cystic fibrosis a target for bullying.

The health of such children and young people in these circumstances is likely to be adversely affected and, therefore, nurses need to listen to be able to assess and plan care that will help the child to cope.

It is possible that you may have chosen to focus on listening to other family members, who are also living with a chronic condition. Foster et al (2001) identifies that treatments are becoming increasingly demanding, are largely performed in the family home and that mothers are often reported to experience greater stress and poorer adjustment than mothers of well children. Hodgkinson and Lester (2002) performed a study exploring current stresses and coping strategies used by mothers living with a child with cystic fibrosis and implications for nurses. The major stresses identified in the study were feeling in the middle in terms of decision-making particularly about the genetic implications of cystic fibrosis and the burden of responsibility for parenting a child with a chronic illness and a change in personal identity. Listening to the perspectives of Ben's mother you may have concluded that she was stressed and have intervened to support her. Hodgkinson and Lester (2002) found evidence that nurses need to adopt roles that involved them being holders of hope, bridge builders and providers of continuity of care. All these roles would require nurses to listen to the mother's perspectives and that has the potential to strengthen the nurse–patient relationship and to promote maternal health.

Alternatively you may have chosen to focus on listening to siblings in your answer. From listening to Ben's older sister's perspectives on living with cystic fibrosis it is clear that she is trying her best to help her mother, but caring for Ben is interfering with her social life. Siblings may receive less attention, because the 'patient's needs' take priority and parents give the ill child preferential treatment (Foster et al 2001). It is important to listen to siblings who are trying to cope with a sick brother or sister and may have difficulty in adapting. Siblings should not go unnoticed because the impact of having a brother or sister with cystic fibrosis should not be underestimated (Foster et al 2001).

Whatever the focus of your answer was it is apparent that listening is an important aspect of care to promote the health of the child/young person and individual family members that are living with a chronic illness.

Trigger 11.2

What respite provision is there for families of children and young people with profound disability in your locality from the following?

- Health services;
- Social services;
- Education services; and
- Voluntary organisations.

The feedback here is going to differ because readers are investigating respite provision by different services in their own localities. The fixed resource session about respite care identified three types of available respite care, institutional, shared care and home-based care. You are likely to find some of these types of care in your own locality provided by the different services.

Your briefing paper will identify these services in the locality and their strengths and weaknesses. For the meeting you should be prepared to discuss how easy or difficult it was to find out about these respite services. This is to enable the working group to gain some insight into the problems that families may be experiencing when trying to get this information.

You may also develop some recommendations for the meeting about how this information may be disseminated to colleagues and/or families requiring respite care if it is not readily available. You may suggest a written source of information in the form of a leaflet, a website, fact sheet or as part of a resource pack.

Trigger 11.3:

Figure 11.4 is an example of a 'Transition protocol' based on the answers to the questions that you are likely to have formulated for this trigger. It is based on the key elements of the effective transition programme developed by Viner and Keane (1998). Whatever you develop should be based on local conditions.

Children's Hospital NHS Trust

Transition protocol

1. Timing of transition
Transition should be completed by the age of 17 years. Exceptions may be made when special individual circumstances prevent completion by this age.
(*There is no 'right time' for transition, but a target transfer age is desirable for both staff and the young people involved (Viner and Keane, 1998)*)

2. Preparation for transition
- Preparation will begin in early adolescence to ensure that the young person is capable of independently managing his or her own condition.
- Planned programmes will be developed to educate the young person about the disease, rationale for treatment, recognition of deterioration and how to respond, how to get help from health professionals and how to operate within the medical system (Viner and Keane 1998).
- Provision of a 'Making the Transition' booklet which will answer frequently asked questions.
- Through the education process the adolescent will be empowered to make autonomous decisions and to become competent in performing nursing/medical care.
- The adolescents' feelings and concerns about transition to adult health services will be explored during consultations in order to provide appropriate support to enable them to cope.
- A support programme for parents will be planned to prepare them alongside the young person for transition.

3. Co-ordinated transition: Adult and child health services
- Selection of an appropriate transition model: Primary care based; generic adolescent health service or disease-focused transition model.
- Every adolescent will be allocated a key worker to co-ordinate an effective transition.
- Gradual clinic transfer: Paediatric service to adolescent clinic to young adult clinic to adult service.
- Child and adult health services (including the primary health care team) work together in partnership with the young person and his or her family to plan the transition by developing joint care plans.

4. Administrative support
- Administrative co-ordinator and clerical support to ensure the efficient organisations of appointments and the transfer of medical records (Viner and Keane 1998).
- Administrative co-ordinator to ensure that all the health care professionals involved in the young person's care are kept informed of his or her transition programme.
- To provide a summary of the young person's medical and nursing records for the adult healthcare team.

5. Evaluation of transitions
- To evaluate the transitions of young people continually and to provide an annual written report.

Figure 11.4 Transitions protocol

Reflect on your learning

- Provide holistic physical, psycho-social nursing care for specific chronic conditions in order to meet the long-term care needs of individual children, young people and their families.
- Use a family-centred care approach to work in partnership with the child, young person, family and multi-disciplinary team in the hospital and community to develop care packages.
- Promote optimum health and compliance for the child/ young person/family by information giving, teaching and facilitating learning about the condition, preventing complications and developing skills for care.
- Support the child and all the members of the family (including siblings) in adapting and coping with ongoing stress and periodic crises.
- Negotiate and plan care with the child/young person/family using theoretical frameworks (Practice Continuum Tool/Negotiated-Empowerment Framework) to underpin the process.
- Use strategies to empower the child/young person/family to develop competencies to manage the physical care and to make autonomous decisions.
- Consult and listen to the child/young person with a chronic condition.
- Promote and monitor growth and development.
- Advocate for resources including adequate respite care provision.
- Plan educational programmes to prepare young people and their families for transition to adult health services.

References

Alderson, P., Montgomery, J. (1996) *Health Care Choices – Making Decisions with Children*. London: Institute for Public Policy Research.

Bradford, R. (1997) *Children, Families and Chronic Illness*. London: Routledge.

British Heart Foundation (2005) http://www.bhf.org.uk (accessed 28 October 2005).

Carter, B. (2000) Ways of working: CCNs and chronic illness. *Journal of Child Health* 4 (2), Summer, pp. 66–71.

Coleman, V. (2002) Empowerment: Rhetoric, reality and skills, in Smith, L., Coleman, V., Bradshaw, M. (eds) *Family Centred-Care: Concept, Theory and Practice*. Basingstoke: Palgrave, Chapter 5, pp. 85–113.

Coleman, V., Smith, L. Bradshaw, M. (2003) *A Toolkit of Skills for Multi-Professional Partnerships*, paper presented at Completing the Circle: Child and family partnerships in practice, RCN and Yorkhill NHS Trust Conference, 11–13 September 2003, Glasgow.

Contact a Family: For families with disabled children http://www.cafamily.org.uk (accessed 24 January 2005).

Cooper, C. (1999) *Continuing Care of Sick Children: Examining the Impact of Chronic Illness.* Dinton: Quay Books.

Coyne, I, (1997) Chronic Illness: The importance of support for families caring for a child with cystic fibrosis. *Journal of Clinical Nursing* 6 (2), March, pp. 121–9.

Cystic Fibrosis Trust http://www.cftrust.org.uk (accessed 2 January 2005).

Department of Education and Skills, *Quality Protects* http://www.dfes.gov.uk/qualityprotects (accessed 24 January 2005.

Department of Health (1989) The Children Act (London: HMSO).

Department of Health (1999) *The Quality Protects Programme: Transforming Children's Services.* London: HMSO. (London: HMSO).

Department of Health (2001) *The Expert Patient: A New Approach to Chronic Disease Management for the 21st Century.* London: DoH.

Department of Health (2003) *Getting the Right Start: National Service Framework for Children Standard for Hospital Services.* London: DoH.

Department of Health (2003) *Emerging Findings.* London: DoH (Transition and Growing Up pp. 20–1).

Department of Health (2003) *National Service Framework for Diabetes.* London: DoH.

Department of Health (2004) *National Service Framework for Children, Young People and Maternity Services.* London: DoH.

Eaton, N. (2000) Children's community nursing services: Models of care delivery. A review of the United Kingdom literature, *Journal of Advanced Nursing* 32 (1), July, p. 49–56.

Eaton, N. (2001) Models of community children's nursing. *Paediatric Nursing* 13 (1), February, pp. 32–6.

Eiser, C. (1990) *Chronic Childhood Disease: An Introduction to Psychological Theory and Research.* Cambridge: Cambridge University Press.

Eiser, C. (1993) *Growing up with a chronic disease; the Impact on Children and their Families.* London: Kingsley.

Escolme, D., James, C. (2004) Assessing respite provision; The Leeds Nursing Dependency Score. *Paediatric Nursing* 16 (2), March, pp. 27–30.

Esmonde, G. (2000) Cystic fibrosis: Adolescent care, *Nursing Standard* 14 (52), 13 September, pp. 47–52, pp. 54–5, 57.

Fisher, H. (2001) The needs of parents with chronically sick children: A literature review. *Journal of Advanced Nursing* 36 (4), November, pp. 600–7.

Flatman, D. (2002) Consulting children: Are we listening? *Paediatric Nursing* 14 (7), September, pp. 28–30.

Fleming, E., Carter, B., Gillibrand, W. (2002) The transition of adolescents with diabetes from the children's health care service into the adult health care service: A review of the literature. *Journal of Clinical Nursing* 11 (50), September, pp. 560–7.

Foster, C., Eiser, C., Oades, P., Sheldon, C., Tripp, J., Goodman, P., Rice, S., Trott, J. (2001) Treatment demands and differential treatment of patients with cystic fibrosis and their siblings: patient, parent and sibling accounts. *Child: Care, Health and Development*, 27 (4), July, p. 349–.

Fulton, Y. (1996) Children's rights and the role of the nurse. *Paediatric Nursing* 8, pp. 29–31.

Gibson, C. (1991) A concept analysis of empowerment. *Journal of Advanced Nursing* 16, pp. 354–61.

Hall, S. (1996) An exploration of parental perception of the nature and level of support needed to care for their child with special needs. *Journal of Advanced Nursing* 24 (3), September, pp. 512–21.

Health Committee (1997) *Health Services for Children and Young People in the Community: Home and School*. Third Report London: Stationery Office.

Hodgkinson, R., Lester, H. (2002) 'Stresses and coping strategies of mothers living with a child with cystic fibrosis: Implications for nursing professionals. *Journal of Advanced Nursing* 39 (4), August, pp. 377–83.

Houghton, J. (2004) Diagnosis and management of Type 1 Diabetes, *Paediatric Nursing* 16 (10), December, pp. 22–3.

Kyngas, H. (1999) 'A theoretical model of compliance in young diabetics', *Journal of Clinical Nursing*, 8 (1), January, pp. 73–80.

Kyngas, H., Rissanen, M. (2001) Support as a crucial predictor of good compliance of adolescents with a chronic illness. *Journal of Clinical Nursing* 10 (6), November, pp. 767–73

Lowden, J. (2002) Children's rights: a decade of dispute. *Journal of Advanced Nursing* 37 (1), January, pp. 100–7.

Lowes, L. (1997) Evaluation of a paediatric diabetes specialist nurse post. *British Journal of Nursing* 16 (11), pp. 625–33.

Madge, S. (2002) National consensus standards for nursing children and young people with cystic fibrosis. *Paediatric Nursing* 14 (1), February, pp. 32–5.

Madge, S. et al (2001) *National Consensus Standards for the Nursing Management of Cystic Fibrosis*. London: Cystic Fibrosis Trust.

Marshall, M., Fleming, E., Gillibrand, W., Carter, B. (2002) Adaptation and negotiation as an approach to care in paediatric diabetes specialist nursing practice: A critical review, *Journal of Clinical Nursing* 11 (4), pp. 421–9.

McWilliam, C., Stewart, M., Brown, J., McNair, S., Desai, K., Patterson, N., Del Maestro, N, Pittman, B. (1997) Creating empowering meaning: An interactive process of promoting health with chronically older Canadians. *Health Promotion International* 12 (2), pp. 111–23.

Miller, S. (1996) Transition of care in adolescence. *Paediatric Nursing* 8, November, pp. 14–16.

Miller, S. (2000) Researching children: Issues arising from a phenomenological study with children who have diabetes mellitus. *Journal of Advanced Nursing* 31 (5), May, pp. 1228–34.

Miller, S. (2002) Respite care for children who have complex healthcare needs. *Paediatric Nursing* 14 (5), June, pp. 33–7.

Morris, J. (1998) *Still Missing, vol. 2. The Experience of Disabled Children and Young People Living Away for their Families.* London: The Who Cares Trust.

Muir, J., Dryden, S. (2000) Collaborative planning for children with chronic, complex care needs, in Muir, J., Sidey, A. (eds) *Textbook of Community Children's Nursing.* London: Bailliere Tindall. Chapter 22, pp. 216–32).

Muir, J., Sidey, A. (eds) (2000) *Textbook of Community Children's Nursing.* London: Bailliere Tindall.

National Children's Bureau (1992) http://www.ncb.org.uk (accessed 24 January 2005).

National Health Service Executive (1998) *Evaluation of the Pilot Project Programme for Children with Life Threatening Illnesses.* London: The Stationery Office.

National Institute of Clinical Excellence (2004) *Type 1 Diabetes: Diagnosis and Management of Type 1 Diabetes in Children, Young people and Adults,* Clinical Guideline 15 http://www.nice.org.uk (accessed 24 January 2005).

Nursing and Midwifery Council (2004) *Standards of Proficiency for Pre-registration Nursing Education.* London: NMC.

Olsen, R., Malsin-Prothero, P. (2001) Dilemmas in the provision of own-home respite support for parents of young children with complex health needs: Evidence from an evaluation. *Journal of Advanced Nursing* 34 (5), June, pp. 603–10.

Pillitteri, A. (1999) *Child Health Nursing: Care of the Child and Family.* Philadelphia: Lippincott.

Proctor, S., Campbell, S., Biott, C., Edward, S., Redpath, N., Moran, M. (1999) *Preparation for the Developing Role of the Community Children's Nurse,* Research Support Series Number 11. London: English National Board.

Rosen, D. (1994) Transition from paediatric to adult-orientated health care for adolescents with chronic illness or disability. *Adolescent Medicine* 5 (2), pp. 241–8.

Ross, A., Parkes, J. (2004) Making doors open; Caring for families with severe cerebral palsy. *Paediatric Nursing* 16 (5), pp. 14–18.

Royal College of Nursing (2004) *Adolescent Transition Care.* London: Royal College of Nursing.

Rudolf, M. C. G., Levene, M. I. (1999) *Paediatrics and Child Health.* Oxford: Blackwell Science.

Samwell, B. (2000) Creating an effective community children's nursing service in Muir.J., Sidey, A. (eds) *Textbook of Community Children's Nursing.* London: Bailliere Tindall, Chapter 32, pp. 295–302.

Sartain, S., Clarke, C., Heyman, R. (2000) Hearing the voices of children with chronic illness. *Journal of Advanced Nursing* 32 (4), pp. 913–21.

Smith, L. (2002) Negotiation of care, in Smith, L., Coleman, V., Bradshaw, M. (eds) *Family Centred-Care: Concept, Theory and Practice*. Basingstoke: Palgrave, Chapter 6, pp. 114–30.

Smith, L., Coleman, V., Bradshaw, M. (eds) (2002) *Family Centred-Care: Concept, Theory and Practice*. Basingstoke: Palgrave.

Smithies, J. (1998) *Pulling it all together in empowerment, participation and health: Involving children and their carers*, Report of National Seminar, 3 April, London: Save the Children.

Stewart, K., Dearmun, A. (2001) Adherence to health advice amongst young people with chronic illness. *Journal of Child Health* 5 (4), Winter, pp. 155–62.

Treneman, M., Corkery, A., Dowdney, L., Hammond, J. (1997) Respite care needs-met and unmet: Assessment of needs for children with disability, *Developmental Medicine and Child Neurology* 39 (8), pp. 548–59.

United Nations (1989) *Convention on the Rights of the Child, United Nations* cited in Newall, P. (1993) *The UN Convention and Children's Rights in the UK*, 2nd edn. London: National Children's Bureau.

Viner, R. (1999) Transition from paediatric to adult care, Bridging the gaps or passing the buck? *Archives of Diseases in Childhood* 81, pp. 271–5.

Viner, R., Keane, M. (1998) *Youth Matters: Evidence-Based Best Practice for People in Hospital*. London: Caring for Children in the Health Services/Action for Sick Children.

Warner, H. (2000) Making the invisible, visible. *Journal of Child Health Care* 4 (3), Autumn, pp. 123–6.

WHO (1998) Health 21: An Introduction to the Health For All Policy Framework for the WHO European Region, European Health For All Series, No 5. Copenhagen: WHO.

Winter, A., Teale, J. (1997) Construction and application of paediatric community nursing services. *Journal of Child Health* 1, pp. 24–9.

Continuing Professional Development in Children's Nursing

12

Valerie Coleman and Maureen Bradshaw

Learning outcomes

- Demonstrate understanding of the Nursing and Midwifery Council Code of Professional Conduct 2004 and its application in contemporary children's and young people's nursing practice.
- Discuss team working (including inter-professional working) and leadership.
- Demonstrate your understanding of decision-making processes.
- Explain the change process and how you would use it to manage change to promote quality care in practice.
- Explore the role of the mentor.
- Develop a Personal Development Plan acknowledging the role of clinical supervision in lifelong learning.

Introduction

This chapter focuses on continuing professional development for children's nurses in order to promote fitness for practice on initial registration, and lifelong learning.

Continuing professional development is:

A process of lifelong learning for all individuals and teams which meets the needs of patients and delivers the health outcomes and healthcare priorities of the NHS and which enables professionals to expand and fulfill their potential. (Department of Health 1999, p. 2)

Clinical supervision is an integral part of lifelong learning for nurses because it can help to develop skills and knowledge throughout their careers (Nursing and Midwifery Council 2002). It is a practice focused professional relationship to enable nurses to reflect on their practice with the guidance of an appropriate skilled supervisor. The Nursing and Midwifery Council (2002) does not support a specific model of clinical supervision, instead it identifies a defined set of principles that should be developed at a local level to meet local needs. In preparation for your future nursing careers you should find out how clinical supervision is developed in your local area and read the fixed resource sessions for Trigger 12.3 about this subject.

It is likely that at the point of registration, to be a children's nurse, individuals may well be anxious about whether they are 'fit for practice' in the role of a qualified nurse and will be fully exploiting learning opportunities on their final clinical placements. There is likely to be a keenness to ensure that clinical skills have been learnt for safe practice and also that other skills for 'managing' are developed. An awareness of professional accountability in relation to the Nursing and Midwifery Code of Professional Conduct (NMC 2004) needs to be present as well. It is suggested that this may be the time for you to review this code and discuss the implications of it for practice in your role as a registered children's nurse.

Many professional issues impact on the practice of children and young people's nursing and child health care, and individual practitioners should be aware of these. *The National Service Framework for Children, Young People and Maternity Care* (Department of Health 2004; Welsh Assembly 2004), for example, has been referred to throughout this book. The implementation of the standards in this *National Service Framework* are likely to be a key feature of child health care and nursing for several years to come. Therefore familiarity with this policy is essential to be able to function effectively in contemporary children's and young people's nursing practice, providing a high standard of care.

Problem-based learning is an approach that helps to develop transferable key skills, such as problem solving, self-enquiry and communication, for engagement in lifelong learning. Throughout this book a problem-based learning approach has been used to facilitate the development of skills for lifelong learning.

The triggers in this chapter provide further opportunities to develop these skills with an emphasis on professional accountability, leadership and team working (including inter-professional working), mentorship, personal development and clinical supervision.

❗ Trigger 12.1: Leading and Managing in Practice

This trigger is intended to encourage you to develop your leadership and management skills.

The Trigger

An extract from Student Nurse Emily Jakes' Learning Diary:

Tuesday 8th

That was a really good day. I was really anxious about it, but I feel much more confidant about 'managing' now. I had to do it because it is only a few weeks until I qualify (hopefully!). Then off course there was the Standard of Proficiency, about managing 'Manage oneself, one's practice and that of others in accordance with the Nursing and Midwifery Council's Code of Professional Conduct, recognising one's own abilities and limitations' that I have to achieve to pass my course and go on the Nursing and Midwifery Council Professional Register. Jenny my mentor was really supportive and she said that I already had management skills and we had already worked together managing throughout my placement. Today I would just be using the skills I have already developed to look after more patients with her supervision and anyway nobody knows everything in managing 'one of the most important things is to know who to ask'.

The whole day seemed to be about making decisions including allocating staff to look after individual children, working out break times, prioritising work and dealing with unexpected events like one staff nurse going off sick, a complaining father and the 3 year old brother of a new admission fell over and banged his head.

I couldn't believe it 'me being in charge' delegating, leading the team, although Jenny was always there and communicating with the multi-disciplinary team. The children got their nursing care all right, so my organisation must have been OK. I was pleased also because it's a difficult time on the ward, the staff are changing to work 12-hour shifts and it's not a popular change with everyone. Jenny, my mentor says that there is always change happening.

Situation

Student Nurse Emily Jakes is a third year nurse undertaking the final clinical placement of her child branch course on a children's medical ward. Students sometimes refer to this to as 'the management placement' because it is the last one. Students are required to achieve specific Standards of Proficiencies that demonstrate their ability to manage. To successfully complete the child branch programme these standards of proficiency and others have to be achieved for entry to the Nursing and Midwifery Council Professional Register. Therefore Emily has negotiated the learning opportunity described in her diary extract.

Feedback

Emily has to write a reflective account for her portfolio about an aspect of this 'management experience'. She has chosen to write about team working, inter-professional working and leadership. She will review the notes that she made about management taken on her study days because she now realises that you use so many different skills to manage and that they are inter-linked. It is suggested that you write a reflective account based on your own experience of 'managing'.

The facts

> What are the main facts in this trigger? Make a list.

Hypotheses: What may these facts mean?

- Student nurses have to be proficient to be entered on the Nursing and Midwifery Council Professional Register.
- Management skills develop throughout a nursing course.
- Managing involves making decisions.
- Team leadership includes delegating staff, prioritising work and communicating with the multi-disciplinary team.
- Leaders have to deal with unexpected events as well as planned ones.
- Change is a common occurrence in the healthcare services.

Questions developed from the hypotheses:

1. How is proficiency defined in terms of the NMC?
2. What processes are involved in decision-making?
3. What effect does a leader have on a team and their work?
4. What is the nurse's role in implementing and managing change?

The answers to these questions should inform the written reflective account.

Trigger 12.1: Fixed resource material

Read the following to help you answer the questions. (You may also wish to search and review other up-to-date research and evidence-based literature and seek other relevant resources to provide you with answers to your questions.)

Bernhard, L., Walsh, M. (1995) *Leadership: The Key to the Professionalization of Nursing*, 3rd edn. St Louis: Mosby.

Broome, A. (1998) *Managing Change*, 2nd edn. Basingstoke: Macmillan.

Buckingham, C., Adams, A. (2000) Classifying clinical decision making: interpreting nursing intuition, heuristics and medical diagnosis. *Journal of Advanced Nursing* 32 (4), October, pp. 990–8.

Dowding, L., Barr, J. (2002) *Managing in Health Care: A Guide for Nurses, Midwives and Health Visitors*. London: Prentice Hall.

Marriner-Tomey, A. (2000) *Guide to Nursing Management and Leadership*, 6th edn. St Louis: Mosby.

Thompson, C., Dowding, D. (eds) (2002) *Clinical Decision Making and Judgement in Nursing*. Edinburgh: Churchill Livingstone.

Trigger 12.1: Fixed resource sessions

Nursing and Midwifery Council Standards of Proficiency for entry to the Branch Programmes and the Professional Register

The Nursing and Midwifery Council is the regulatory body for nursing. The Nursing and Midwifery Council has previously used the term competency to describe: 'The skills and ability to practice safely and effectively without the need for direct supervision' (United Kingdom Central Council 1999, p. 38). These competencies following consultation have been adopted as Standards of Proficiency by the Nursing and Midwifery Council. Students on a 3 year pre-registration nursing programme in the United Kingdom are required to achieve the Standards of Proficiency that have been established by the Nursing and Midwifery Council. 'The standards define the overarching principles of being able to practice as a nurse; the context in which they are achieved defines the scope of professional practice' (Nursing and Midwifery Council 2004a, p. 4).

Students are required to achieve the first year outcomes (Table 12.1) to proceed on to one of the four branch programmes: adult; children's; mental health; learning disability. To be entered on to the different parts of the Nursing and Midwifery Council Professional Register students have to achieve the branch Standards of Proficiency (Table 12.2), to demonstrate that they are proficient to practice as registered nurses in respect of the branch programme undertaken. All nurses, midwives and specialist community public health nurses who wish to practice in the United Kingdom must be on the Nursing and Midwifery Council Professional Register.

The Standard of Proficiency statements are listed under four domains as follows:

- Professional and ethical practice.
- Care delivery.

- Care management.
- Personal and professional development.

Table 12.1 Nursing and Midwifery Council Standards of Proficiency for entry to the Branch Programme

1. Professional and ethical practice
1.1   Discuss in an informed manner the implications of professional regulation for nursing practice.
1.2   Demonstrate an awareness of the Nursing and Midwifery Council Code of Professional Conduct: standard for conduct, performance and ethics.
1.3   Demonstrate an awareness of, and apply ethical principles to nursing practice.
1.4   Demonstrate an awareness of legislation relevant to nursing practice.
1.5   Demonstrate the importance of promoting equity in patient and client care by contributing to nursing care in a fair and anti-discriminatory way.

2. Care delivery
2.1   Discuss methods of, barriers to, and the boundaries of, effective communication and interpersonal relationships.
2.2   Demonstrate sensitivity when interacting with and providing information to patients and clients.
2.3   Contribute to enhancing the health and social well being of patients/clients by understanding how to; assess health needs; identify opportunities for health promotion; and identify networks of health and social care services.
2.4   Contribute to the development and documentation of nursing assessments by participating in comprehensive and systematic nursing assessment of the physical, psychological, social and spiritual needs of patients/clients.
2.5   Contribute to the planning of nursing care, involving patients/clients and where possible carers, demonstrating an understanding of helping patients/clients to make informed decisions.
2.6   Contribute to the implementation of a programme of nursing care, designed and supervised by registered practitioners.
2.7   Demonstrate evidence of a developing knowledge base that underpins safe and effective nursing practice.
2.8   Demonstrate a range of essential nursing skills, under the supervision of a registered nurse, to meet individuals' needs, which include: maintaining dignity; privacy and confidentiality; effective observational and communication skills, including listening and taking physiological measurements, safety and health, including moving and handling and infection control; essential first aid and emergency procedures; administration of medicines; emotional, physical and personal care, including meeting the need for comfort, nutrition and personal hygiene.
2.9   Contribute to the evaluation of the appropriateness of nursing care delivered.
2.10 Recognise situations in which agreed plans of nursing care no longer appear appropriate and refer these to an appropriate accountable practitioner.

3. Care management
3.1   Contribute to the identification of actual and potential risks to patients/clients and their carers, to oneself and to others and participate in measures to promote and

ensure health and safety.

3.2 Demonstrate an understanding of the role of others by participating in inter-professional working practice.

3.3 Demonstrate literacy, numeracy and computer skills needed to record, enter, store, retrieve and organise data essential for care delivery.

4. Personal and professional development

4.1 Demonstrate responsibility for one's own learning through the development of a portfolio of practice and recognise when further learning is required.

4.2 Acknowledge the importance of seeking supervision to develop safe and effective nursing practice.

Source: NMC (2004a): © Nursing and Midwifery Council

Table 12.2 Nursing and Midwifery Council Standards of Proficiency for the entry to the Professional Register

1. Professional and ethical practice

1.1 Manage oneself, one's practice and that of others in accordance with the Nursing and Midwifery Council's Code of Professional Conduct: standards for conduct, performance and ethics, recognising one's own abilities and limitations.

1.2 Practice in accordance with an ethical and legal framework, which ensures the primacy of patient and client interest and well-being and respects confidentiality.

1.3 Practice in a fair and anti discriminatory way, acknowledging the differences in beliefs and cultural practices of individuals or groups.

2. Care delivery

2.1 Engage in, develop, and disengage from therapeutic relationships through the use of appropriate communication and interpersonal skills.

2.2 Create and utilise opportunities to promote health and well being of patients, clients and groups.

2.3 Undertake and document a comprehensive, systematic and accurate nursing assessment of the physical, psychological, social and spiritual needs of patients, clients and communities.

2.4 Formulate and document a plan of nursing care, where possible in partnership with patients, clients, their carers and family and friends, within a framework of informed consent.

2.5 Based on the best available evidence, apply knowledge and an appropriate repertoire of skills indicative of safe and effective nursing practice.

2.6 Provide a rationale for the nursing care delivered which takes account of social, cultural, spiritual, legal, political and economic influences.

2.7 Evaluate and document the outcomes of nursing and other Interventions.

2.8 Demonstrate sound clinical judgement across a range of differing professional and care delivery contexts.

3. Care management

3.1 Contribute to public protection by creating and maintaining a safe environment of care through the use of quality assurance and risk management strategies.

3.2   Demonstrate knowledge of effective inter-professional working practices, which respect and utilise the contributions of members of the health and social care team.

3.3   Delegate duties to others as appropriate, ensuring that they are supervised and monitored.

3.4   Demonstrate key skills.

4. Personal and professional development

4.1   Demonstrates a commitment to the need for continuing professional development and personal supervision activities in order to enhance knowledge skills, values, attitudes needed for safe and effective nursing practice.

4.2   Enhance the professional development and safe practice of others through peer support, leadership, supervision and teaching.

Source: Nursing and Midwifery Council (2004a) © Nursing and Midwifery Council

Decision-making

decision-making is associated with problem solving, but it is a much broader concept. It involves deciding on a particular option to problem solve. Decision-making is a process that can be complex. A right decision is not always made because it depends on the position from which you are looking at the problem and what you want to achieve from the situation. The decisions taken in clinical practice may be personal, clinical and managerial.

Suggested Activity

Reflect on a personal or professional decision that you have taken recently

- What type of processes did you use to make this decision?
- Identify sources of evidence/information that you used to inform your decision.

Approaches to decision-making

Nurses use prescriptive and descriptive approaches to decision-making approaches in practice. The prescriptive approach focuses on the outcome of the decision and it is grounded in the application of systematic, scientific reasoning. This approach may be used to select the best intervention or treatment option.

The descriptive approach is concerned with the processes of decision-making. Both formal and informal knowledge play a part in the decision-making process in the descriptive approach. Benner (1984) particularly in relation to decision-making along a continuum from a novice to expert practitioner is associated with the study of intuition and experience in nursing practice.

Clinical decision-making has been reduced to certain types of reasoning, which have then become associated with particular professional groups (Buckingham and Adams 2000). Therefore, traditionally a doctor has tended to use rational scientific reasoning and conversely a nurse used intuition in decision-making. There may be a switching from one type of reasoning to another though in both professional groups in contemporary practice. Hamm (1988) suggests that rational scientific reasoning and creative intuitive reasoning could be seen as both ends of a continuum with decision-making occurring at some point along that curriculum. These differences in reasoning have been instilled through individual professional education. However, all decision-making is based on the same cognitive functions that both professions share. If this shared system of cognition is acknowledged, differences can be respected and multi-professional collaboration facilitated (Buckingham and Adams 2000). The move towards inter-professional education in modern health and social care has the potential to promote this collaboration.

Inter-professional education is:

Informal and formal opportunities for members of two or more professions to learn with and from each other, involving patients/users of health and social care where possible with the aims of improving the effectiveness of care delivery and increasing collaborative practice. (United Kingdom Central Council 2001, p. 33)

Inter-professional education has the potential to break down traditional professional boundaries to facilitate cross boundary working, which improves the quality of care to children, young people and families (Bradshaw et al 2003). A wide range of professional knowledge may be used in decision-making using problem-solving approaches when professionals work collaboratively together (Miller 1999).

Decision-making process

Marriner-Tomey (2000) states that the decision-making process is a systematic process that is not unlike the nursing process. It involves:

1. Identifying the problem and analysing the situation;
2. Exploring the alternatives;
3. Choosing the most desirable alternative;
4. Implementing the decision; and
5. Evaluating the results.

There are various decision-making models that follow a similar framework to the one offered by Marriner-Tomey (2000).

Identifying the problem

Several factors including; past experiences, education, professional issues in the work setting, control issues, ambiguity, and level of personal involvement identify the problem in the first place (Walton 1995). The steps taken to resolve an identified problem are dependant upon factors such as the importance of the problem, risk issues and urgency of response required, alongside external pressures and constraints (Walton 1995).

Analysing the problem

Different people may interpret the same facts differently, for example, different managers may interpret the reasons for resistance to the change to 12-hour working shifts on Emily's clinical placement differently. This is problematic because different diagnoses of the rationale for resistance to 12-hour shifts will lead to different decisions being taken to address the problem. Frameworks and guidelines may be used to clarify what is going on to help the decision-making. A problem analysis grid is offered by Walton (1995), which has the potential to provide a complete picture of a situation for decision-making. This grid comprises several boxes headed up by the questions concerned with 'what, where, when, whom, and size' in relation to the problem with the question 'why' being asked about all the answers given. An example from the grid is:

What:
- What is the problem?
- What isn't the problem?
- What are the problem's distinctive features?

Suggested Activity

The purpose of the grid is to make you think more broadly about difficulties and problems you may encounter.

- Think of a situation that you could explore using a problem analysis grid and use it.
- You do not have to put an answer in every box, but look at all the questions to clarify the chosen situation that is a problem.

Categorising issues and concerns

Walton (1995) suggests that the following are possible categories that may emerge from a problem analysis:

- The same people are always involved.
- The same department, ward or professional group emerge.
- The same professions, for example nurses or pathologists are involved.
- Repeating operational issues such as procedures/budgets/resources.

If there are no repetitive issues arising you need to look deeper below the surface. Blake and Mounton (1976) suggest that differences and conflicts may be about: power or authority; morale or cohesion; standards or norms; or goals or objectives.

Information to use in decision-making may include

- Policies;
- Protocols;
- Procedures
- Research studies;
- Codes of professional conduct;
- Evidence-based literature;
- Charters;
- Information technology;
- Ethical guidelines;

Emily would have used some of these sources of information to inform the decisions that she made with the supervision of her mentor during her shift as team leader. Her learning diary extract identified that she had to make decisions for example about dealing with unexpected events like one staff nurse going off sick, a complaining father and the 3 year old brother of a new admission who fell over and banged his head. There would be policies and procedures available that could be implemented to help with decision-making for all these issues.

The Change Process

Change has a powerful impact on people (Broome 1998) and it may be destabilising (Upton and Brookes 1995). Destabilisation seemed to be happening in Emily's clinical placement area in relation to the staff changing to working 12-hour shifts, because it was 'not a popular change with everyone'. This shift change may be causing cognitive dissonance; conflict between an individual's behaviour and attitudes (Bernhard and Walsh 1995). The staff will change their behaviour to comply with the managerial decision to work these new shifts, but their attitude towards the change is not favourable and this may cause resistance.

Change is:

> An attempt to alter or replace existing knowledge, skills, attitudes, norms and styles of individuals and groups, which involves the discontinuity of past behaviors and the perceptions of that discontinuity held by both individuals and groups. (Wright, 1989 p. 6)

Change will affect all those that are involved with it, often provoking fear, worry and anxiety (Walton 1995) regardless of whether it is viewed as a positive or negative change in practice. Negatively perceived changes are more likely to result in people moving through three stages associated with the change process; shock and detachment; defensive retreat and confusion; acknowledgement and adaptation (Broome 1998).

In Emily's diary extract she mentioned that her mentor stated that there were always changes happening in the health care services. Curtis and White (2002) would support this view articulating that nurses work in a rapidly changing work environment and that they need to be knowledgeable and skilled facilitators of the change process. Hence the need for this fixed resource session with its aim of providing this knowledge for skilled facilitation of change.

There are many drivers for change within the National Health Service, including the *National Service Framework for Children, Young People and Maternity Care* (Department of Health 2004; Welsh Assembly 2004), which sets out clear national quality standards to be met, that are likely to result in changes in the patterns of local service delivery (Scott 2001). One tool for assessing the scope of change is 'PEST'; political, economic, social, technological. This tool demonstrates the areas for change and can be used to identify the broad national issues driving change that impact at local levels (Upton and Brookes 1995).

Change that is planned according to Bennis et al (1976) is a conscious, deliberate and collaborative effort to improve practice utilising evidence-based knowledge. Conversely unplanned change is likely to prove less successful in the long term because it lacks clear purpose or goals. Change may be imposed from outside an organisation or alternatively it may be internally generated. Walton (1995) identifies that internally generated change is usually viewed more positively than change that is externally imposed, which causes greater resistance.

Change occurs due to innovation that involves the introduction of new ideas, methods or devices such as policies, procedures and equipment (Wright 1989). Social change, such as a change to 12-hour shift working patterns and other ones that are very different from established traditions in nursing practice create resistance from staff. There is less resistance to change created by the introduction of technological innovations (Bernhard and Walsh 1995) that will improve the care of children and families and also save time for nurses.

Suggested Activity

Reflect on your own experience of innovation and change in practice:

- What innovations have you seen implemented?
- Were they social or technological innovations?
- Distinguish between unplanned and planned change that you have been involved in?

I What were the effects of these changes on yourself and colleagues?

Change as a Systematic Process

To facilitate this process an internal or external change agent may be allocated (or alternatively emerge informally) in the situation where the change is to be introduced. The change agent is integral to the process because of his/her role in changing the knowledge, attitudes and behaviour of the staff. An effective change agent is a problem-seeker, problem-solver, innovator and a leader (Dowding and Barr 2002). To do this effectively the change agent has to develop good working relationships with all the nursing staff involved in the change so that everyone is clear about what is expected of them during the change process (Bernhard and Walsh 1995).

The use of a model of change should be used throughout the systematic process of change. The Lewin (1951) Model of Change is one such model.

The model comprises three stages:

- Stage One is *Unfreezing*: it involves identification of problems and forces that need to be addressed to be able to move through the change process. It involves changing attitudes, behaviours and creating feelings of ownership for the individuals or groups involved.
- Stage Two is *Change*: this occurs during the implementation stage when strategies are used to bring about change.
- Stage Three is *Refreezing*: this is about stabilising the change as a permanent position.

> ### Suggested Activity
> - What do you think about this model?
> - What other models of change are there?

Assessment

Proposed innovations ideally should be assessed to determine their likely implementation success, prior to implementing the change process. This is because some innovations are more acceptable than others. The attributes identified by Roger and Shoemaker (1971) may be used to assess an innovation. These attributes are:

- *Relative advantage*: will this innovation result in an improvement compared to maintaining the status quo?
- *Compatibility*: does the proposed innovation for change match up with the existing ethos and values of the staff?
- *Communicability*: how easily is it to articulate the need for change and for it to be understood?

- *Simplicity*: can the change be easily implemented?
- *Trialability*: what is the potential for piloting the innovation on either a small or large scale?
- *Observability*: would the benefits of the innovation be observable?
- *Relevance*: will the change be seen as meaningful?

A scale (1–5) devised by the English National Board (1987) may be used to determine the likelihood of an innovation being adopted or not. Innovations are assessed for each attribute on the 1–5 scale and those with an overall score of 21 or less are unlikely to be adopted.

If the innovation is to be adopted the change agent during the assessment stage needs to identify the existing strengths and/or weaknesses of the nursing staff to determine how these may be best used or developed for a successful change. Roger and Shoemaker (1971) developed a continuum of behaviours of individual's responses to change. It ranges from those who reject change preferring to maintain the status quo to those who welcome change. The continuum is shown in Figure 12.1.

Change (Progressivism)

Innovator
↓
Early Adopter
↓
Early Majority
↓
Later Majority
↓
Laggards
↓
Rejecters

Status Quo (Traditionalism)

Figure 12.1   Continuum of behaviour in response to change

Planning

In the planning stage the change agent has to identify progressive individuals in order to use their support in bringing about the change. The rejecters need to be identified so that negative reactions to the change may be contained. Time scales for change also need to be planned, however, these will vary dependent on the nature of the change.

The force field analysis of Lewin (1951) can be used in the process of planning change. This analysis identifies areas for action so that forces driving against change may be weakened and forces driving to support the change may be strengthened.

Implementation

Chin and Benne (1976) describe three change strategies:

1. *The Power-coercive Strategy*: This is based on the assumption that people with less power will always comply with the plans of those with more power. This strategy can cause cognitive dissonance and conflict, which may be the situation on Emily's ward with the change to 12-hour working shifts.
2. *The Rationale-empirical Strategy*: This is based on the assumption that people are rational and will act according to self-interest. Therefore people will change their behaviour providing that they can see the benefit in doing so. Research recommendations are often associated with this strategy with regard to implementing them in practice to bring about change.
3. *The Normative re-educative Strategy*: This is based on the assumption that the people concerned are, and need to be, involved with all aspects of the change process, including the impetus for change in the first place to it's eventual implementation. A sense of ownership of a proposed change through being actively involved in the process throughout is often seen as vital for success (English National Board 1987).

The power-coercive and rationale-empirical strategies are top-down approaches to change. Those in positions of power will identify the need for change, the focus of change, the implementation and evaluation of change.

The normative re-educative strategy, conversely, is a bottom-up approach, which is reliant upon an individual's or group's perceptions of the need for change and their own desire to implement it in their daily nursing practice. Similarly, a six-step process of managing change identified by Teasdale (1992) also stresses the importance of involving staff and enabling them to develop as change is implemented.

An eclectic strategy for change that combines elements of all three of the strategies described by Chin and Benne (1976) is often adopted to be responsive to the needs of individuals and groups at different points in the change process.

Evaluation

This should be ongoing with the change agent responding to individual's and group concerns, demonstrating a willingness to listen and to overcome problems.

Resistance to the proposed change should be identified in the ongoing evaluation process and strategies to handle it developed. Resistance factors have to be addressed to prevent the change process being undermined. Clarke (1994) listed seven major resistance factors; loss of control; questioning about why change; uncertainty and ambiguity; unexpected surprises; loss of face; fear of not coping; and more work.

An evaluation process as a final outcome will identify when the change is fully adopted by the individual or group and 'frozen' into practice.

Change in the current health service is a constant feature. For change to be lasting it needs to be planned and the process of implementation carefully managed (Department of Health 2002).

→ Trigger 12.1: Feedback

Go to Chapter 12 trigger feedback on p. 414

! Trigger 12.2: Mentorship and Assessment

This trigger is intended to facilitate learning about mentorship and assessment in clinical practice.

The Trigger

Jenny is the mentor of these two student nurses. She is responsible for completing their assessment of practice.

Student 1

Student nurse Tina Jones is a child branch student on your ward for four weeks. It is her first placement in the branch programme. She is keen to be involved in all aspects of care on the ward. She is very friendly with everyone; staff, children and parents alike. In fact she is so busy trying to see, meet and do everything that you wonder how much she is actually taking in.

Student 2

Student nurse Jack Dean is in the common foundation part of the course. He is on your ward for a four week child placement, but will be following the adult branch programme. He has had three days off sick so far, so time together has been limited. You are however receiving feedback from colleagues that he appears lazy and disinterested.

Situation

Jenny is mentor to the two student nurses identified in the trigger. She is supporting them and developing their knowledge and understanding of the nursing care required by children, young people and families on the children's ward. Jenny provides learning opportunities to enable to them to develop practical nursing skills that are appropriate to meet their individual needs and to pass the assessment of practice.

Feedback

Write a short account about:

- How might mentorship progress for these students?
- How would you enable these students to maximise their placement experiences?
- What approach would you take to mentoring these students?

The facts

What are the main facts? Make a list:

Hypotheses. What may these facts mean?

- Student nurses from different years work on children's wards.
- Mentors receive feedback from colleagues about the progress of students that they are responsible for.
- Student nurses may present challenges to the mentor.
- Mentors assess student nurses in practice.

Questions developed from the hypotheses

1. How might mentorship progress for these students?
2. How would you enable these students to maximise their placement experiences?
3. What approach would you take to mentoring these students?

Trigger 12.2: Fixed resource material

Read the following to help you answer the questions. (You may also wish to search and review other up-to-date research and evidence-based literature and seek other relevant resources to provide you with answers to your questions.)

Nursing and Midwifery Council (2003) *NMC Requirements for Mentors and Mentorship*, QA Factsheet 0/2003. http://www.nmc-uk.org (accessed January 2005)

Stuart, C. C. (2003) *Assessment, Supervision and Support in Clinical Practice: A Guide for Nurses and Midwives*. Edinburgh: Churchill Livingstone.

Trigger 12.2: Fixed resource sessions

Mentor's role

The *Concise Oxford English Dictionary* (2004, p. 833) describes a mentor as an 'experienced and trusted advisor . . . in an organisation or institution who trains and counsels new employees or students'. Rogers (2001) talks about mentorship in terms of the accumulated wisdom of a senior person being made available to someone junior, but suggests that it is most powerful when combined with a coaching approach, which aims to release the student's own resourcefulness in order to progress to the next level of effectiveness.

In a nurse education context the mentor will be a registered nurse with the equivalent of one years full time qualified experience (Nursing and Midwifery Council 2003). New mentors should have successfully completed a mentorship programme, and thereafter receive support from both experienced practitioners and nurse teachers when performing their mentorship role. Regular opportunities then need to be provided for mentors to update their mentoring knowledge and skills on a regular basis (United Kingdom Central Council 1999).

Mentors are often described as 'role models' with the idea that they accurately represent the knowledge, skills and attitudes that professional nursing comprises. Students can observe, capture and aspire to emulate these professional requisites by 'modelling' themselves on their mentor. Darling (1984) sees mentors as energisers and envisioners who enthusiastically kindle student's interest, thus helping them to catch the vision and hold the dream containing all the possibilities and opportunities that nursing encapsulates. Stuart (2003) points out that mentors require a mixture of both personal and professional attributes in order to fulfil their mentoring role successfully. These include the attitude of being genuinely interested in and respectful towards the student, and demonstrating good interpersonal skills, which among other things signal the mentor's approachability to the student. A mentor who is a self-confident, competent and enthusiastic practitioner will have much to contribute to the student's learning environment and experience.

Student's evaluative comments indicate that when they start on a new ward placement, they require the mentor to be someone who looks out for them, helps them settle into the culture of the new learning environment, and shows them the ropes. Students feel safe when the required standards are made clear to them. They are spurred on by accurate feedback, praise and encouragement from mentors. At the end of the day, students want to feel useful, that they belong; that they've made a worthwhile contribution in terms of patient care and team effort, and that personal growth has taken place through a variety of learning opportunities offered to them by their mentor.

Although students are responsible for their own learning, mentors have much influence on enhancing the learning process when they invest time and effort in their relationship with the student. While there may be an element of mentors 'taking students by the hand' to lead them through new learning experiences initially, mentors have to develop skill in assessing what has been learnt under supervision and then trusting students to do appropriately delegated care on their own. As mentors encourage students to 'fly on their own', that experience can still be deepened by next exposing students to increasingly complex situations where their problem-solving and critical, analytical thinking skills can be further developed through examining and discussing the theory and evidence that relates to clinical practice.

Mentors have a lot of nursing expertise to share with students but it is important in mentorship terms that mentors are not seen and used as *the* expert because mentorship is about the *process* of coaching not the subject. Mentors can't possibly be the fount of all knowledge that the student can drink from at will, and indeed if this was the case then Marton and Säljö (1984) would argue that this tends to lead to surface rather than deep learning taking place. Instead mentors use risk assessment and discernment skills to decide when it is appropriate to show or instruct students exactly what to do and when it is safe to simply open doors for students to find out for themselves.

As well as being a rewarding activity, mentoring can include numerous challenges as students with their unique strengths and weaknesses are supported and counselled towards successful achievements in their clinical placements. Mentors who successfully grapple with this challenging aspect of their own professional role, gain satisfaction from knowing that they have been instrumental in opening doors to rich learning experiences for students, and that student eyes have been further opened to appreciate an even bigger picture of what professional nursing comprises.

Assessment

Part of a mentor's responsibility is continuous assessment of the performance of their students. The Nursing and Midwifery Council (2004a) has laid down the standards of proficiency that the student is required to fulfil for entry to the Branch Programme and for entry to the Professional Register. Currently students are assessed in four 'domains' (spheres of activity) comprising: Professional and ethical practice; Care delivery; Care management; and Personal and professional development. These domains are further broken down into outcomes that students are required to demonstrate competence in at the required level at the end of the Common Foundation Programme and the Branch Programme (see Tables 12.1 and 12.2).

These requirements and how they might be achieved, form the basis of the initial interview between student and mentor preferably on the first day (but certainly within the first week) of placement. After reflecting on any previous clinical assessments, students may wish to discuss strengths and weaknesses highlighted therein with their new placement mentor. These can be used to influence the action planning process where student and mentor consider the learning opportunities offered by the placement that will assist students to gain relevant experience leading to the demonstration of competence in all four domains.

Throughout the placement there is opportunity for formative reviews of student progress to take place (e.g., fortnightly), however the mid-placement review requires formal documentation to give clear feedback to students regarding their progress with each learning outcome. New action plans can be formulated at this stage for different learning outcomes. For those where strengths are already being displayed the mentor may for example discuss plans to expose students to more complex care situations for experience enrichment. The mentor will need to show evidence for judging certain areas of the student's practice to be weak or demonstrating little progress. Discussion will need to be opened up so that the student's perspective on areas of struggle can be appreciated. As part of their normal support role for mentors, senior nurses or clinical link teachers may also be involved in such discussions and the setting of appropriate action plans to help the student achieve competence in the highlighted areas by the end of the placement. It is then only fair to ensure further feedback for students on their progress (or lack of it) before the final summative assessment of clinical practice takes place during the final week of the placement. Hopefully by this time previous areas of weakness will have been strengthened sufficiently to demonstrate competence. If this is not the case mentors must not be frightened of failing students.

Duffy (2004) reveals a number of reasons why mentors do not fail incompetent students and instead give them the 'benefit of the doubt'. These include: believing it to be uncaring, believing students will improve thus picking up the required skills in future placements, and not wishing to jeopardise the future of senior students approaching registration. Regardless of the reasons however, the consequences are serious in terms of patients, the students themselves, future mentors and the nursing profession. Duffy (2004, p. 9) emphasises that 'passing students who should have failed does not protect the interests of the public and puts the patients who will be under their care at risk.' This clearly has to be considered from a professional stance but if mentors are not confident to fail incompetent students, then perhaps considering more personal scenarios may assist in ramming the point home. Consider this. If you as a mentor pass an incompetent student, in reality this means that you have no objection to having him or her back on your ward as a staff nurse and trusted professional colleague. Your actions also imply that you are quite content for him or her to be responsible for the nursing care of anyone you personally care about (for example *your* child, nephew or niece) while still displaying the level of incompetence that *you* would not speak up about! Could it be that *your* lack of professional responsibility and accountability in this area is just as likely to bring the profession into disrepute as that of the incompetent student that *you* will not fail?

→ Trigger 12.2: Feedback

Go to Chapter 12 trigger feedback on p. 414

! Trigger 12.3: Personal Development Plans

This trigger encourages you to formulate a Personal Development Plan in preparation for your first job application as a registered children's nurse and lifelong learning.

The Trigger

Reflect on your problem-based learning from reading and working on the triggers in this book:

- What have you learnt about child health and nursing?
- What skills have you developed for future independent learning?
- What other learning opportunities do you need to plan for your future nursing practice and further independent learning about child health and nursing?

Situation

You are preparing your curriculum vitae and applying for your first post as a staff nurse at the end of your three year nursing course to become a Registered Nurse (Child). Your tutor has discussed personal development plans with your group and suggested that to help you prepare for the job application process, interviews, and then preceptorship and clinical supervision in due course that you do a 'SWOT Analysis' (Strengths, Weaknesses, Opportunities, Threats), and develop a personal development plan. (The Nursing and Midwifery Council advises that all newly registered nurses should have a period of formal support under the guidance of a preceptor for about four months).

Feedback

You are required to do a 'SWOT Analysis' (Strengths, Weaknesses, Opportunities, Threats), and then develop a Personal Development Plan, taking into account the questions in the trigger.

The facts

What are the main facts? Make a list:

Hypotheses: What may these facts mean?

- Learning about child health and nursing has occurred as a result of using this book.
- Skills for independent learning have been learnt through using a problem-based approach to learning.
- There is still more to learn for practice as a registered children's nurse.

Questions developed from the hypotheses

1. What is a Personal Development Plan?
2. What is a SWOT analysis (Strengths, Weaknesses, Opportunities, Threats)?
3. What knowledge and skills do I need to develop for my future nursing practice, and further independent learning?

Trigger 12.3: Fixed resource material

Read the following to help you answer the questions. (You may also wish to search and review other up-to-date research and evidence-based literature, and seek other relevant resources to provide you with the answers to your questions.)

Department of Health (2004) *Agenda for Change*. London: The Stationery Office, http://www.modern.nhs.uk/agendaforchange (accessed 24 January 2005).

National Competence Framework for Children's Services (2004) http://www.skills-forhealth.org.uk (accessed 24 January 2005).

Nursing and Midwifery Council (2002) *Supporting Nurses and Midwives Through Lifelong Learning*. London: NMC, http://www.nmc-uk.org (accessed 24 January 2005).

Trigger 12.3: Fixed resource sessions

Personal development plans

Throughout your three year nursing course you will have maintained a personal professional profile in a portfolio to provide evidence of your learning and achievement. The Nursing Midwifery Council requires registered nurses to maintain a profile as a record of career progress and professional development. It has to be more than a record of achievement though; it should be based on a regular process of reflection and recording of your learning from everyday practice as well as planned learning activity. The Nursing Midwifery Council describe three broad inter-related steps for building a profile:

- Step One: Reviewing experience to date;
- Step Two: Self-appraisal;
- Step Three: Setting Goals and action plans.

Personal development plans were required to be in place for the majority of health professional staff by April 2000. All National Health Service employees have access to training and development opportunities and are required to build personal development plans (National Health Service Jobs 2005). Higher education institutions are also advocating the use of personal development plans for students to enable them to get the most out of their undergraduate studies. Maintaining a personal professional profile, as a student and a registered nurse, will inform the formulation of personal development plans.

Personal development plans are personal records that identify an individual's current skill gaps, learning objectives and an agreed action plan following an in depth discussion between a member of staff and his/her direct line manager at a personal development review (Department of Health 1999; 2004a).

Personal development reviews for the nursing student with a personal tutor may identify strategies to help to improve study skills, identify opportunities for theoretical learning and developing practical skills, and personal development outside the curriculum.

The 'National Health Service Knowledge and Skills Framework' is a tool developed as part of the *Agenda for Change* (Department of Health 2004a). It provides a means of recognizing the skills and knowledge that an individual requires to be effective in a particular National Health Service post. It is envisaged that the framework will ensure better links between education and development and career and pay progression. One of the main aims of the framework is that it will help to identify and develop knowledge and skills that will support career progression and encourage lifelong learning. An annual personal development review meeting with your manager is where personal development plans are agreed. The plan will identify developmental needs and describe how learning will be supported (Department of Health 2004a). All National Health Service staff are expected to develop their knowledge and skills for the benefit of patients. It will also ensure that by the time they reach certain pay bands known as gateways they are applying the appropriate knowledge and skills to move on.

It is useful for students preparing to apply for their first posts as registered nurses to devote sometime to identifying their future development needs in the form of a personal development plan. The three inter-related steps described by the Nursing and Midwifery Council form the basis for developing a personal development plan.

SWOT Analysis (Strengths, Weaknesses, Opportunities, Threats)

This is an analysis (Figure 12.2) of an individual's strengths and weaknesses. This analysis enables an individual to then identify opportunities for self-development and threats that might prevent them from achieving their goals (Dowding and Barr 2002). Undertaking a SWOT Analysis will help you to complete a personal development plan and is ' also most impressive when this exercise forms part of your application for jobs in the future' (Dowding and Barr 2002, p. 6).

Clinical supervision

Clinical supervision is one approach to developing professional expertise and enhancing clinical practice to ensure that quality high standard nursing care is provided (Bishop and Scott 2001; Lyle 1998). Winstanley (1999) found that when clinical supervision was implemented nursing staff reported improved care, skills and increased job satisfaction.

The aim of clinical supervision is to bring practitioners together for reflection on practice in order to identify solutions for problems, to increase awareness and

What are your **strengths**?	What are your **weaknesses**?
What **opportunities** are there for your development?	What **threats** are there to your development?

Figure 12.2 SWOT analysis

understanding of professional issues and to improve standards of care (Nursing and Midwifery Council 2002).

It was identified in the introduction to this chapter that the Nursing and Midwifery Council (2002) believe that clinical supervision is best developed at a local level in accordance with local needs. The Nursing and Midwifery Council (2002) defined a set of principles that should be used to underpin any system of clinical supervision that is used in practice.

Suggested Activity

Access Nursing and Midwifery Council (2002) to identify these defined principles for clinical supervision:

Nursing and Midwifery Council (2002) *Supporting Nurses and Midwives through Lifelong Learning*. London: NMC

There are several clinical supervision models and approaches that may be used to provide a framework to meet clinical supervision needs in local clinical areas. The one developed by Proctor (1986) is a well-known model with three interactive elements:

1. *Formative*: to highlight professional development needs for registered nurses in relation to maintaining and developing skills, and integrating theory to practice.
2. *Restorative*: the identification of emotional needs for the supervisor to help the practitioner(s) to deal with negative experiences and stressful situations.
3. *Normative*: the identification of management needs for the supervisor to facilitate and to support the development of practitioner(s). (Proctor, 1986).

Clinical supervision may be implemented on a one-to-one basis with a supervisor working in the same practice location or alternatively the supervisor may be external to the practitioner's area of practice. Group clinical supervision may be the approach taken in some local areas.

It is suggested that you consider your future clinical supervision needs in your personal development plan.

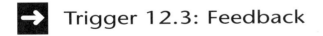 Trigger 12.3: Feedback

Go to Chapter 12 trigger feedback on p. 414

Chapter 12 Trigger feedback: What do you know?

Trigger 12.1: Leading and managing in practice

This is a reflective account that Emily Jakes may have written after her shift as a team leader. Your reflective account will be personalised to your own experience.

Reflective account of team leadership: Introduction

I am going to reflect on my experience of team leadership, using the Gibbs (1988) reflective cycle. At the end of my shift I wrote in my learning diary that I had become more confident as a result of this experience. I am now going to reflect on this experience, linking theory to practice in relation to leaders and managers; leadership styles, team and inter-professional working. I will use my lesson notes about leadership styles (Table 12.3)

Description

This is my final clinical placement on the three year Registered Nurse (Child) course. I am working on a Children's Medical Ward. My mentor has been very supportive throughout my placement and most days I have worked with her. She has encouraged me gradually to take on more responsibility for my own work and that of others, with appropriate supervision from her. During the shift that I am reflecting on I was the 'team leader'. My mentor was there to help as always, but she encouraged me to make most of the decisions that day.

It was not a particularly busy day, but there were lots of decisions to make, for example: prioritising work, delegating staff, working out break times, and dealing with unexpected events like one staff nurse going off sick, a complaining father and the 3 year old brother of a new admission who fell over and banged his head.

Feelings (Good)

The children all got their nursing care all right, so my organisation must have been satisfactory. I felt that my confidence increased as the day passed. So I felt really good about this. It is a difficult time on the ward because of staff changing to work 12-hour shifts and it's not a popular change with everyone. However, the team's morale was good during this shift, which was a great help. I felt that I learnt a great deal about decision-making.

Feelings (Bad)

I was really anxious at the start of this shift. I doubted my ability to be able to 'manage'. I was lacking in confidence, although there was no reason why I should be, because my mentor has been developing my management skills throughout the placement. My worst fear was about asking nursing colleagues to do things and communicating with some members of the multi-disciplinary team. On reflection, I wish I had reviewed my lesson notes on some aspects of being a team leader before the shift to allay my anxiety, especially those about team working.

Analysis of key issues

I am going to discuss team and inter-professional working as one of the issues in this section. First I will try and distinguish between managers and leaders, and then leadership styles so that I am clear about my responsibilities in the future as a team leader.

Leaders and managers

Leaders are concerned with people power and managers with position power (Sofarelli and Brown 1998; Walton 1995).

Managers delegate, control situations, human and material resources, plan, organise, achieve organizational outcomes, and enforce policy and procedures from a position of legitimate power (Sofarelli and Brown 1998). Excellence in communication is also required from managers in the twenty-first century to enable them to be sensitive to patient needs and to anticipate patients and families expectations of the [health care] service in advance (Department of Health 2002). Managers are characterised as being reactive promoting stability (Sofarelli and Brown 1998), as opposed to leaders who are characterised as being proactive and risk takers.

Leadership occurs at many levels in nursing and the *NHS Leadership Qualities Framework* (Department of Health 2002) is to be used to support the personal and professional development of practitioners in preparation for taking on leadership roles. The framework of qualities is arranged in three clusters:

1. *Personal qualities*: Self-belief/self-awareness/self-management/drive for improvement/personal integrity;
2. *Setting direction*: Seizing the future/intellectual flexibility/broad scanning/political astuteness/drive for results;
3. *Delivering the service*: leading change through people/holding to account/empowering others/effective and strategic influencing/collaborative working.

Nurses are now being encouraged to take on new leadership roles such as modern matrons and nurse consultants (Department of Health 2000) and they should integrate these qualities into their roles. Every nurse has the potential to be a leader though and to use leadership qualities and skills in practice at all levels, including that of a nurse functioning as the team leader like myself on the shift that I am reflecting on.

Leaders are involved with empowerment and change, while managers bring about order and consistency (Kotter 1990; Sofarelli and Brown 1998). However, contemporary health service policy now suggests that managers must lead change as well as managing it according to the National Health Service Chief Executive (Department of Health 2002). However, leaders do not always have to be managers.

Leadership styles

A review of my lesson notes suggests that during my shift I was trying to use a trans-actional style of leadership because my main objective for the shift was to ensure that the children safely received appropriate nursing care and prescribed treatment. I had to delegate team members appropriately to provide this care and in doing so I surveyed their abilities and status so that I was aware what I could expect of them as individuals. I also checked which parents were present during the shift engaging in family-centred care and I assessed the amount of support that they required. The team members for the shift comprised first and second year student nurses, staff nurses (D and E grades) and Health Care Assistants. I did not seek to bring about change, but maintained the status quo, acting in the caretaker role described by Cook (2001).

The 'Maturity Model' offered by Cook (2001) suggests that the starting point for those taking on leadership roles is as a transactional leader, which supports me adopt-ing this type of leadership. My mentor appears to be a transformational leader who empowers the team. She really does treat me (and others) with respect and values my input into care. She provides me with positive feedback on my work, and my confi-dence is growing with her teaching and mentorship.

It has been useful reviewing these leadership theories (see Table 12.3). It has helped me to appreciate the leadership role more fully and the different approaches taken by 'team leaders' I have worked with on my clinical placements.

Table 12.3 Leadership theories

These theories have developed from early efforts to identify key characteristics and styles of individual leaders, to focusing on specific situations and/or the tasks to be achieved and the role of the team (King and Cunningham, 1995)

Early theories

Great man theory
This theory, based on Aristotelian philosophy, proposed that leadership is an innate quality that cannot be learned. Therefore some people are born to lead and others are born to follow (Bernhard and Walsh 1995). Good leaders cannot be made, only chosen (Beech 2002).

Trait theories
This theory of leadership attempted to identify the special traits or qualities that set leaders apart from other people (Bernhard and Walsh 1995). Initially traits were believed to be inherited, however, subsequent theory suggested that leadership traits might be developed through learning and experience (Marriner-Tomey 2000). Leader traits include intelligence, initiative, self-assurance, decisiveness, enthusiasm, certain physical attributes, dominance, self-confidence and knowledge of the task (Beech 2002; Clegg 2000).

Style theories
Bernhard and Walsh (1995) identified the following three styles of leadership:

1. The autocratic leader who is powerful, controlling and sole concern is to complete tasks.
2. The democratic leader who shares power and responsibility with the team. Promoting effective teamwork.
3. The laissez-faire leader who abdicates all their responsibility and devolves decision-making to the team with no interest in promoting effective team working.

It is assumed that teams will work harder for leaders that adopt one particular style of leadership as opposed to another. Teams have been found to perform more effectively with a democratic, rather than an autocratic, style of leadership (Clegg 2000; Handy 1993). The laissez-faire style does not promote effective leadership.

Situational theory
Situational theory proposes that the traits required of the leader differ according to the situation. Different individuals will, therefore, emerge as leaders in different situations (King and Cunningham 1995). Although an effective leader does not emerge in every situation (Bernhard and Walsh 1995). Emergent leaders are unlikely to be effective in nursing practice, because no ongoing direction or strong leadership would be provided (Murphy 2001).

Contingency theory
Leaders are those who can establish a fit between tasks to be done, the team performing the tasks and the environment in which the tasks are to be undertaken (Dowding and Barr 2002). This theory is based on Fielder's Contingency Model (Fielder 1967), which suggests leadership characteristics and styles are stable, but as the context changes different leaders emerge in response to new demands.

   King and Cunningham (1995) state that these earlier leadership theories are no longer appropriate in contemporary ever changing health care environments.

Contemporary theories of leadership

Transactional leadership
Transactional leadership is about the impact of the leader on the team members (Clegg 2000). It is orientated towards achieving daily goals and maintaining the status quo (Bernhard and Walsh 1995). The transactional leader surveys the team's abilities and sets goals that are based on what can be expected from those individual team members (Cook 2001).

Transformational leadership
Transformational leadership is different because it focuses on the team as well as the leader. Team members are valued for their strengths and there is a fostering of mutual respect and understanding for empowerment. Transformational leaders have the ability to motivate others to achieve higher standards and long-term goals for the improved care (Clegg 2000) of children and their families.

Renaissance leadership
A renaissance leader uses persuasion and communication skills to take charge at both national and local levels of areas work that impact directly on the quality of patient care (Cook 2001). Renaissance nursing leaders are likely to have participated in the development of the *National Service Frameworks for Children, Young People and Maternity Care* (Department of Health 2004) or the setting up of new services in response to meeting the specific needs of a local population.

Connective leadership

Connective leadership creates a bridge between transformational and renaissance leadership (Cook, 2001). The leader uses persuasion and influence to affect productive collaborative relationships with key stakeholders at all levels of the health service.

Maturity model of leadership

Cook (2001) offers a maturity model of leadership because leadership moves through different phases along a continuum: from transactional leadership, through transformational leadership and connective leadership, to renaissance leadership. These different types of leadership are associated with different modes of care provision: task allocation; nursing process; clinical pathways, and holistic care. The careers of individual leaders, too, tend to develop along the same continuum from transactional leadership to renaissance leadership (Cook 2001).

Team working

A team is set of people working together to achieve common goals. Effective teamwork seems to be characterised by good communication skills, listening, respect, sharing and support. One of the most significant factors for effective team working is that of good team leadership, inadequate team leadership causes more team problems than any other single factor (Clegg 2000; Ovretvat 1993). A transformational leader is likely to provide purpose and direction for the team thus motivating the members for effective team working (Clegg, 2000).

The Seven 'S' Framework offered by Handy (1993) provides an illustration of the leader's contributions to team functioning. Leaders tend to adopt a soft approach to team functioning that involves:

- *Style*: that directs how things are done (e.g., transformational leadership);
- *Staff*: valuing and respecting the team members and the work they do;
- *Skills*: the competencies of the team members. Promoting personal and professional development;
- *Shared goals*: the beliefs, principles and priorities of the team are shared and owned.

Conversely, managers tend to rely on a harder approach that involves employing:

- *Strategy*: plan of action that facilitates resource management in an organisation.
- *Structure*: the fitting together of different parts of the organisation.
- *Systems*: information collection in databases.

Inter-professional working

Miller (1999) found that collaborative inter-professional working enhances the continuity and consistency of care from professional to professional with a reduction in ambiguous messages being passed between the different professionals themselves, and also to their clients/carers. Inter-professional education can make a valuable contribution to professionals sharing with each other the concepts of their own discipline;

understanding each other's beliefs and value systems to reduce the potential for professional conflict in health and social care practice (Reeves and Freeth 2000; Warner 2001).

Conclusion

This reflection has enabled me to link theory to practice in relation to team leadership. The role of the leader in promoting effective teamwork and inter-professional working for the optimum care of children and their families is important. A transformational leader is most likely to motivate the team to work well together. The manager's role differs from the leaders and relies on a harder approach, which appears to be happening in relation to the introduction of 12-hour working shifts on my ward.

Future Practice

I will try to apply theoretical principles of leadership and management to my future practice of team leading and management. My mentor was a good role model and I will aspire to become a transformational leader like her in the long term. However in the meantime I will communicate with, listen to, respect, and value colleagues in teams that I work in, to be supportive.

Trigger 12.2: Mentorship and assessment

Question 1: How might mentorship progress for these students?

Question 2: How would you enable these students to maximise their placement experience?

Question 3: What approach would you take to mentoring these students?

Potential answers to all three of these questions are addressed together in the accounts that follow.

With regard to *Tina*, Jenny is likely to arrange a progress discussion with her as soon as possible. Jenny could ask Tina to self-assess her progress in relation to the specific requirements of her continuous assessment of practice document. Torrance and Pryor (1998) suggest that it is only by involving students directly in self-assessment, that we achieve truly formative assessments that have meaning for them, and that profoundly influence student's professional development. Concentrating on the document may help Tina to realise that she hasn't got a very focused approach to her learning. In the ensuing discussion, Jenny may need to convey to Tina that while she respects Tina's enthusiasm to see, experience and help with everything, it isn't a particularly useful strategy for helping her learn in any depth or in a structured way that can be built upon later. Tina may be spreading herself too thinly and trying to run before she can walk, so it's time to refocus. Jenny can help Tina re-establish what specific learning outcomes do need to be achieved on this placement and discuss a time frame for achieving first some then others, with reference to the ward's learning opportunities.

Their discussions may include the importance of concentrating on and honing what are often described as 'basic' skills in order to build firm foundations for future practice. Infection control measures for example can appear fairly simple, obvious and routine when first considered, but Tina needs to spend time and effort watching and looking for the subtle ways in which we can easily fall short of not maintaining required standards. Situations that Jenny may challenge and encourage Tina to think about might include: when disposing of paper towels for example, is Tina convinced that she always uses the foot pedal to elevate the lid of the refuse bin or does she sometimes forget and touch the bin lid with her hands? When nursing or medical staff call her over to help with an aspect of care or to show her something new, does Tina in her eagerness arrive at their side instantly, or explain that she will be there just as soon as she has washed her hands? How clean and short are Tina's nails?

The apparent drama of observing qualified nurses and doctors respond astutely and skilfully with complex measures to a patient whose condition is deteriorating due to an overwhelming hospital acquired infection, may initially seem exciting to Tina, however, the 'back to basics' focus should help her to appreciate how much more exciting it is to prevent such infections in the first place and that she has a major role to play in this. Getting the basics right often has dramatic, favourable outcomes and research demonstrates this clearly to us, so Jenny may also encourage Tina to find and read one of the research articles that underpin the ward's infection control policy. Jenny will want to ensure Tina receives appropriate feedback on her progress following this interview so will remind Tina of the date set for her formal mid-placement review .

With reference to *Jack* it's important not to make assumptions and, therefore, a progress discussion with him would be in order as soon as possible. Genuine concern for Jack's welfare will lead Jenny to enquire about his health. If there are health issues, he needs to know that Jenny can not remain silent about them and that his tutor will be contacted for appropriate counsel and support. Professional decisions would then need to be made regarding the personal and patient safety aspects of Jack remaining on the placement.

Otherwise Jenny has to recognise that she doesn't know how Jack is feeling about the placement until she asks him. She needs to get Jack's perspective on how he's settling into the placement, what he feels he is learning quite easily and what he feels uncertain about or perceives as difficulties. 'If assessment is to be a true learning process, the student should be an equal partner' (Stuart 2003, pp. 159–60). Any number of scenarios may unfold at this point and Jenny needs to listen carefully.

Jenny may, for example, be astonished to find out that Jack feels frightened of working with such tiny children, he has no younger family members and doesn't know how to communicate with them. Also the child protection lectures in school appeared to counsel male students not to get themselves into potentially vulnerable situations that could be misconstrued by being left alone with children, so Jack hangs back rather than approaching children to comfort them when distressed or play for example.

Jenny will, therefore, need to clarify these issues and negotiate altering the action plans in order to help Jack feel more at ease, and communicate more easily and appropriately. Conversations about the ward's philosophy of family-centred care and the need to interact with the whole family may be useful here. Encouraging Jack to talk with parents is likely to lead to conversations including the children and insight into the things that children like to do and talk about. Jenny may initiate plans for Jack to spend time with the ward's nursery nurse who is well skilled in sharing her expertise on child development and linking this to appropriate communication and therapeutic play for sick children. So much can be done to help if Jenny elicits what the problem actually is.

In a converse scenario however, Jack may indicate that he can't see the relevance of this placement with children and young people for an adult branch student. Also, if he gets out of bed too late to be on duty punctually, he's unsure what to do so he 'phones in sick'. When on duty he doesn't see much that needs doing for the children because their parents are often there. Jenny has different issues to deal with this time but again a progress discussion is in order. Jenny has the role of opening Jack's eyes to the fact that although he has chosen to nurse adults, this doesn't mean that he will never encounter children and their care requirements in his future practice. For example, there are few accident and emergency departments in the UK that are specifically dedicated for children. Children and young people requiring such care will usually arrive at a department that treats a mixture of adults and children. Most accident and emergency departments attempt to comply with recommendations for having a minimum of one children's nurse on duty per shift to lead the care of attending children. With holidays and sickness this is a difficult standard to maintain for some departments and inevitably children end up being cared for by adult trained nurses even if it is only in the capacity of assisting the children's nurse on duty. Should Jack choose to work abroad when he is qualified, he may find adults and children being nursed in the same care environment and he would, therefore, need to be able to use skills learnt in both of these areas of practice.

Jack needs convincing that his time is not being wasted here and that skills learnt in nursing children will also be directly transferable to adult care environments. For example, if an adult nurse learns to recognise the non-verbal cues of a 13 month girl for signalling pain or wanting a toy she can't reach, then these same skills can be used to recognise cues about discomfort or the desire for help to sit up in an aphasic, hemiplegic, adult patient following a cerebro-vascular accident (stroke).

Jenny may wish to consult the clinical link teacher or Jack's tutor to clarify the sickness and absence policy and discuss with Jack that saying he is sick (not late) is not truthful. Checking that he knows where to refer to this policy in his course handbook may be useful. With reference to required competence in the assessed domain of professional and ethical practice, Jack needs to be aware that telling the truth and arriving punctually for duty is a professional requirement that he has to satisfy, so greater efforts will have to be demonstrated in this area. He could think about using the alarm on his mobile phone as well as his usual alarm clock to help him wake in time to be on duty punctually for example.

In the midst of everything being rather new at Jack's initial interview with Jenny, explanations about the ward's philosophy of care may have got a bit crowded out. In response to Jack's comments about not seeing much that needs to be done for the children because parents are present, Jenny is likely to encourage Jack to look deeper and observe how most children and parents are inextricably linked, therefore, when children's nurses think about care required by sick children, they cannot ignore that the main supporters of those children will also require care, hence the philosophy of family-centred care. Smith et al (2002, p. 22) define family-centred care as 'the professional support of the child and family through a process of involvement, participation, and partnership underpinned by empowerment and negotiation'. Jenny may challenge Jack to explore the complexities of this highly skilled way of working with children, young people and their families, and negotiate that he be ready to discuss his insights and supervised participation in family-centred care at their next progress discussion.

Finally Jenny may wish to speak with her colleagues who had passed their concerns about Jack on to her. Getting this information to the designated mentor was appropriate, however Jenny may wish to explore with them why in her absence, they didn't in the first instance discuss their concerns or observations directly with Jack. For the first scenario involving Jack where he was frightened, they are likely to have been able to offer appropriate help more quickly than he received it in this instance. For the second scenario, where more effort is required from Jack, it may be helpful that he receives the message about professional standards and requirements from more than one registered member of the nursing team.

Trigger 12.3: Personal Development Plans

The feedback for this trigger is going to differ from the perspective of the content of your personal development plan and SWOT analysis. Individuals will have different strengths and weaknesses and hence opportunities and threats will not be viewed the same by everyone.

The plan should provide evidence that you are thinking long term as well as short term in your action plan. It is worthwhile considering the direction in which you want your nursing career to develop and to identify the experiences, knowledge, skills and clinical supervision that will support this career progression.

You are likely to have already developed skills for lifelong learning through engaging in problem-based learning in this book and in your plan you should consider how best to use these skills for lifelong learning. Problem-based learning is very much about developing skills for independent learning and therefore it endeavours to cover some issues in depth as opposed to superficially covering many more issues. In your personal development plans it is suggested that you give some consideration about what else there is to learn about child health and nursing to enable you to achieve your action plan.

Reflect on your learning

- Understand the Nursing and Midwifery Code of Professional Conduct and its application in practice.
- Develop an awareness of the implications of contemporary issues for children and young people's nursing.
- Be well prepared for leadership and mentorship roles; team and inter-professional working.
- Utilise the change process effectively.
- Engage in independent lifelong learning.
- Use Personal development plans acknowledging the role of clinical supervision.

References

Beech, M. (2002) Leaders or managers: The drive for effective leadership, *Nursing Standard* 16 (30), pp. 35–6.

Benner, P. (1984) *From Novice to Expert*. Menlo Park: Addison Wesley.

Bennis, W., Benne, K., Chin, R., Corey, K. (1976) *The Planning of Change*, 3rd edn. New York: Holt, Rinehart and Winston.

Bernhard, L., Walsh, M. (1995) *Leadership: The Key to the Professionalizationof Nursing*, 3rd edn. St. Louis: Mosby.

Bishop, V., Scott, I. (eds) (2001) *Challenges in Clinical Practice: ProfessionalDevelopments in Nursing*. Basingstoke: Palgrave.

Blake, R., Mounton, S. (1976) *Consultation*. Reading MA: Addison-Wesley.

Bradshaw, M., Coleman, V., Smith, L. (2003) Inter-professional learning andfamily-centred care, *Paediatric Nursing* 15 (7), September, pp. 30–3.

Broome, A. (1998) *Managing Change*, 2nd edn. Basingstoke: Macmillan.

Buckingham, C., Adams, A. (2000) Classifying clinical decision making: Interpreting nursing intuition, heuristics and medical diagnosis. *Journal ofAdvanced Nursing* 32 (4), October, pp. 990–8.

Chin, R., Benne, K. D. (1976) General strategies for effecting changes inhuman systems, in Bennis, W., Benne, K. D., Chinn, R., Corey, K. (eds) *The Planning of Change,* 3rd edn. New York: Holt, Rinehart and Winston.

Clarke, L. (1994) *The Essence of Change.* London: Prentice Hall.

Clegg, A. (2000) Leadership: Improving the quality of patient care'. *Nursing Standard* 14 (30), pp. 43–5.

Concise Oxford English Dictionary (2004) 14th edn. Oxford: Oxford University Press.

Cook, M. (2001) The renaissance of clinical leadership. International Council of Nurses. *International Nursing Review* 48, pp. 38–46.

Curtis, E., White, P. (2002) Resistance to change: Courses and solutions. *Nursing Management* 8 (10), March, pp. 15–20.

Darling, L. A. (1984) What do nurses want in a mentor? *Journal of Nursing Administration,* 14 (10), pp. 42–4.

Department of Health (1999) *Working Together with Health Information Annex: Other Important Recent Initiatives in NHS Education, Training and Development and Related Actions for this Strategy and Local Implementation Strategies,* http://dh.gov.uk/policyandguidance (accessed 14 January, 2005).

Department of Health (2000) *The NHS Plan, A Plan for Investment, A Plan forReform.* London: DoH, www.nhs.uk/nhsplan (accessed 14 January, 2005).

Department of Health (2002) *Managing for Excellence in the NHS.* London: DoH, www.doh.gov.uk/managingforexcellence/index.htm (accessed 14 January, 2005).

Department of Health (2004) *National Service Framework for Children Young People and Maternity Care.* London: DoH.

Department of Health (2004a) *Agenda for Change* http://www.dh.gov.uk/Policy AndGuidance/HumanResourcesAndTraining/ModernisingPay/AgendaForChange/fs/en (accessed 25 January, 2005).

Dowding, L., Barr, J. (2002) *Managing in Health Care: A Guide for Nurses, Midwives and Health Visitors.* London: Prentice Hall.

Duffy, K. (2004) Failing students – should you give the benefit of the doubt'? *N&MC News* (8), July, p. 9.

English National Board (1987) *Managing Change in Nursing and Education, Pack One: Preparing for Change.* London: ENB.

Fielder, F. E. (1967) *A Theory of Leadership Effectiveness.* New York: McGraw Hill Book Company.

Gibbs, G. (1988) *Learning by Doing: A Guide to Teaching and LearningMethods.* Oxford Further Education Unit: Oxford Polytechnic.

Hamm, R. M. (1988) cited by Dowding, L., Barr, J. (2002) *Managing in Health Care: A guide for Nurses, Midwives and Health Visitors.* London: Prentice Hall. Chapter 2, pp. 12–34.

Handy, C. (1993) *Understanding Organisations,* 4th edn. London: Penguin.

King, K., Cunningham, G., (1995) Leadership in nursing: More than one-way. *Nursing Standard* 10 (12), pp. 3–14.

Kotter, J. (1990) *A Force for Change: How Leadership Differs from Management.* New York: Free Press.

Lewin, K. (1951) *Field Theory in Social Sciences.* New York: Harper & Rowe.

Lyle, D. (1998) Is clinical supervision the answer to quality care? *Nursing Management*, 5 (6), October, pp. 5–7.

Marriner-Tomey, A. (2000) *Guide to Nursing Management and Leadership*, 6th edn. St. Louis: Mosby.

Marton, F., Säljö, R. (1984) 'Approaches to learning' in Marton, F., Hounsell, D., Entwhistle, N. J. (eds) *The Experience of Learning.* Edinburgh: Scottish Academic Press.

Miller, C. (1999) *The Role of Collaborative/Shared Learning in Pre-Post Registration Education in Nursing, Midwifery and Health Visiting, Research Highlight Thirty Nine.* London: English National Board.

Murphy, W. (2001) Leadership and community children's nurses. *Paediatric Nursing* 13 (10), December, pp. 36–40.

National Competence Framework for Children's Services (2004) http://www.skills-forhealth.org.uk (accessed 24 January 2005).

National Health Service Jobs (2005) *Working in the NHS,* http://www.jobs.nhs.uk (accessed 24 January 2005).

Nursing and Midwifery Council (2002) *Supporting Nurses and Midwives through Lifelong Learning.* London: NMC, http://www.nmc-uk.org (accessed 24 January 2005).

Nursing and Midwifery Council (2002a) *Requirements for Pre-registration Nursing Programmes, Section 3 Nursing Competencies.* London: NMC, pp. 9–21.

Nursing and Midwifery Council (2003) *Nursing and Midwifery Council Requirements for Mentors and Mentorship, QA Factsheet 0/2003.* http://www.nmc-uk.org (accessed 25 January 2005).

Nursing and Midwifery Council (2004) *Code of Professional Conduct: Standards for Conduct, Performance and Ethics.* London: NMC.

Nursing and Midwifery Council (2004a) *Standards of Proficiency for Pre-registration Nursing Education.* London: NMC.

Ovretvat, J. (1993) *Co-ordinating Community Care: Multi-disciplinary Teams and Care Management.* Buckingham: Open University Press.

Proctor, B. (1986) Supervision: A co-operative exercise in accountability, in Marken, M., Payne, M. (eds) *Enabling and Ensuring.* Leicester: NationalYouth Bureau and Council for Education and Training in Youth and Community Work.

Reeves, S., Freeth, D. (2000) Learning to collaborate, *Nursing Times* 3(96), pp. 40–1.

Rogers, E., Shoemaker, F. (1971) *Communication of Innovations: A cross-cultural Report.* New York: Free Press.

Rogers, J. (2001) *Adults Learning*, 4th edn. London: Open University Press.

Scott, I. (2001) Clinical Governance: A framework of models for practice, in Bishop, V., Scott, I. (eds) *Challenges in Clinical Practice: Professional Developments in Nursing*. Basingstoke: Palgrave, Chapter 2, pp. 37–58.

Smith, L., Coleman, V., Bradshaw, M. (2002) *Family-centred Care: Concept, Theory and Practice*. Basingstoke, Palgrave.

Sofarelli, D., Brown, D. (1998) The need for nursing leadership in uncertain times, *Journal of Nursing Management*, 6 (4), pp. 201–7.

Stuart, C. C. (2003) *Assessment, Supervision and Support in Clinical Practice: A Guide for Nurses and Midwives*. Edinburgh: Churchill Livingstone.

Teasdale, K. (ed) (1992*) Managing the Change in Health Care: An Explanation and Exploration of the Implications for the NHS of Working for Patients*. London: Wolfe.

Thompson, C., Dowding, D. (eds) (2002) *Clinical Decision Making and Judgement in Nursing*. Edinburgh: Churchill Livingstone.

Torrance, H., Pryor, J. (1998) *Investigating Formative Assessment*. Buckingham: Open University Press.

United Kingdom Central Council (1999) *Fitness for Practice: The UKCC Commission for Nurse Education*. London: UKCC.

United Kingdom Central Council (2001) *Fitness for Practice and Purpose: Thereport of the UKCCs Post Commission Development Group*. London: UKCC.

Upton, T., Brookes, B. (1995) *Managing Change in the NHS*. London: Kogan Page.

Walton, M. (1995) *Management and Managing, Leadership in the NHS*, 2nd edn. Cheltenham: Stanley Thornes.

Warner, H. (2001) Children with additional needs: The transdisciplinary approach. *Paediatric Nursing* 13 (6), July, pp. 33–5.

Welsh Assembly (2004) *National Service Framework for Children, Young People and Maternity Services*, http://www.wales.nhs.uk/sites/home.cfm

Winstanley, J. (1999) *Methods of Evaluating the Effectiveness of Clinical Supervision*, Clinical monograph. London: Nursing Times Books.

Wright, S. (1989) *Changing Nursing Practice*. London: Edward Arnold.

Index